WORKING FOR HEALTH

To the memory of Albert Spanswick

Working for Health

The History of the
Confederation of Health Service Employees

Mick Carpenter

LAWRENCE & WISHART
LONDON

Lawrence & Wishart Limited
39 Museum Street
London WC1A 1LQ

First published 1988

Photoset in North Wales by
Derek Doyle & Associates, Mold, Clwyd.
Printed in Great Britain by
Billing and Sons, Worcester.

Contents

PART THREE:
COHSE and the NHS Since 1946

Illustrations

Preface

Working for Health is being published at a challenging, exciting time for COHSE. As we approach the 1990s and take steps to ensure that our union is fully geared to meeting the needs of our members into the next century, it is timely to look back at the struggles of the past, to salute the people who founded and built up the union – to pay tribute to those who have made the Confederation what it is today.

It is a history to be proud of. In an accessible style which makes considerable use of archive material, Mick Carpenter brings to life the early struggles and charts the events that led to the beginnings of health service trade unionism – and the founding of the National Health Service itself.

COHSE, born in 1910 when a small group of Lancashire male asylum attendants met to discuss a common grievance, is now 212,000 members strong. We are now *the* health care union, organising in every place that health care is delivered. Today's membership, comprising over 75 per cent women, embraces the full range of health care jobs – in the hospitals, primary and community services, voluntary and private health sectors, old people's homes and local authority social services.

There is much to be learnt from COHSE's history and much to hold dear – such as the cry that echoes down the years for equality for decent pay and conditions rather than exploiting a caring profession, and for well funded health provision for all.

And the history's title, *Working for Health*, could not be more appropriate, looking back as it does to the pioneers who sacrificed so much to establish the union, and pointing to the future battles ahead to safeguard the service and ensure its survival.

We must carry on where our predecessors left off, looking to the future with courage and conviction and continuing the enormous responsibility of working for health, and for the right of all people to free and equal health care.

Hector MacKenzie,
General Secretary

Introduction

This history is a record and celebration of more than 75 unbroken years of trade union organisation in the health and social services, as represented by the unremitting efforts of members, activists and officials of COHSE and its predecessors to improve their lot and the service as a whole. It portrays the problems which successive generations of health workers have experienced and the aspirations for change that arose among them. It traces the emergence and development of the collective organisation they constructed to pursue their aspirations and assesses the extent to which they were realised.

There have been victories, some temporary, some more enduring, and these are worth describing in order to show that improvements rarely came as acts of benevolence bestowed from above but had to be fought for. In the process risks were taken and sacrifices were made, often without thought of material gain but because the workers involved believed they had a duty to improve conditions for those coming after them. This history is first and foremost a tribute to their efforts, a declaration that theirs is a story worth telling, and I am grateful to COHSE for providing me with the time and resources to research and write it, and patience in waiting for the final product to emerge. I was often moved by what I found, by the foresight, courage, perseverance and humanity of successive generations of health service trade unionists, traditions which I know continue to this day.

Despite what some of its critics have argued, trade unionism is not foreign to the health and social services but can demonstrate long and proud traditions of betterment for both workers and the service as a whole.

The knowledge of this can be a source of strength and inspiration today, as we confront anew many of the same dilemmas and difficulties which previous generations faced and surmounted with both courage and ingenuity. If they did so, so can we. Yet both as a tribute and as a practical tool in present struggles, it cannot simply be a chronicle of progress made. Gains were not always easy to come by. Tactical errors were inevitably made on occasion, and these must be honestly appraised.

In more general terms, the story of COHSE shows an unfamiliar side of the history of the health and social services, one that has been ignored for too long. The collective efforts of health workers to change the circumstances of their lives contributed every bit as much, if not more, to the development of the service, as those of the famous individuals like Florence Nightingale who dominate most historical accounts. This discovery inevitably challenges the traditional stereotypes of health workers which for too long have been accepted as the reality. In place of the celebrated 'angels' – contented, submissive and self-effacing – we will find discontented, assertive and even, on occasion, militant individuals, who rather than giving in to circumstances believed it was possible to change them. They may not at all times have been in the majority, but there were many more of them than is commonly admitted, and they made their mark.

The other myth that will be shattered is the more recent portrayal of health service trade unionists as selfish and uncaring 'bullies', willing at the drop of a hat to put the interests and even the lives of patients at risk in search of a material or power advantage. In most instances health workers have only resorted to industrial action under conditions of extreme provocation, and even then have usually conducted themselves in such ways as safeguard patients' well being. Nor have health service trade unionists exerted pressure or taken action solely on their own behalf. They were in the forefront of the campaign to establish the National Health Service in the first place, often in the teeth of opposition from those who described themselves as 'caring professionals'. They have also served as the first line of defence for a service whose fundamental principles have increasingly been under attack in recent years.

Above all, health service trade unionists continually fought against the mistaken notion that health workers had no right to think of their own material needs and must always put the needs of the patients and the service first. They argued that it was a false choice, that a service which cared about one would care about the other – an argument that has obvious modern relevance. In other words COHSE, in campaigning against the traditional self-sacrificing angel, was also seeking to bring into being a 'new model' health worker, one who cared about the patients and the service, but who was prepared to assert her or his own needs as well. It disputed the claim long held to by professional associations like the Royal College of Nursing that decent wages and conditions might attract the 'wrong type' into the health service. The union claimed, I think rightly, that material improvements for workers would lead to a better service for patients and the development of a staff with a more balanced outlook rather than one whose horizons were often neurotically limited to the hospital walls.

The union's motto since its inception, 'All For One and One For All', expresses its basic outlook well, especially when we remember that it was originally followed by 'Thou Shalt Love Thy Neighbour as Thyself'. Behind it lies a commitment both to workers' solidarity and the 'good Samaritan' socialism that underpins the NHS. On the one hand it expresses the union's belief in the comradeship and interdependence of all workers in the health team against a narrow professional elitism that would favour advances for some at the expense of others. On the other it insists that ill health and the care of the sick should be a public not a private responsibility. Both are inseparable parts of COHSE's traditions of caring trade unionism, and there is no better way of describing what the union stands for.

In the pages which follow we trace the emergence and unfolding of these ideals in practice. Part One traces the birth and growth of trade unionism in the mental health services. Part Two describes parallel struggles to establish trade unionism in the Poor Law service and general hospitals. Part Three shows the coming together of these separate traditions with the creation of COHSE in 1946, and follows its course to the present day.

I would finally like to acknowledge the support and assistance given me by COHSE officials, activists and members throughout the period of my research into the union's history, not least by the generous funding of a Research Fellowship at the University of Warwick. COHSE head office staff have been particularly helpful, but I would like to single out Albert Spanswick for special mention. He believed, as I do, in the necessity of the study of history for an understanding of the present, and he encouraged me to develop my own, independent assessment of COHSE's problems and achievements. I am sorry that he did not live to see the final result, and this book is therefore dedicated to his memory.

Mick Carpenter
University of Warwick

Chronology

1909	Asylum Officers' Superannuation Act passed
1910	*National Asylum Workers' Union* (NAWU) formed
1914	NAWU affiliates to the Labour Party
1918	Asylum workers' strikes
	Poor Law Workers' Trade Union (PLWTU) formed
1919	Joint Conciliation Committee established between NAWU and employers
1921	PLWTU Brentford dispute
1922	PLWTU becomes *Poor Law Officers' Union* (PLOU) after failure to amalgamate with National Poor Law Officers' Association
	NAWU Radcliffe dispute
1923	NAWU affiliates to TUC
1930	PLOU changes name to *National Union of County Officers* (NUCO) after Poor Law system dismantled
1931	NAWU becomes *Mental Hospitals and Institutional Workers' Union* following 1930 Mental Treatment Act
1933	NUCO affiliates to TUC
1937	TUC Nurses' Charter launched, Guild of Nurses set up within NUCO
1938	Guild of Nurses masked march for 48-hour week for LCC nurses
1943	NUCO becomes *Hospitals and Welfare Services Union* (HWSU)
1946	*Confederation of Health Service Employees* (COHSE) is born from merger of MHIWU and HWSU

1948   National Health Service Whitley Council system established.
              Student nurses march for £5 minimum wage
1957   Mental nurses' overtime ban
1959   Mental Health Act passed
              COHSE head office moves to Banstead
1962   Battle against the 'Pay Pause'
1965   Campaign for nationalised ambulance service
1972   COHSE leaves TUC
1973   Ancillary workers strike
1974   COHSE rejoins TUC
              Halsbury campaign for nurses' pay
1978-79   'Winter of Discontent'
1982-83   Campaign for 'Common Core' claim
1985   COHSE members vote to retain Political Fund

Part One

Trade Unionism in the Mental Health Services, 1910-46

Chapter 1
The Roots of Unrest

> In my old days we used to work about a hundred hours a week, and we had a slogan which, fortunately, does not apply today. It was 'Cheer up, you'll soon be dead.'
> George Vernon, former Union President, 1931

Trade unions are not created in a vacuum. They arise to deal with particular sets of pressing problems. Some features of unionism are probably universal: a need shared with others to work in order to live, and to combine with them to overcome individual weakness in the face of a powerful employer. And along with the feeling that something *needs* to be done, must go the conviction that something *can* be done. But the actual circumstances in which these tendencies are made real varies enormously. They are affected by chance occurrences, the times in which people live, the personalities involved, and much else besides. Most important, however, are the constraints imposed by the power structure in which emerging trade unionists must intervene, so that is where we will begin.

The Victorian Legacy

The intention of early nineteenth century reformers was that an 'asylum' should provide a 'refuge' for the mentally afflicted, but by the end of the century county insane asylums for the pauper lunatics had departed considerably from this ideal. The late Victorian reality closely resembled a penal colony, with staff in sombre uniforms, keys clanking at their hips, closely regulating the lives of the unfortunate inmates. The system was governed by the

19

precepts of the complicated legal code established by the 1890 Lunacy Act.

Such asylums were, in theory, places of treatment where inmates would be helped back to sanity and returned to society. Increasingly, however, as pessimism set in about the possibility of curing insanity, the sober regimes of asylum life, regarded originally as a form of treatment for 'excited passions', became more and more simply a means of controlling permanently captive populations. The resulting prison-like regime inevitably proved extremely resistant to change.

The emphasis upon security, order and discipline, as ends in themselves, gave rise to a further requirement: economy. The social function of the asylum was not so much to effect cures, but to segregate permanently the mad from the sane, at the lowest possible cost. The chief measures of any asylum's success followed from its central objectives. One was achieving the lowest possible escape rate, but the most commonly referred to measure of success was keeping the average weekly cost of maintaining each patient as low as possible.

Economy in all things – provisions, accommodation and so on – was one means of pursuing this goal. Another was ensuring that patients contributed to their keep by working. This also had a profound effect on staff roles. Some 'indoor' staff 'attended' on 'refractory' inmates, which meant the patients, i.e. the most disturbed and difficult, as well as watching over physically debilitated patients, or those taking exercise on outside 'airing courts'. The remainder of the indoor staff and all of the 'outdoor' staff spent much of their time supervising the daily labours of patients who were expected to work in order to contribute to their upkeep.

In theory, central government (through the Board of Control), and local councils (through Visiting Committees) could exercise wide powers over asylums, but in practice these were rarely exercised. In most matters it had, by the beginning of the twentieth century, become customary for most day-to-day matters to be left to the discretion of the medical superintendent, the Visiting Committee endorsing whatever decisions he had deemed necessary to make in the previous month.

It is hard for us to envisage the degree of power exercised by the medical superintendent. By the early twentieth century he appears to have become virtually an absolute monarch in the closed kingdom over which he ruled. Increasingly, he devolved the actual care of the patients upon assistant medical officers who, aspiring one day to achieve the same dizzy heights, themselves left as much as possible of the daily work to ill paid and overworked attendants and nurses. Visiting Committees increasingly found this to be a convenient arrangement. Thus an extraordinary degree of power was concentrated in the hands of the medical superintendent, but – it must always be remembered – only if it was exercised within the constraints of order, security and minimum cost that had been imposed from the outside.

Life and Labour

If order and security, at minimum cost, were the main principles governing the treatment of patients, it is hardly surprising that they were also applied rigorously to asylum employees. Since the authorities regarded the asylum as a necessary but unproductive burden on the rates, it would be unrealistic to expect them to be generous employers of labour. Thus, for example, the Wages Book of Lancaster County Asylum shows that for the year 1887 the highest paid attendant, one John Stavely, received £40 and the lowest paid, R.S. Farrer, £28 a year. The highest paid day nurses, like Mary and Agnes Denny, received £22 a year, while Alice Hayes apparently only merited £16. Reliable wage data for this period are difficult to obtain, but a few comparisons show that asylum nurses' and attendants' wages were close to the bottom of the league.[1]. For men, the most comparable wages were those of agricultural labourers (though artisan attendants received more for their possession of a craft); for women, those of domestic servants.

Another area where asylum work often compared unfavourably with most other forms of employment, was in hours of work. In the last quarter of the last century, considerable pressure was mounted from within the labour movement to achieve reductions in the working week. Legislation, by the late 1870s, restricted the number of hours worked by women in manufacturing industries to ten hours a day, but public and professional employment was excluded. Unionised male employees were able to use more traditional means of pressure. Where neither legislative protection nor union strength existed, as in the health services, hours of work continued to be excessively long well into the twentieth century.

Hours of work, therefore, remained long, even by the standards of the time. In the 1840s, according to Dr Connolly, 'The duties of an attendant in an asylum begin early in the morning, are incessant during the day, and end late.'[2] How little things had improved since the 1840s can be seen from the survey of 31 mental hospitals conducted by COHSE's predecessor, the National Asylum Workers' Union (NAWU) in 1912, as part of its (unsuccessful) agitation for legal reductions in hours, of which we shall hear more later. With two exceptions, the working week for men and women was found to be in excess of 70 hours a week, exclusive of mealtimes, and in some cases more than 80 or even 90 hours a week. The effect of long hours, living-in and geographical isolation was to exclude staff from participation in a wider society, to almost the same degree as asylum inmates.

Given the low wages, long hours and poor conditions, widespread fears that sustained contact with the insane was contaminating, and the increasing general prosperity, it is not surprising that asylum work was often regarded as an occupation of last resort. Dr Browne in 1837 described attendants as

the unemployed of other professions ... if they possess physical strength and a tolerable reputation for sobriety, it is enough; and the latter quality is frequently dispensed with.[3]

Medical superintendents often took those they could get: on the male side, ex-servicemen and policemen, whose pensions made them less reluctant to accept low wages; otherwise, especially in rural areas, they competed in the market for farm labourers.

It was quite apparent to the asylum authorities that rarely did anyone seek to enter asylum employment from a sense of vocation to help the mentally afflicted. As Henry Burdett commented in 1891:

> Higher motives than those of earning a livelihood have not as yet induced many, if any, to adopt asylum nursing.[4]

As a result, medical superintendents did not believe that attendants and nurses would perform their duties conscientiously, unless they were compelled to do so by constant surveillance and harsh disciplinary measures. Such low trust led to military, even penal, discipline being imposed on staff by the superintendent or his senior nurses and attendants. Ordinary attendants and nurses were contemptuously regarded as 'subordinate staff', with the medical superintendent the equivalent of a commanding officer. The doctor's own Handbook to asylum nurses, first issued in 1885, but still in use (in only a partly revised form) in the 1950s, made matters plain when it listed 'discipline' as first and foremost of an attendant's 'varieties of duty', both 'as it is imposed upon the attendant, and as he should impose it upon his patients'.[5] We can obtain a more detailed understanding of what this meant in practice from an examination of the 'Regulations and Orders' (note the military terminology) of individual asylums. These were often issued in booklet form to staff on joining the service. They were long and detailed, often covering every conceivable eventuality such as: the conduct of mealtimes, behaviour of patients at divine service, the marriage of staff, the depth of water in patients' baths, the distribution of medicines, the conduct of patients' working parties, and many other things, including (for the London County Asylums) the rules and regulations covering the asylum fire brigade.

The rules of particular asylums naturally varied, but there were many similarities between them. Security occupies a central place in all those I have been able to examine.[6] The counting of patients, care of keys, tools and cutlery were usually given particular emphasis. For example the Manual of Duties for the London County Asylums in 1906 specified that:

Attendants and workmen shall see that all ladders, steps, or other things used by them, which may enable patients to escape ... are carefully guarded, and directly the work is performed, removed out of their reach.

The Staff Regulations for the Metropolitan Asylums Board 'Imbecile Asylums' at Leavesden and Caterham detailed 15 rules for preventing escape including:

The charge attendant of each ward is to examine, at least once a week, all screws and fastenings which are accessible to patients.

It was a legal offence for nurses to help patients to escape, leading on conviction to a fine not exceeding £20, i.e. half an attendant's annual salary. Where escape occurred by negligence, the attendant responsible had to pay for the cost of recapture, sometimes including a reward to the police constable or an additional fine by the asylum authorities.

Care of keys – more than anything else the symbol of asylum authority – attracted almost obsessive attention. Thus, at the London 'Imbecile Asylums', 'taking key off a chain' merited a fine of 1 shilling, while 'neglecting to wear chain, with keys attached, while on duty' led to a fine of 5 shillings. The loss of a key involved a fine of 10 shillings. Violating the sacred principle of economy, such as not turning a light off at a particular time, was also liable to lead to a fine or disciplinary action. Thus, from an examination of which rules were emphasised, we can begin to discern the main priorities of asylum authorities.

Although particular rules were given more weight than others, staff could be punished or dismissed for infringing any regulation in the rulebook including, in some instances, not being able to produce the book of regulations! On joining the service, staff were often compelled to sign 'Obligation Forms' which granted virtually absolute power to the medical superintendent to punish or dismiss a member of staff at whim. A typical form in the early twentieth century, for Napsbury Asylum, near St Albans, ran as follows:

I acknowledge the right of the Superintendent to suspend me without warning for acts of unkindness, harshness or insolence, violence to patients, disobedience of elders, trangression of rules or negligence; also for intemperance or immorality, whether occurring within or without the asylum boundaries; in any of which cases the wages due to me will be paid only up to the day of suspension.

Subsequent dismissal by the Visiting Committee was merely a formality for those 'sent down the drive' by the superintendent. Through such provisions, his authority spread into every aspect of employees' lives; for example, they usually had to ask his permission to marry, or risk dismissal.

Not only were the off-duty lives of staff subject to a host of petty restrictions – off-duty time itself was typically treated as an act of generosity by the medical superintendent rather than as a right. As the Regulations and Orders for Wakefield Asylum in Yorkshire put it, 'no leave of absence can be claimed as a right.'

Until well into the twentieth century, staff (especially male staff) slept in rooms adjacent to the wards, and were expected to deal with emergencies in the middle of the night.

There is evidence that these wide-ranging disciplinary powers were often exercised in arbitrary ways. For example, at Lancaster Asylum – which will figure again later on – the Charges Book gives an indication of the reasons why staff were dismissed by the medical superintendent. On 4 May 1892, C. Dean, an attendant with nearly two years' service was dismissed summarily 'for sitting up playing cards'. Staff were expected to be in their beds by 10.30 pm and failure to do so was a dismissable offence. Fanny Walker, a housemaid with nearly three years' service was dismissed on 6 February 1896 'for carelessly leaving a door open'. In 1897, the services of Martha Clarke, a kitchen maid, were dispensed with 'for quarrelling', and James Murphy, an attendant with more than four years' service, was 'discharged for staying out without leave'.[7]

In short, for most intents and purposes, staff were as

confined to the asylum as if they too had been certified. The same management objectives of security and order, with the greatest economy, were applied to them almost as ruthlessly as they were applied to the lives of the patients. It was against the background of this harsh reality that a movement arose among 'subordinate staff', which sought to challenge such abysmal conditions of employment and the tyrannical exercise of authority. This chapter has shown why such a challenge was justified. The next chapters will show how it was made possible, by men and women who believed that, through joint action, they could remedy the grievances and redress the injustices to which they were subjected.

Notes

[1] For a comprehensive discussion, see my chapter, 'Asylum Nursing Before 1914', in C. Davies (ed.), *Rewriting Nursing History* (1980).

[2] J. Connolly, *The Construction and Government of Lunatic Asylums and Hospitals for the Insane* (1847).

[3] Quoted in K. Jones, *Lunacy, Law and Conscience 1744-1855* (1955), p.159.

[4] H. Burdett, *Hospitals and Asylums of the World* (1891), Vol. 1, p.215.

[5] Medico-Psychological Association, *Handbook for Attendants on the Insane* (1908 edition), p.323.

[6] My main source is the collection which forms part of the COHSE archive, Modern Records Centre, University of Warwick.

[7] Records of Lancaster Asylum, County Records Office, Preston.

Chapter 2
The Roots of Unionism

There is no reason why the conditions described in the previous chapter should automatically lead to trade unionism among asylum employees. The most oppressed, overworked and economically exploited workers are not necessarily in the forefront of the labour movement. More often than not, they become easily demoralised, or their discontent may be expressed in individual forms of action, such as high turnover. When such a pattern sets in, trade unionism will not easily take root.

Yet rarely do such groups of workers surrender permanently to apathy. When wider political and economic conditions are favourable, movements often arise from below to emulate the example of more organised groups of workers. Gains still do not come automatically but need to be struggled for, and courage, imagination, judgement and luck are all necessary for success. It was such a combination of circumstances which made it possible for asylum workers to establish – albeit rather precariously – a union in 1910. The right issues existed, the wider economic and political conditions were favourable and, above all, there existed a group of activists who saw and grasped the opportunities open to them.

Foundations of Solidarity

There had been previous attempts to form a union of asylum workers, but these had not proved successful. In the 1890s, a short lived attempt by attendants in London County Asylums came to nothing. However, London asylum workers continued to put informal pressure on the authorities and this culminated in a petition for reduced hours, submitted jointly in 1899 by male and female attendants. Although this was turned down by the Asylums Committee, for reasons of expense, faltering steps were taken to improve the lot of LCC asylum staffs. The *Medical Press and Circular* commented at the time that the petitioning was indicative 'of an unrest and anxiety as to the future of their [workers'] asylum service which was bound to manifest itself sooner or later'.[1] It went on to argue that the 'keeper' image was increasingly an anachronism, and that staff demanded official recognition for 'brains which can be educated and exercised' and 'manners which can be polished'. It also connected asylum workers' agitation to the growth of the 'New Unionism' which was extending the base of the trade union movement beyond privileged groups of skilled workers. London was one of the centres of the New Unionism and, after Lancashire, was the largest concentration of asylum employment. But the agitation was not restricted to London. It surfaced in the West Country and Yorkshire, and in Ireland in 1896 there was even an attempt to establish a National Union of Asylum Attendants. It was immediately suppressed by militarily minded authorities who regarded the formation of such an organisation as virtually an act of mutiny. As the medical superintendents' house journal put it:

> A trade union is as impossible in an Asylum as in the Army or Navy. Discipline would be impossible, and no confidence could be placed on a staff which would at any moment be paralysed by the action of an irresponsible and often tyrannously autocratic trade union committee.[2]

Medical superintendents did not consider it possible, of course, that their actions in denying rank and file workers the right to organise, might also be regarded as 'tyrannously autocratic'.

Repression might temporarily stem the movement towards trade unionism, but was not a long-term solution. Staff felt that they had interests in common which were distinctly different from those of their superiors. This lay in the realisation that they, the humble nurses and attendants, and not the doctors, were most important in keeping the institution going. Dr Mercier, an eminent medical superintendent, frankly admitted that:

> The attendants are the backbone of a lunatic asylum ... To the comfort of ninety-nine out of a hundred patients in the asylum the removal and replacement of the Medical Superintendent is a matter of no moment at all in comparison with the removal or replacement of the attendant who has immediate charge of them.[3]

Yet at the same time as attendants and nurses received only between £40 and £50 a year for their many and unremitting duties, it was not uncommon for the medical superintendent of a large asylum to earn £800 a year and, in addition, to live in a fine house with servants and the pick of the asylum farm's produce.

A mutual sense of injustice, combined with a feeling of exclusion from the rest of the community, and the close bonds formed among those carrying out socially despised and sometimes dangerous work, formed the basis for the creation of strong ties of solidarity among asylum nurses and attendants. They formed what has been called an 'occupational community', where 'members of the same occupation or who work together have some sort of common life together and are, to some extent, separate from the rest of society'.[4] In such circumstances, people's shared work identity often forms the basis of a whole way of life; mining communities are, of course, the most obvious and well known example, of this, and asylum workers are in many ways comparable. For example, the work could be dangerous and workers relied on each other to ensure others' physical safety. Moreover, asylum nursing cut a person off from the rest of society – *geographically*, because of the physical isolation of the institutions, and *socially*, partly because of the long hours and the restrictions placed upon their lives by the authorities, and partly because of society's widespread fear and loathing of the insane, and the strong suspicion that those who worked in close contact with them had become somehow tainted.

Asylum workers therefore tended to associate with each other, to live in communities closely hugging the asylum, and to receive their own sense of worth and pride from each other, in a society which despised them only a little bit less than it despised 'lunatics'. Asylum nursing became a way of life, passed down through generations as children followed their parents into 'the trade', a tradition which, though not so pronounced, still survives to this day.

Even before the advent of trade unionism, then, asylum workers provided each other with mutual support. A culture of resistance to the harsh discipline imposed by higher authority became established, with a strong emphasis upon loyalty and helping one another out. Such support flourished whether the authorities banished it or not. Because doctors were so few and far between, many of their theoretical powers were in practice exercised by nurses and attendants. They became particularly influential in decisions regarding the giving of sedatives. By the end of the nineteenth century 'medicinal restraint' – as it was called – was replacing the 'mechanical restraints' of the past, such as straitjackets. It was the cheapest and easiest solution to the problem of maintaining order among large numbers of patients, where staffing levels were minimal, and medical opinion was pessimistic regarding chances of recovery. For, as Dr Mercier put it, patients in asylums were managed by 'the gross' rather than as individuals.

This indicated the existence of a very different set of power relations to the official one. The disparity between the two – the fact that attendants and nurses could still be fined or dismissed, arbitrarily, and received pitifully small rewards in relation to their contribution to the institution – all served to heighten their sense of grievance. This germinated and took root in the collective culture of the asylum workers' community. Out of it, sooner or later, would grow permanent trade union organisation.

The Doctors' Crusade for Staff Loyalty

Some far-seeing medical superintendents were able to

grasp that an entirely repressive approach to managing their staff, ruthlessly economising wherever possible, could not in the long run be completely successful, and was not entirely in their own professional interests. From among their ranks developed proposals for reforming the recruitment, training and conditions of employment of attendants and nurses, some of which were implemented. It would be uncharitable not to accept that many of these proposals were genuinely motivated by a concern for the welfare of patients and staff, but they were also seeking to wrest back some of the control they knew had been surrendered to ward staff. They wanted also to uplift the status of attendants and nurses so that their own image would be enhanced in relation to medicine as a whole. They knew also that 'subordinate staff' were often more loyal to their own peer group than to their superiors, and were even threatening to adopt trade unionism.

In 1859 central government Commissioners had argued that improvements in the quality of care would only come when nurses and attendants received decent pay and conditions. Because this conflicted with management's imperative of 'economy' some medical superintendants, particularly in Scotland, sought the cheaper alternative of attracting greater numbers of women nurses inspired by vocational ideals, along the lines pioneered by Florence Nightingale in general nursing. On the whole this was not successful, but more success was had in attracting general-trained nurses to asylums with the promise of a rapid rise through the ranks.[5] By 1910, nursing on the female sides of asylums had become a recognised part of the general nursing universe. Its extension to the separately administered male sides was, however, quite another matter. Attempts were made, especially in Scotland (where many of the attempts to reform asylum nursing can be traced), to introduce female nursing into the male sides of asylums. The motives were various. One theory was that male patients would co-operate more readily with female nurses. Dr Robertson, a leading proponent, claimed that

The presence of good women always has a refining influence on male society ... Excited patients who are ready to fight any

man who comes near them, will often do anything they are
told by a nurse, and they will become calm if they receive a
word of sympathy from her.[6]

Yet considerations of economy were not far from the
surface, as their lower wages enabled staffing ratios to be
improved and for more night staff to be taken on. The
employment of female nurses on male wards became
widespread in Scotland, but it did not become common in
England and Wales until much later; as we shall see, this
was in large part because of the resistance of male
attendants.

The introduction of training schemes for nurses and
attendants by medical superintendants was, in similar
fashion, partly motivated by concern for the welfare of
patients and staff, and partly from self-interest. In the
1840s and 50s some far-seeing medical superintendents
introduced lectures for attendants and other staff, notably
Dr Browne at the Crichton Royal Asylum. However, it was
not until much later in the nineteenth century that any
positive steps were taken nationally, though a number of
asylums experimented with training schemes. The first
step was the publication of the first edition of the *Handbook
for Attendants on the Insane* in 1885. This created a uniform
curriculum so that national training in 1890 was a natural
next step. By 1899, 100 asylums were participating in the
two-year training scheme (three years from 1908) and
500-600 certificates were granted each year.[7] The
curriculum was modelled very closely upon general
nursing (itself slavishly imitative of medical students'
training), with heavy doses of anatomy and physiology
during the first year. Actual care of patients was regarded
as an issue of only secondary importance. The certificates
were awarded by the psychiatrists' own professional body,
the Medico (later Royal) Medico-Psychological Association
(MPA/RMPA).

This system was very different to that which had been
achieved by general nurses. There, due to the efforts of
non-medical reformers such as Florence Nightingale,
training schools had been established under the firm
control of nurses, though doctors might be brought in as

'guest' lecturers. In the asylums training schemes were a paternalistic innovation by doctors. As a result they defined the nature and content of asylum nursing, and typically gave all the lectures. However, with the influx of general trained nurses to matron positions in the first decade of the twentieth century, it later became common for medical superintendants to delegate control of the training school to them. Thus asylum nursing, dominated by psychiatrists, became mental nursing, dominated by former general nurses.

In the subsequent years this was to prove particularly divisive, because it provided the means by which the matrons extended their power and influence to male sides of mental hospitals. Men were discriminated against in general nursing and could not obtain double qualifications. As a result the chief male nurse did not usually wield influence over the training school, and his power as 'only' a MPA/RMPA certificate holder was restricted to the male side.

The major aim of this unprecedented initiative from above could be said to be, in the speech of Dr Clouston of the Royal Edinburgh Asylum to the annual meeting of the MPA in 1876, the creation of an 'ideal attendant'. He was alarmed by the high turnover in Scottish asylums of around 60 per cent a year. It had become common for 'roving attendants' to travel from asylum to asylum, staying a few months in the job before leaving and, it was said, spreading dissatisfaction among existing staff. Training would be a means of stabilizing the workforce and instilling loyalty to 'the doctors' point of view'. He also made other far-reaching proposals for achieving a stable and loyal workforce, including substantial improvements in pay and conditions, provision of suitable accommodation and opportunities for male attendants to marry, greater possibilities for promotion, more off-duty time and holidays and pensions on retirement.[8]

Some of these objectives were more realisable than others – particularly those involving only limited expenditure, otherwise Visiting Committees would not sanction them. Thus some progress could be made in improving promotion opportunities, though the superintendents themselves fuelled the dissatisfaction of their own trained staff by allowing many of the higher positions to be annexed by general trained nurses. Pensions were also an issue on which some advances were made. Under the Lunacy Act of 1890, Visiting Committees were allowed, if they wished, to grant discretionary pensions to long-serving members of staff. Thus medical superintendants, despite their apparent power, were unable to secure significant material improvements for the staff serving under them. Furthermore, they made no attempt to recognise the central place of attendants and nurses in the asylum by decentralising some of the power which they held. Awarding certificates of proficiency might increase a worker's sense of professional 'dignity', but did not lead in most cases to any real improvement in the material or social conditions of work. Asylums were not in any fundamental sense changing from custodial to treatment based institutions. In fact, one authority has claimed that by the end of the nineteenth century, with custodialism in the ascendant, mental *nursing* was an occupation in decline.[9]

Holders of the MPA Certificate received no extra pay for their efforts. They were frequently passed over for promotion by general trained nurses, had no more real influence in the power structure of the asylum, and they could still be arbitarily dismissed. In short, the doctors' crusade offered nurses and attendants the trappings of professionalism without any of the substance: certificates, prize-giving ceremonies and a greater sense of 'dignity', but no real uplift in their material conditions, job satisfaction or recognition of an associated right to exercise professional autonomy.

Notes

[1] 'The Future of the Asylum Service – I', *Medical Press and Circular*, 21 March 1900.
[2] *Journal of Mental Science*, July 1896.
[3] Dr C. Mercier, *Lunatic Asylums, Their Organisation and Management* (1895).
[4] G. Salaman, *Community and Occupation* (1974), p.19.

[5] *Asylum News* (1918), p.35.

[6] Ibid., (1916), pp.7-9.

[7] A. Walk, 'History of Mental Nursing', *Journal of Mental Science* (1961), pp.1-17.

[8] Dr Clouston, 'On Getting, Training and Retaining the Services of Good Asylum Attendants', *Journal of Mental Science*, October 1876.

[9] R.A. Hunter, 'The Rise and Fall of Mental Nursing', in *The Mental Hospital: Articles from the Lancet* (1955).

Chapter 3
Association or Union?

The development of trade unionism among asylum workers can thus be regarded in part as a result of the failure of the doctors' own crusade for staff loyalty. The poor pay, working conditions and low status of asylum work failed to attract significant numbers of staff who would be likely to defer completely to doctors. Training was only partially successful in lifting standards and status, and in indoctrinating ward staff with the values of their superiors. It made no real difference to the workers' material position. As one attendant expressed it ironically in the *NAWU Magazine* in 1912:

> Why should you grumble because a tradesman works 50 hours a week and you 80 or 90 or more? Cling to that precious position; feed the wife and children with it when pay-day is approaching; when the coalman comes with his bill, try paying him with a 'dignified' look. If the 'Super' has you up for some little offence, ask him how he dare meddle with one engaged in a 'dignified profession'. Grievances vanish and sorrows fade before the wonderful zephyr of dignity.

It is true that with the growth in size of the asylums from the second half of the nineteenth century, some growth of middle management grades created promotion opportunities. These perhaps helped to defuse the growing discontent. On the male side, however, promotion was extremely slow, because of a relatively low turnover of staff. Either the 'eye colour' method of promotion ('blue-eyed boys') operated, or else the 'dead man's shoes' principle of seniority blocked the rise of ward staff. On the female side high turnover. rates seemingly offered promotion for those who remained. Yet, as we have seen, higher positions were from the beginning of the twentieth century increasingly monopolised by 'high flyers' from general nursing.

These changes created a major split in the workforce. On the one hand a small minority of relatively more privileged staff who had escaped (and in some instances had never been exposed) to the harsh realities of miserable low pay and appalling working and living conditions. On the other hand the majority, whose life and livelihood has been portrayed in the two previous chapters. This division in the work-force enabled the doctors' to play their 'trump card' with some initial success. This was the encouragement of a 'loyal' professional association which would be led by themselves, with the assistance of middle and senior management, who would in turn 'influence' their subordinates to become members. For a time, the strategy appeared to be winning. The organisation concerned – the Asylum Workers' Association – attracted at its peak some 5,000 members, nearly half of all asylum employees. But its mishandling of the pensions issue in 1909 led to its demise and eventual disappearance by 1920. As we shall see this was not entirely unconnected with the appearance on the scene, in 1910, of the National Asylum Workers' Union.

The Rise of the Asylum Workers' Association

First we must understand why the Asylum Workers' Association (AWA) enjoyed such an influence for so long. It would be tempting to suggest that asylum workers were either hoodwinked or bullied into joining. This may have been so in certain cases, but the split in the workforce created a group for whom a professional association commanded some loyalty. Others simply deferred to the seniors, or were out one day to occupy the same position. But the AWA also probably included some more trade-union minded attendants and nurses, who joined because there was no 'real' union around. When one did appear on the scene, however, this last group proved to be potential defectors.

In his speech of 1876 Dr Clouston had envisaged the formation of a professional association for attendants to be central to his crusade. As he made clear to his fellow doctors, he wished to

> ... develop an *esprit de corps* among attendants as a class, making them proud of their profession as we are of ours. I should like to see them get diplomas from the asylums where they were trained, and get up an association of attendants all over the kindgom.[1]

Since they were unlikely to get one up for themselves, it was apparent that they needed a little help from some friends.

The AWA was very close to being what in private industry would be described as a company union, that is, an organisation set up with the express intention of preventing independent organisation by rank-and-file workers. While giving the appearance of advancing the interests of employees, the main purpose of a company union is to protect management's power. The AWA was formed in 1895, a time when, as we have seen, it looked as if trade-union organisation might grow among asylum workers, and when many psychiatrists were showing concern at possible 'mutiny' in the ranks. It cannot, therefore, be regarded as purely coincidental that doctors chose this particular time to promote an alternative professional association to 'look after' asylum workers' interests.

The AWA was set up only after the British Nurses' Association (BNA), then the leading professional association for general nurses, had rejected the proposals of several leading MPA doctors, that asylum nurses should be allowed to join the BNA. The 'ladies' of the BNA were aghast at the prospect of having to associate themselves with male, working class, insane attendants. Mrs Bedford Fenwick, the BNA's leading light declared.

> Everyone will agree that no person can be considered trained who has only worked in hospitals and asylums for the insane.

The scheme also proposes to open the register of trained nurses to men as well as to women, and, considering the present class of persons known as Male Attendants, one can hardly believe that their admission will tend to raise the status of the association, while we foresee considerable trouble for the executive council from such members.[2]

And that was the end of the matter.

The MPA doctors then set up the Asylum Workers' Association, closely modelled upon the BNA in its aims and constitution. The organisation hastily sought to reassure some worried asylum authorities that 'the Association has in it nothing of the nature of a trade union: it does not presume to dictate in the matter of wages.'[3] It also encouraged members to obtain the MPA Certificate in order to lift themselves above the generality of workers, as 'professional qualifications' should suggest to all asylum workers the desirability of differentiating themselves from mere domestic servants.[4] The organisation became dominated by the elite of medical superintendents who had formerly campaigned within the BNA. Its Honorary Secretary and leading light was Dr G.E. Shuttleworth, the retired Medical Superintendent of the Royal Albert Institution, Lancaster. Its Vice-Presidents included most leading medical superintendents, as well as the Archbishop of Canterbury and the Chief Rabbi. Even a sympathetic medical historian was forced to admit that the AWA was far from being a democratic organisation:

> Its constitution and government were entirely paternal ... and the Annual General Meetings ... consisted largely of uplifting speeches by distinguished Honorary Vice-Presidents; no mental nurse seems ever to have spoken and it is doubtful if any attended.[5]

This would accord with the view of the AWA projected by an anonymous 'dissillusioned member', in the *NAWU Magazine* of May 1912, who claimed that the AWA

> is nothing more nor less than a despotic oligarchy and a showy sham, an ingenious *imitation* of a trade union, but a real death trap for progress ... It is an instrument framed for keeping the subordinate staffs 'in its place'.

Thus it was an organisation claiming to speak for all asylum staff, yet dominated by medical superintendents. Of the nurses and attendants involved at all in the organisation, all were senior managers, with a particularly strong representation of the ex-general nurses who had entered the asylums in the twentieth century.

The one 'union' issue which the AWA pressed was that of pensions, which provided the basis for a common interest between managers and workers. It studiously avoided such issues as pay or discipline, over which there were bound to be conflicts of interest. Pensions, as we saw, might be a way for management to achieve a greater stability in the workforce. They would serve as an inducement to attract and keep staff, as well as damping down militancy. Workers might think twice about disobeying orders or organising among themselves, if they risked losing their pension rights through being dismissed.

One of the first acts of the AWA was to organise a petition to change the law to make the granting of pensions obligatory upon employing authorities. A Private Member's Bill succeeded in the House of Lords, but was thrown out by the House of Commons. The obstacles, as always, lay in the objections of some county councils, as ultimate employing authorities, to the expense that might be involved. Therefore the unsatisfactory situation continued with some asylum workers enjoying pension rights and others none, as annual Private Member's Bills were dutifully put and rejected by Parliament.

Changes more favourable to the working class generally, and from which asylum employees might benefit, were in the air. In 1906 a Liberal government was elected but at a time when the working-class electorate was increasingly turning to the Labour Party, which had won 30 seats in the new Parliament. In order to keep the working-class vote, the Liberal government had to address itself directly to solving working-class discontents. In this more favourable atmosphere, the AWA's frequent attempts to achieve compulsory pensions stood a much greater chance of succeeding. The AWA was not without friends in high places. Its President in 1909 was Sir William Collins, MD, FRCS, Liberal MP for St Pancras West, who submitted a

Private Member's Bill before the House. To his surprise it was passed in a single session and became the Asylum Officers' Superannuation Act 1909. The scheme was based broadly on that operating within the poor law service. The qualifying age was 55 to 60 years with 20 years' minimum service for a pension of 1/50th of total pay for each year of service, while incapacity after ten years qualified an employee for a pension.

The AWA hailed the Act as a great victory, a vindication of its patient effort and non-militant efforts over the years. Its leaders little dreamt that unfavourable reaction to the Act from many asylum workers would, within the space of a decade, lead to the ultimate downfall of the AWA, and its replacement by the National Asylum Workers' Union (NAWU). Yet unrest caused by the effects of certain clauses of the 1909 Act was taken as a wider indication of the inadequacy of an organisation dominated by senior nurses and doctors, dedicated to methods that avoided any taint of conflict.

The Birth of the Union

Unfortunately the 1909 Act had several very painful stings in its tail. For those who already enjoyed the discretionary pensions allowed under the 1890 Act, the new scheme represented a worsening of conditions. Under the old arrangements, no qualifying period was required before a pension could be granted on the grounds of incapacity. Under the 1909 Act, it was necessary to have ten years' service. Under the old arrangements pensions could be granted at 50 years of age, after 15 years' service. Under the new scheme they could not be granted until workers had reached at least 55 years of age, with a minimum of 20 years' service. What rankled most of all, however, was the fact that whatever meagre benefits might be provided for under the Act would have to be paid for by the workers themselves. While under the previous scheme pensions had been non-contributory, asylum employees would have 2-3 per cent of their inadequate pay deducted to pay for pensions that many of them would never receive.

The anger of asylum employees at the 1909 Act was part

of a growing political disenchantment and industrial militancy of manual workers during the Edwardian period, one of the most turbulent periods in recent British history. Labour was becoming increasingly restive. The means for improvement existed in growing national prosperity, as Britain remained, throughout this period, the world's leading trading nation, at a time when retail prices were rising faster than money wages. Particularly from 1910 to 1913, when the level of unemployment fell, there was an upsurge of militancy in many industries: strikes took place among miners, dockers, seafarers, transport workers and on the railways.

These were some of the features of the wider social context in which NAWU was formed. Asylum workers in England and Wales formed a tiny section of the working class:

Male attendants	5,687
Female nurses	6,445
Total	12,132*
Number of patients	102,000

*This figure does not include craftsmen, kitchen staff, etc.
(*Source*: Commissioners in Lunacy: Annual Report for 1910)

Nor could they be said to possess significant industrial muscle. Yet, as we have already seen, they possessed a keen sense of mutual support and a communal way of work and residence which reinforced it. They therefore were able to identify with the rising working-class movememt, if at first in a rather cautious and hesitant manner.

Lancashire was the centre of the protest movement that would rapidly lead to permanent, national trade union organisation. It had one of the highest concentrations of asylum employment in the country, and its five huge asylums were grouped into a single employing authority, the Lancashire Asylums Board (LAB). Lancashire was also a predominantly working-class county, with trade union organisation almost second nature to its inhabitants. Most significant of all was the fact that Lancashire asylum workers were particularly badly affected by the 1909

Asylum Officers' Superannuation Act. Previously the
Board had used its discretionary powers liberally, to grant
non-contributory pensions. What would happen now?

A group of eight charge attendants from the Lancashire
asylums were invited to a meeting convened by Martin
Meehan of Winwick Asylum in December 1909. Visiting
Committees were petitioned, with a view to gaining wage
increases to cover the compulsory deductions required by
law. Eventually the matter came before the Lancashire
Asylums Board on 26 May 1910 where petitions signed by
attendants at Lancashire asylums were presented. In the
absence of a union, petitioning was the traditional means
for workers to make their views known. When the motion
was presented that the Board increase wages to cover
pension contributions, only six councillors voted for the
proposal, while 44 voted against. It was this refusal of the
Lancashire Asylum Board to protect their employees that
encourage the informal pressure group around a single
issue to turn itself into a trade union. The events of those
early days were recalled to the union's 1931 anniversary
Conference by Martin Meehan:

> In Lancashire, when the Asylum Officers' Superannuation
> Act of 1909, with its glaring anomalies and defects came
> along, I thought 'Now is the time to form a union; this is a
> great chance, and something must be done.' Having been a
> member of a trade union since I was five years of age (that's
> funny isn't it?) I thought to myself, now is the time to get a
> union of asylum workers started. Well we succeeded, but not
> without an effort ... I thought to myself, now is the time when
> we have a national grievance, if we can only get a union
> started now, so much the better. I called a meeting at Winwick
> and after that we had other meetings. I was instructed by
> several charge attendants to send out little circulars to other
> institutions in Lancashire.

As a result of Martin Meehan's 'little circulars' a meeting
was called for Saturday 9 July 1910 at the Masons Arms
Hotel in Whitefield, Manchester. Three delegates from
each of the five Lancashire asylums attended. Unfortunately, Martin Meehan was not himself able to attend.

I was one of the representative delegates who was chosen ... but the chief came round at 7.15 at night and said 'Your day off tomorrow is stopped; you cannot go to that meeting.' I made a fairly big outcry against this. However, seeing I could not go, I said to the other members: 'Well I think we have a bright lad in Gibson.' He was only a lad. I said to him: 'Look here, George, my day's leave is stopped tomorrow, and we are determined to form an organisation on trade union lines ... When you go there what I want you to do is to move a resolution that there shall be a union formed of asylum workers, and if there is a job offered you as secretary, accept it.'

Another individual keen to form a union was, according to his own account, the Rev H.M.S. Bankart, the recently appointed Chaplain at Lancaster Asylum, at a stipend of £250 a year, plus emoluments to the value of £120. As he stated in the *NAWU Magazine* for January 1912:

I very quickly learnt for myself, at first hand, that the conditions of the staff generally were far from ideal, though I was not aware then that that asylum is by no means the worst. As time went on I often had complaints poured into my ears and many a time I said: 'The only way to remedy your grievances is to form a union; one individual needs to be backed up by all the others; one asylum needs to be supported by all other asylums, or each single one is helpless.' The time, long overdue as it was, was not yet ripe.

The agitation and unrest over the 1909 Act provided such an opportunity especially when invitations arrived for delegates to attend the meeting at Manchester of 10 July. The Rev Bankart repeated his advice:

'The only thing to do is to form a union.' 'A very good idea; we'll form one for the men,' was the reply. 'No you don't, if I have anything to do with it,' I answered; 'it must be for *all* asylum workers – girls and men, inside and outside – or you won't get my help in the matter.'

Given, however, that asylums were strictly divided into male and female sides, there were practical problems in seeking to spread the movement to the female sides.

Fortunately, Bankart, as Chaplain, could move freely throughout the asylum and collected, on a sheet of foolscap, names of 250 male and female staff prepared to join a union. When this list was presented to the Manchester meeting on 10 July it had a profound impact. A resolution was carried 'to form an organisation for asylum Workers, and to ask for 4d a month to defray initial expenses'. George Gibson, the young attendant from Winwick, was duly elected to the post of Honorary General Secretary.

Events moved rapidly from then on. Bankart enlisted the support of a prominent Christian Socialist, the Rev Samuel Proudfoot. A co-founder of the Church Socialist League he had, as curate of Westhoughton in Lancashire, helped to obtain the return of its first Labour MP in the 1906 election. He had also been active in encouraging a strike of mill girls at Hulton Mills, on the River Lune. The mills were owned by Sir Norval W. Helme, Liberal MP for Lancaster and Chairman of the Lancashire Asylums Board. Proudfoot initially became involved with the campaign to establish a trade union for asylum workers as a result of an invitation by Bankart to preach a sermon to the workers of Lancaster. He and Bankart toured the Lancashire asylums in the wake of the Manchester meeting, drumming up support for the new union. This led to a meeting to 'christen' the new union, held on Saturday 24 September 1910, at the Boar's Head Hotel, Preston. The chair was taken by Mr Williamson, the President of Preston Trades Council. Fortunately we have Proudfoot's own account of that meeting as recollected at the Union's Anniversary Conference in 1931:

I knew that trade unionism was the only hope for humanity, and I spoke to that audience for one hour. At the conclusion of the meeting I got up and asked if there were any questions they would like to put, or if they had any grievances they would like to mention. There was absolute silence for a considerable time, no one venturing to come forward. After what appeared to be an eternity one man got up and broke the silence. I thanked God for that man. (Laughter). Then he blurted out: 'We're starving. It is time things were remedied, but they cannot be remedied and never will be. We are only slaves, and can only be slaves.' You know the story! Now the climax of that meeting was when a woman got up (God bless that woman!) and said: 'Mr Proudfoot, you have spoken the truth, and we shall all be fools if we do not join this union.' (Applause.) I am wholehearted in my belief that women will send forward trade unionism with a far greater impetus than we men can do. I know that their ingenuity can win through where men will stand agape. A resolution was then put to the meeting to support the movement for a trade union and this was supported.

The suggestion then was that the union should be called the National Asylum Workers' Union, and this was unanimously agreed. Bankart suggested that its motto should be 'All for One and One for All: Thou Shalt Love Thy Neighbour as Thyself'– which seems highly appropriate for a union christened in an atmosphere highly charged with both trade union and religious fervour. A committee of five, consisting of one from each asylum, was appointed to draft provisional rules, and to approve the text of a recruiting pamphlet, to be written by the Rev Proudfoot. 30,000 were printed and widely distributed throughout Great Britain and Ireland.

The next and third meeting in the formation of the union, held at the Victoria Hotel, Rainhill on 18 February 1911, was in some respects the most important. For the first time delegates came from outside Lancashire, from Yorkshire asylums and Chester. The meeting approved an amended version of the draft constitution and then turned to consider the appointment of a paid officer. The chief candidate for the post of paid secretary was George Gibson, previously the unpaid General Secretary. However, during the meeting news arrived by telegram that Bankart had been dismissed from his position as Chaplain. He had committed the cardinal sin of 'putting up notices in the institution without the permission of the Medical Superintendent', Dr Cassidy, who had reported him to the Visiting Committee. When the meeting heard of this, George Gibson withdrew his candidature, and the Rev H.M.S. Bankart was unanimously elected to the position of

General and Organising Secretary of the National Asylum Workers' Union of Great Britain and Ireland. His yearly salary was to be £104, somewhat less than he had previously received.

Bankart took charge of the union's administration in March 1911. In April, Herbert Shaw, the acting Secretary of the NAWU at Wakefield Asylum, was dismissed for unauthorised use of an envelope belonging to the West Riding County Council. He had used it to post circulars to other asylums asking workers there to join the union. Shaw was appointed as an official of the NAWU, to work with Bankart at the union's Manchester office. Thus both the first full-time officials of the union occupied their posts as a result of victimisation by employers.

The circumstances under which the NAWU was born indicated that some difficult battles lay ahead if the union was to survive, let alone realise any wider objectives. After all, some previous attempts to establish unionism had got almost as far, yet ultimately failed. It was by no means a foregone conclusion that the present agitation would be any more successful than previous ones, especially since the authorities seemed as determined as ever to put down any signs of 'insubordination' in the ranks.

Notes

[1] Clouston, op. cit.
[2] Quoted by F.R. Adams, 'From Association to Union', *British Journal of Sociology* (1969), pp.11-26.
[3] Quoted in 'Trade Unionism in Mental Hospitals', *The Hospital*, 11 October 1913, pp.49-50.
[4] *Asylum News*, 5 March 1900.
[5] Walk, op. cit.

Chapter 4
Years of Frustration, 1911–17

Despite the formidable obstacles in its way, the union quickly established a solid base of support throughout England and Wales. By the time of the National Asylum Workers' Union's first Annual Conference, held in Birmingham on 8 July 1911, membership had soared to 4,400 in 44 institutions. Delegates attended from as far afield as Lancaster in the North, Maidstone in the South, and Bodmin in the West. The NAWU had rapidly become a truly 'national' union of asylum workers.

The chief casualty of this success was the AWA, and Dr Shuttleworth admitted in an internal memorandum that compulsory pensions deductions had led to the defection of 1,000 members to the NAWU, mainly in London and Lancashire.[1] The AWA sought to rally support to its flagging cause. Its journal published a 'Plea for Cohesion amongst Asylum Workers' by Dr Doherty of Armagh Asylum. In it he accused the NAWU of fermenting division among the ranks when unity was required. While he admitted that the AWA had not enjoyed a great deal of success in obtaining improvements for asylum workers, Dr Doherty denied that trade unionism would prove any more successful. Asylum workers were chastised for being 'too prone to build castles in the air', and he pointed out to them that

> Lunacy is the Cinderella of the services; it is a dead weight; it is unremunerative; expenditure on asylums is like so much money thrown into the sea; and consequently the Government is slow to move in increasing that dead weight.[2]

He undoubtedly had a point. Despite the initial successes against the AWA, the NAWU had an uphill task. Its finances were precarious. At the end of 1910 its first accounts showed the balance of income over expenditure to be exactly 1s 6d. The first offices, at 174 Egerton Road, Manchester were hardly stylish. As the union's auditor, Mr A. Yearsley recalled in 1931:

> In my young days I went to Sunday School and was taught to see how a great flame arose kindled by a spark of love. I have seen the union grow from very small beginnings ... When I first knew the union it did not even have an office, it only had half an office, for the other half was leased to a jeweller.

Before they could even think of doing battle with the employers, union activists had also to win the support and loyalty of those they sought to represent. The first years of campaigning on behalf of asylum employees did not, generally speaking, result in significant improvements in pay and conditions of employment, but a base of support was laid, from which later more successful campaigns for improvement could be launched.

The Cul de Sac of Legislative Reform

Partly because of these difficulties, the NAWU was not from the outset a particularly militant body, either on industrial or wider political fronts. The union's leadership at this stage took a *tactical* rather than *principled* position towards political parties, and sought allies among MPs in all parties, as did some other organisations, like the National Association of Local Government Officers (NALGO). On the industrial front, strikes were also deprecated.

There were, however, critics from the ranks who felt the union's Executive Council was treading too cautiously. An anonymous correspondent from Hanwell Asylum complained in *NAWU Magazine* of June 1912 of the leadership's 'antique and slow' methods, and called for a more 'vigorous forward movement'. The 'methods' referred to were those sometimes resorted to by groups of workers who lack the strength and confidence to secure their ends by pressure at the place of work: legislative change. This had the advantage of not requiring nurses and attendants to risk victimisation and, if successful, might obtain conditions that would apply universally, despite the uneven membership strength at different institutions.

George Gibson succeeded in persuading the Conservative MP for Newton-le-Willows, Lord Wolmer, to introduce a Private Member's Bill to amend the 1909 Act. This became the Asylum Officers' (Employment Pensions and Superannuation) Bill of 1911. Its central clause sought to enforce a maximum working week of 60 hours for asylum workers. Other clauses sought to abolish the upper age limit of eligibility for pensions, and to remove the power of summary dismissal from medical superintendents. This would have given staff a statutory right of appeal to Visiting Committees.

Initially the Liberal government promised support for the Bill if it reached a second reading. The AWA however, had considerable support in Parliament. It lobbied heavily, forcing the government to establish a select committee and making sure that the AWA had the decisive representation on the Committee so that the Bill could be amended to conform with AWA policy. This is indeed what happened.

Of the 20 witnesses called to give evidence to the committee, eleven were members of the AWA, and most of these were medical superintendents. Only two rank-and-file asylum attendants were called, neither members of the union. Only the Rev Bankart was permitted to give evidence for the NAWU. Only after much pressure from the NAWU was a survey which it conducted, showing hours in excess of 80, 90 and even 100 hours a week, allowed to be published as part of the Committee's minutes of evidence. When the medical superintendents gave evidence to the Committee, they were outspoken in condemning the proposed 60-hour week, mainly on grounds of expense. Questions to Dr Cassidy, the man who had sacked Bankart, revealed in his evidence that hours were extremely elastic for nurses and attendants. As well as their official hours of duty, they were expected to attend entertainments, play cricket if they were in the asylum team, practise an instrument if they were in the band, and be available to deal with any emergency. None of this merited extra pay, and it led to a very wide disparity between nurses and attendants, and other staff, such as craftsmen.

The latter were typically employed for between 54 and 56 hours a week, in line with general trade union conditions. At Lancaster, as elsewhere, the hours of women nurses tended to be even longer than those of men, with greater restrictions placed on their freedom during their off duty hours. Even after finishing duty at 6 am the night nurses at Lancaster were not allowed out of their rooms until 2 pm in the afternoon, which Dr Cassidy justified on the grounds that:

> I think the effect of too much leave, too much freedom, too many hours off duty, would be distinctly demoralising, especially to the female staff ... They have the leisure within certain bounds, within the bounds of the nurses' block or within the bounds of the Asylum grounds and so forth; but it is absolute freedom to run away down into town where nurses can do as they like at all hours, that I think would be dangerous. I would not myself feel happy about it.[3]

Bankart, as the only witness associated with the NAWU, not surprisingly painted a rather different picture of asylum work than other witnesses. He justified the case for a shorter working week, not so much on the grounds that the work was hard physical labour, but that it was 'trying'. He spoke of the 'fearful monotony' of the work, and that

> The staff are not even allowed to speak to each other during the 14, 16 or 18 hours of inside work, except at meals; they are not allowed to sit down.[4]

He went on to describe how staff might be spat at, have chamber pots thrown at them, and be 'liable to all sorts of disagreeables like that'. In short, he described asylum work as 'loathsome' which, though it horrified many members of the Select Committee, probably struck a chord with many asylum workers. One of them, who described herself as a 'Lunar Laureate', subsequently expressed such feelings in verse in the *NAWU Magazine* of February 1914:

> We work for fourteen hours a day, and sometimes even more,
> But we are under discipline throughout the twenty-four.
> It's naughty to complain about the fourteen hours a day,
> Because, you know, we're told our work is only so much play.
> We look quite nice, and comely in our uniforms, 'tis true,
> To see us none would realise the *dirty* jobs we do.
> And we are told we must possess a temper like a saint
> (If they would practise what they preach, I wouldn't make complaints.)

Bankart then went on to accuse asylum authorities, since the 1909 Act, of deliberately employing younger men so that, taking advantage of the age limit, they would not have to pay them pensions until long after they had completed the required 20 years' service.

Given the forces ranged against the NAWU's proposals, it came as little surprise that the AWA's compromise of a 70-hour maximum week, exclusive of mealtimes, became the main recommendation of the Select Committee.

The Report also recommended a reduction in the retirement age for women, and that staff should have a right of appeal to a Visiting Committee against dismissal by the medical superintendent. The recommendations never became law, primarily because of lack of Parliamentary time, but despite the dilution of the original Bill, it did indicate the amount of pressure which the AWA (and hence the authorities), were coming under from the fledgling NAWU. Not long after the report was published the membership of the NAWU had increased to 6,000, well in excess of that of the AWA. The Bill to reduce hours had fallen, but the NAWU had shown itself to be the champion of ward nurses and attendants. It therefore came out of this first test with considerable credit, if little to show materially for its encounter with the legislative process.

Campaigning for Asylum Workers, 1911-14

Following this 'defeat' the union's attention shifted to increasing membership in the localities, and pursuing a more active policy, if not immediately of confrontation, then of pressure at particular asylums. In the process the no-strike policy was inevitably placed under strain and also, as support was increasingly sought from the wider labour movement, its neutral political stance.

The first kind of pressure exerted was simply publicly to criticise and ridicule asylum officials in the *NAWU Magazine*. In the absence of material gains, this at least allowed asylum workers to vent their grievances, and convince them that someone was championing their cause. In regular features such as 'The Pillory', the *NAWU Magazine* drew attention to grievances at particular asylums. For example, one case reported in October 1912 was the dismissal of James Brennan, a second-charge attendant with seven years' service at Winwick Asylum, Lancashire, 'for taking home a piece of butter which formed part of his own rations'. Another case concerned the attendant at Caerlon Asylum, Cardiff, who was sacked 'on suspicion' of leaving a door open. Another series, 'We Have Our Eye On ... ', warned asylum authorities that their acts and omissions would not go unnoticed. Among the 'watched' included:

> – the Matron 'who wished to know how any nurse at Cardiff *dared* to sign a petition to the Committee without first asking her permission',
> – the Matron who pays the AWA subscriptions of the girls under her and then goes round demanding repayment; the girls have to pay if they are to get any days off or other privileges from the female at whose mercy they have the misfortune to be.

Such items, mocking figures in authority, allowed rank-and-file asylum workers to use the *NAWU Magazine* as a kind of graffiti board, ventilating grievances without fear of reprisal.

The letters page also provided a means by which staff

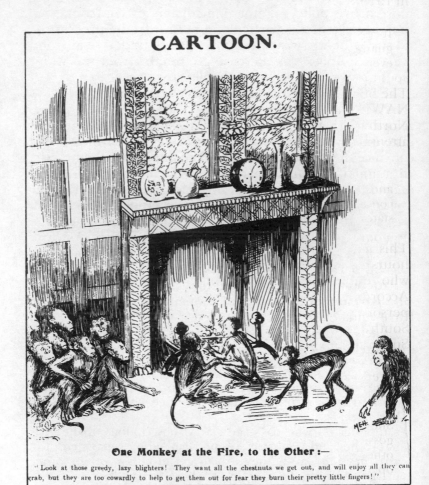

CARTOON.

One Monkey at the Fire, to the Other :—

" Look at those greedy, lazy blighters! They want all the chestnuts we get out, and will enjoy all they can grab, but they are too cowardly to help to get them out for fear they burn their pretty little fingers!"

Cartoon from National Asylum Workers' Union/*NAWU Magazine*,
February 1912

could announce any grievances, and express support for
the union. 'Sir, your union is an ideal one from the
workers' point of view', wrote a Waterford City Attendant
in 1912:

> It is officered purely from the ranks, which is a sure
> guarantee that our interests will be closely looked after in
> every respect.

The failure of the medical superintendents to support the
NAWU's campaign for the 60-hour week, led 'Langcliffe
North' (as he colourfully called himself) to draw readers'
attention to

> ... the oft-repeated remark, that 'the staff have the sympathy
> and help of the Med Supers in all things'. I have for some
> considerable time past had my doubts about the truth of this
> statement. Today I have no doubts.

This letter writer complained of the poor pay and long
hours he had to work, and of the plight of married men,
who only received 3 shillings a week towards rent.
According to Maud Pember Reeves in 1913, a 'poor'
person's rent, rates and taxes came to 8 shillings a week in
South London, though it would be less in the provinces.[5]
Such rallying cries were clearly designed to draw others to
the union. Other letter writers, on the other hand, had
matters to get off their chest – like 'Liza Jane' from
Winwick, Lancashire, who complained in April 1912 that

> She [the Matron] selects those who are likely or given to
> gossip, and encourages them to chatter, either in her office or
> other secluded places. Extremely nice girls they are. First
> opening for promotion that occurs these are the ones selected
> ... As for myself, I am clearing out; but I hope before I do to
> let some light into the state of affairs here.

As well as these kinds of issues, the *NAWU Magazine*
detailed attempts to exert real pressure to obtain much
needed improvements. In a number of instances it seems
that improvements occurred as a result not so much of
indirect intervention of the NAWU, but as a result of a

hope to forestall a move towards unionisation on the part of staffs.

Not all authorities were hostile to trade unionism. Here and there we find an accepting and even sympathetic response, especially in the Midlands, for example at Lichfield and Barnsley Hall in 1912. Sometimes senior officials were praised, despite being disciplinarians, so long as they combined it with 'fairness'. For example, the late Chief Attendant of Durham County Asylum was praised for having risen from the ranks and though 'a rigid disciplinarian, whose word was law in matters of duty', he did not prevent staff from exercising 'the fullest liberty of action in regard to securing improvements in the conditions of service' – and was even a regular contributor to union subscriptions. The most striking success was at Portsmouth in mid-1913 where the union branch, which claimed to represent 96 per cent of the staff, won not only concessions but full recognition from the Visiting Committee.

In other asylums recognition was usually only granted after concerted pressure. In the West Riding of Yorkshire, recognition for the NAWU branches in March 1914 only came after a threat of strike action.

Such breakthroughs were rare. More usually, petitions for substantial improvements and recognition of the union met with no success. Or else trivial concessions were granted, as at Lincoln, where the Visiting Committee granted two bars of soap a month to each member of staff instead of meeting the union's demands! Progress was slow even at the London County Asylums, where the Visiting Committee and its sub-committees for individual asylums (if not all of the medical superintendents) had hitherto established a progressive, sympathetic reputation since the turn of the century. The image of the London County Council as a 'model' employer was becoming somewhat tarnished. In Lancashire, too, the Lancashire Asylums Board remained obstinate in its refusal to recognise the union. Elsewhere union activists faced more than obstruction. Direct intimidation and victimisation occurred, for example, in Ireland, where conditions were among the worst anywhere. At Portrane Asylum in 1913, the staff were forced to sign, on pain of dismissal, a document declaring that they were not members of a union.

One of the most significant disputes during this period, which eventually became an issue of victimisation, was centred on Cardiff Asylum. The Visiting Committee – in a rather typical way – had refused to consider a petition from staff late in 1911, because it had not come through Dr Goodall, the Medical Superintendent. The union had requested increases in ration money and made complaints about the quality of food given to staff. The workers also called for the abolition of all fines for breaches of discipline, claiming they contravened the Truck Acts. The nature of the dispute changed when Attendant D.G. Williams, the NAWU Secretary, was sacked in February 1912 for having been responsible for an item in the *NAWU Magazine* claiming that the asylum butter was really margarine. The dispute was also significant in that it led to the active intervention of Cardiff Trades and Labour Council, but the Mental Hospitals Committee of Cardiff Council refused to receive a deputation from them.

It must be remembered that disputes over diet were about the real material wage of asylum employees. Discontent over food also served as a symbol of how double standards operated, for it was often noted with resentment that higher officials enjoyed a vastly better diet, gleaning the best produce from the asylum farm.

The failure of the legislative road to reform, the growing membership strength of the NAWU and the raised expectations caused by its campaigning activities were leading to a growing restiveness among the branches.

The First Strike

The first actual 'strike' occurred in Lancashire at Rainhill Asylum – over diet, significantly enough. After the substitution of oatmeal porridge for meat on the breakfast menu for Monday 6 April 1914, the normal work of the asylum stopped. 35 attendants occupied the breakfast room from 7 am refusing either to eat the porridge or to go to their wards. The medical superintendent, Dr Cowen, visited the scene of the trouble three times throughout the morning, but despite thinly veiled threats of disciplinary action, the attendants refused to budge. By mid-morning the mood of revolt had spread throughout the asylum where staff kept their eye on patients but would perform none of their normal duties. At midday Dr Cowen had agreed to revise the old diet sheets. The strike was over and the attendants left the breakfast room. The action appears to have been spontaneous and unofficial, and did not entirely meet with the Executive Council's approval. Ten days later, the attendants concerned were hauled before the Visiting Committee and threatened with disciplinary action unless they apologised for taking such 'drastic' action without first consulting them. This they agreed to do.

Such restiveness led to the more adventurous policy of putting pressure on individual asylums which the union leadership sought to develop whilst seeking to maintain its central authority over industrial action. The increasing membership strength – nearly 8,000 by 1914 – and growing confidence also led to a more open commitment to the wider labour movement.

As we have seen, the NAWU was originally a non-political union. In 1912 it also declined to seek affiliation to the Trades Union Congress, not as a matter of principle but because the union could not afford affiliation fees. By 1914, it was reviewing its stance, in the light of the Trade Union Act of 1913 which established the right of unions to set up political funds. The NAWU had come into closer contact with the wider labour movement, through assistance received by local trades councils (for example at Cardiff). Its attempt to seek individual allies in all parties, such as Lord Wolmer, had not yielded any material results. The motion to affiliate to the Labour Party was put to the NAWU's Annual Conference in August 1914 by Councillor Mactavish, prospective Labour candidate for Portsmouth, who mocked the union's past reliance on Lord Wolmer, who had recently sought to prevent the Trade Union Act becoming law.

The speech was decisive, and the NEC was empowered

to affiliate to the Labour Party, but the proposal to affiliate
to the TUC was 'left on the table'. Thus, unusually in the
trade union movement, the NAWU sought affiliation to
the Labour Party before seeking affiliation to the TUC.

Organising the Members, 1911-14

The first and most important battle for the NAWU – as
for any other union – was to secure the loyalty of those it
sought to represent. At first this was rather shaky.
Although membership reached 6,000 by mid-1912, it
slumped dangerously during 1913. Lack of recognition by
the authorities and the failure of Lord Wolmer's Bill, was
compounded by an active policy of victimisation by quite a
number of asylum authorities. As a result, the union's
finances became balanced on a knife edge. An unsuccessful legal attempt to get Herbert Shaw reinstated further
drained the organisation's funds. It was this background
that set in train the events which led to the removal from
office of the union's first and most colourful General
Secretary, the Rev H.M.S. Bankart.

Bankart's departure was due to the combination of two
factors: personality clashes between himself and leading
members of the NEC, and his own organisational and
financial ineptitude. Bankart's pride and joy was the
NAWU Magazine of which he was editor, and on which he
lavished considerable expense. Large numbers were sent
free to asylums where the NAWU did not yet have
branches. It not surprisingly lost considerable amounts of
money. The low and inadequate subscription rates could
not be raised without fear of losing more members. At the
same time victimised members needed assistance and
organising visits had to be arranged to the far flung
membership in Great Britain and the whole of Ireland.
Bankart was asked to resign in 1913, a decision confirmed
by Conference in July. George Gibson was subsequently
unopposed when he stood for the position of General
Secretary, and Herbert Shaw became his assistant and
editor of the journal. They both remained in post until
after the amalgamation in 1946 which created the
Confederation of Health Service Employees.

Union activists often had some difficulty in securing the support of the members. The key figure was the branch secretary, but in those days to take office was often to be placed in an extremely exposed position. Quite early on, the *NAWU Magazine* observed that there were different types of members, with varying degrees of loyalty to trade unionism. For example, an editorial in January 1913 differentiated between 'true unionists', who joined from 'principle' out of a sense of 'duty to help in the work of improving the service for others – for those who will come after'; 'selfish' members 'who joined merely because they hoped for some *personal* gain'; and 'discontented grumblers' who, it argued, are 'more ready to criticise than sacrifice themselves', and were felt to be 'generally blacklegs at heart'.

The major recruitment problem lay among women asylum workers. In 1914 overall membership was 7,900, of whom 5,200 were men, while women only totalled 2,700. One of the most important reasons for the disparity was the higher turnover among female staff. They were not any less dissatisfied than the men, but at that time their response was more often to 'vote with their feet' (like Liza Jane) than to 'dig in their heels' and try to change things by joining the NAWU. Those who were long-serving tended more often to be unmarried women with a 'professional' outlook, and hence more likely to be members of the AWA. Furthermore, though the pensions issue was central to many men, it did not excite the majority of women, only a minority of whom stayed long enough to collect one. High turnover created other problems. A continual emphasis had to be placed on recruitment, as staff left. So since men generally stayed longer, recruitment was usually a once-and-for-all question – though getting them to pay their dues regularly was not always an easy matter. Yet this needs putting in its proper context. Large numbers of women employees did join the union and were every bit as committed as the majority of men, but because of the barriers that existed to their participation, no women during these early years came to hold office in the union. However, as we shall see, the influence of women was to be decisive in the gains made by the union after the First World War.

The War Years

The onset of war in Europe in August 1914 led to a general lessening in industrial and political conflict. The bulk of the labour movement came out in support of the war effort, and the NAWU was no exception. Along with this, at least initially, went a new acceptance of the need for economy. As the *NAWU Magazine* put it in September 1914:

> In common with other sections of the community we shall have our burdens to bear ... It is imperative, however, that Visiting Committees should be compelled to shoulder their share.

The main concern at that stage was that authorities would not replace staff who enlisted, including, in May 1915, the union's General Secretary, George Gibson. In many cases, however, the authorities took on 'temporary' staff. These were encouraged to join the union and many subsequently became 'established' officers after the war, because many of those joining up were killed in action.

Conditions in the asylums deteriorated during the war as the plight of asylum patients fell even lower than normal down the scale of national priorities. Some asylums were requisitioned for use as war hospitals and the evicted patients were crammed into the already overcrowded existing accommodation. The standard of diet for patients was in many cases reduced and little 'extras', like patient entertainments, were often stopped.

These developments set the context for the NAWU's post-war militancy: grievances accumulated among staff which would later erupt into major disputes.

The most immediate effects however, were on patients, with a staggering rise in the death rate. Before 1914 the overall death rate was under 10 per cent a year; by 1917 it had risen to 17.4 per cent overall, and 21.5 per cent among male patients. The biggest killers were dysentry and tuberculosis, associated with poor hygiene, overcrowding and inadequate nutrition which also put staff at risk.

One issue that the union leadership did pursue vigorously during the war was its objection to female nurses working on male wards of asylums. Outside Scotland, this had been virtually unknown, but the pressures of staffing and finance due to war led to the introduction of women nurses on male wards in England and Wales, the first reported instance being at Hull City Asylum in June 1916. The NAWU wrote to the recently established Board of Control calling upon it to halt the practice. The union's official view was not just that employment of poorly paid women on male wards threatened to undercut the price of male labour, but also that working on the male sides was morally degrading to the women concerned, exposing them to unmentionable sexual dangers. The culmination of the campaign was the publication of a 'manifesto' in August 1915 and the publication each month of a 'Roll of Dishonour' listing those authorities who employed female labour on male sides. The strong response probably succeeded in slowing down the increase of women nurses in male wards, but did not eliminate them. The campaign undoubtedly showed the strength of male values within the union, though it had some support among women who did not want to work in male wards.

The other major issue, festering just below the surface, was concern at the rapid increase in the cost of living. Between July 1914 and August 1918 the Ministry of Labour estimated that the price of items included in the working-class family budget (food, clothing, rent, fuel and light, etc.) rose by approximately 110 per cent. Early in the war the union petitioned Boards and committees for 'war bonuses', and in some cases union pressure met with some success. By August 1916 the Metropolitan Asylums Board, covering mental handicap institutions around London, was accepting union delegations and making at least some concessions. In Yorkshire, from 1914, a 'Conciliation Scheme' operated in which full recognition was accorded to the NAWU and 'war bonuses' granted to staff. However, in all such instances, workers were rarely compensated by authorities for the full increase in the cost of living. Elsewhere the NAWU met determined and uncompromising opposition from the authorities, especially from authorities in Lancashire and the London County Council. The reasons were, as always, concern at the expense, and a determination to uphold the authority of the medical superintendents. In July 1917 the Lancashire Federation of NAWU branches was already threatening strike action. Hostilities between asylum workers and employers, suspended for the duration of the war, were about to resume.

Notes

[1] Memorandum by Dr E. Shuttleworth (1911), in Wellcome Library for the History of Medicine (London).

[2] *Asylum News*, (1912), p.12.

[3] *Minutes of Evidence* of the Select Committee on the Asylum Officers' (Employment, Pensions and Superannuation) Bill (1911), paras 1005-1283.

[4] Ibid., paras 586-784.

[5] Maud Pember Reeves, *Round About a Pound a Week* (reprinted 1979).

Chapter 5
The Forward Thrust, 1917–20

The longer the war continued, the more the original ready acceptance of deteriorating pay and conditions began to wear thin. The large drop in unemployment levels, combined with rapid inflation which ate away at the value of money wages, set the scene for a massive rise in trade union activity as the end of the war came in sight. There was an extraordinary growth of the trade union movement, whose numbers doubled from 4 to 8 million between 1914 and 1920. The government, anxious to maintain industrial peace, often brought strong pressure on employers to recognise unions and to set up institutions of collective bargaining which, it was hoped, would canalise the aggressiveness of labour.[1]

Many of the gains made by labour in the immediate post-war years were short lived. With the collapse of the post-war economic boom, and the passing of the (never very great) threat of revolution, the government and employers began to counter-attack. Growing unemployment weakened the trade union movement, which eventually suffered a humiliating defeat in the General Strike of 1926. However, the last year of the war, and those immediately following it, provided a favourable environment for asylum workers to press their claims for union recognition and material improvements in wages and conditions. Although this assertiveness waned as the wider economic situation deteriorated in the 1920s, by no means all the progress made was wiped out.

'Wake up Lancashire!'

In 1910 the asylum workers of Lancashire had been the spearhead of the social movement that had created the National Asylum Workers' Union. In the closing days of the war, they were destined once more to be in the forefront of a renewed and more successful campaign to win real improvements and proper recognition from the authorities. By 1916 the NAWU's national membership had declined from its peak of nearly 8,000 in 1914, to under 7,000. In 1917, however, recruitment picked up, while the *NAWU Magazine* in March noted 'a certain liveliness' among the branches, due to 'an accumulation of grievances'. These included the rapid increase in the cost of living and the inadequacy of 'war bonuses' (or cost-of-living increases), the increased responsibility that had been placed on staff and the reduction in the quality of rations.

The movement in Lancashire dated from October 1916, when branch secretaries met at the union's head office in Manchester to try to find a way to reverse the erosion of membership and commitment to the union. The union's previous acceptance of war economies had evidently led to a decline in membership morale, and means had to be found of restoring confidence in the NAWU. The outcome of the meeting was a programme for recognition, improvement in pay and hours, and uniformity between all Lancashire asylums. During 1917, the workers began to petition the Lancashire Asylums Board with their demands, in the time honoured fashion. In May the Liberal-controlled Board, determined to uphold the authority of medical superintendents, refused to grant recognition to the union.

Following this refusal, the Lancashire Federation of the NAWU met on 4 August 1917 and set in motion moves for a strike ballot among members in Lancashire. In the meantime, Herbert Shaw (the NAWU's Acting Secretary in Gibson's absence) wrote to the Minister of Labour on 24 July 1917 complaining of the Board's 'persistent and stubborn refusal to recognise the union, or to allow any representations on wages and conditions'. The Chief

Government Arbitrator, Sir George Askwith, then wrote and offered his services to the Board, which initially agreed to refer the issue of union recognition to arbitration. When, however, the Board told Sir George Askwith that it was prepared to allow extension of the existing practice of petitioning Visiting Committees by individual members of staff, Askwith wrote to Herbert Shaw, saying he no longer believed that arbitration was necessary.

This was recognition of a sort, even though the union was far from happy at the proposals. The Board was still insisting that all applications be made first to medical superintendents. Neither could the union make an application for staff throughout Lancashire without first submitting simultaneous claims at each asylum, and seeing them referred upwards. Nevertheless, the NAWU's Executive Council recommended that the Lancashire members give the system a trial.

On 7 March 1918, the first union deputation appeared before the Finance Committee of the Board. Consisting of Ted Edmondson (the President) and Herbert Shaw, it presented a list of nine demands (which had already been formally submitted on 7 January). They included a 5 shilling permanent advance for men and women 'indoor staff', the trade union rate for craftsmen, a 60-hour week, £5 a year recognition for MPA Certificate holders, and permission to post union notices in mess rooms. On 30 May 1918, the Board reached a decision. While a war bonus (rather than a 'permanent advance') of 5 shillings a week was granted to all indoor staff, and the minor demand that asylums should keep no more than a week's wages in hand agreed, none of the others was met. As the union put it: 'Verily has the mountain laboured and brought forth a mouse.' In June 1918 membership was reported to be at an all time high of more than 9,000. By the end of July 1918, the NAWU Executive had sanctioned a 14-day ultimatum by the Lancashire branches to the Board to meet its full demands, otherwise a strike would go ahead. The ultimatum was, however, ignored by the Board, which promised only to consider the demands at its next scheduled meeting. Herbert Shaw asked the

Ministry of Labour to intervene but it claimed that it was unable to do so, since the Board did not wish to proceed to arbitration.

According to Shaw's own account in the *NAWU Magazine* of September 1918 he and Edmondson addressed meetings at the end of August at Rainhill, Whittingham, Lancaster and Prestwich, where they sought to calm the situation. However, staff were tired of waiting, and 'at all meetings we found the strike fever raging'. On their visits they discovered through Sir Norval Helme, Chairman of the Board, that a farcical mix-up had occurred: the Board had not refused arbitration at all. Instead the Ministry of Labour had got the NAWU's application for arbitration confused with another, over a completely different dispute, from the National Union of General Workers. However, this did not substantially alter matters. Sir Norval still maintained that the union's ultimatum could not be considered until the meeting of the Finance Committee, which was not due to take place until after the 14-day period.

The national leaders were in no position to hold the membership back until the slow wheels of the Board rolled round. A strike finally broke out in Prestwich on 4 September. The evening before, all paid officials, the President, Secretary, Treasurer (Mr Shanks) and a leading Executive Council member, George Vernon had, according to the *NAWU Magazine*, rushed to Prestwich:

Owing to information which had reached the Head Office of the imminence of trouble. The crowded meeting almost uanimously decided to cease work at six next morning and to leave the institution. The women would hear of nothing else.

The 'necessary arrangements' were therefore made – including provision of a skeleton staff to safeguard patients' welfare. The strike had its humorous side. Some of the resident women were deliberately locked into their accommodation by the authorities to prevent them striking. Yet they got out, by means which 'the ladies themselves could best explain' and joined their brothers and sisters picketing on the gates. Only five members of staff went to work as normal.

Events moved rapidly with telegrams and phone messages passing speedily between the Asylums Board, the Ministry of Labour and the union's leadership. The NAWU wanted immediate arbitration and a promise of no victimisation. By the end of the first day of the strike Sir Norval Helme had agreed to convene a special meeting of the Board for the following day, 6 September. He invited the union officials to address it and urged the staff to call off their strike. This they refused to do. News had reached them that the staff at Whittingham had come out at dinner time. Although they had returned to put the patients to bed at six in the evening, they had promised to come out again at six the next morning. This they duly did. As at Prestwich, support for the strike was solid, 'particularly among the ladies'. Meals and accommodation were provided at the local pub, the Stag's Head at Goosnargh, near Preston. Sleeping accommodation had been arranged by the strikers in readiness for a long dispute – one sign, if it were needed, of the strikers' determination.

On the same day, the specially convened meeting of the Asylums Board met at nearby Preston, and was addressed by Herbert Shaw. After discussion, the Board dropped an original insistence that the nurses return to work immediately. Instead it passed a resolution that the NAWU application be referred to an arbitrator to be decided by the Ministry of Labour. When pressed, Shaw was confident that members would agree to abide by the arbitrator's decision, since the Board had given guarantees that it would not victimise strikers.

Shaw went hot foot to Whittingham and, after telephoning Prestwich, addressed the assembly of Whittingham strikers from the upper storey of the Stag's Head. The strikers applauded him and were back to work within the hour. At Prestwich the President, Mr Edmondson, gave the strikers the news. He was carried shoulder-high by union members, after which a procession formed and they marched triumphantly back to work.

These celebrations were a little premature. The arbitrator allowed only three of the original demands – on the 60-hour week with overtime rates for excess hours, artisan's rates to be increased to within ½d an hour of the prevailing union rate in the borough, and a maximum of a week's wages to be held in hand. All of these, Shaw claimed subsequently, the Board probably would have conceded anyway. Despite widespread disappointment at the results, the prestige of the union had risen considerably. Asylum workers had demonstrated an ability to stand united against their employers. Within two months of the strike, twelve new branches were formed and 2,500 new members enrolled into the union.

There were some accusations in the press that patients had suffered as a result of the strikers' actions, particularly from Alderman Shelmerdine, a die-hard opponent of unionism on the Asylums Board, who was also Chairman of Whittingham's Visiting Committee. His complaints of inadequate cover, were strenuously denied by the union.[2] The union boldly ar, in reply that the authorities were to blame for making the strike necessary:

> Patients' welfare will be better safeguarded and more adequately promoted by the services of free and intelligent men and women, working harmoniously under fair conditions, than it ever has been or could be under the old system of employing underpaid servants for an excessive number of hours on duties exceedingly trying to the nerves and tempers of those engaged in them, and subject to a ruthless discipline, the object of which seemed to be the creation of a class of slaves subservient to those in authority above them, and brutal to those unfortunate enough to be in subjection to them.[3]

Post-War Discord and Development

The unrest among asylum workers in Lancashire was not an isolated phenomenon but ran throughout the service and, as in Lancashire, women were often more prominent in militant activities than were men. Large numbers of women had entered the asylum labour force during the war, and were now flexing their industrial muscles. We have already seen that before the war the NAWU

leadership had identified women as the main problem
area for recruitment. The union's first General Secretary,
the Revd H.M.S. Bankart, had claimed in the *NAWU
Magazine* of May 1912 that this was because of a capricious
female temperament:

> Girls [sic] promise to join – and back out breaking their word
> – having exercised their 'women's privilege' to 'change their
> minds'. Girls remain nominal members and don't pay up their
> just dues ... Another complaint made against women – and I
> fear, not without some show of justice – is that they have no
> sense of unity, and cannot stick together.

He urged women asylum employees to:

> ... show your true womanliness, by joining the Union and
> sticking to it. Rouse ye, womenfolk, and the day of Reform
> and Justice will hasten its coming at your call.

By the end of the First World War, women asylum
workers were apparently heeding the call. By 1920 nearly
7,000 of the NAWU's 16,000 members were women. With
women playing a prominent, often the leading role in
industrial disputes, the male union leadership now
referred admiringly to 'the fighting spirit of the females'.

The militancy initially mounted in Lancashire was
sustained elsewhere. In December 1917 the staff at
London County Asylums presented the Asylums Committee with a long list of demands for improvements,
including the formation of a Joint Committee between the
NAWU and the authority. The management dragged
their heels and workers threatened strike action unless
there was an immediate increase of 11 shillings per week.
A strike was only averted by the intervention of a
deputation led by Ted Edmondson, the union's
President. Mr Carmichael, the Secretary of the London
Trades Council, subsequently acted as mediator and the
concessions started to flow by March 1918; first the
granting of a 60-hour week, then revised scales plus a
substantial 'war bonus' to cover increases in the cost of
living. The revised scales marked a significant shift away

from the widely disliked 'emoluments' system of paying workers in kind, through meals taken at work; henceforth workers would be charged a specified amount for meals taken at work.

In the West Country the spreading unrest caused two famous strikes: one a dazzling victory, the other a bitter defeat. In October 1918 the wearing of union badges on duty was the subject of a hard fought strike among women asylum workers at Bodmin Asylum. The matron, Miss Margaret Hiney, who had been appointed within the previous eighteen months, succeeded in antagonising staff by introducing changes which led to an increased turnover. There were, in any case, many accumulated grievances: a working week of 80 hours or more, no recreation room or even bathroom for staff and, as elsewhere, bitter staff resentment at the quality of the food they were offered. The nurses were not provided with uniforms, only the material with which to make them up. Neither had the women staff received any cost-of-living increase since the beginning of the war.

Enter on to the scene a new nurse, Mrs Hawken. She had been a NAWU member at her previous place of employment, Prestwich Asylum. When the nurses at Bodmin told her of their grievances, she advised them to join the union. 62 had joined out of a staff of 70 within two days, and most of them bought union badges and wore them. They were ordered to 'take off that thing', which they agreed to do at first, but then changed their minds. On 20 October 1918 they were hauled before the matron, who ordered them to take off their badges, the pretext being a rule that nurses were not allowed to wear jewellery. By 22 October, the five 'ringleaders', Nurses Hawken, Hill, Adams, Richards and Whitford, had been dismissed by the medical superintendent. When they went back to the wards 34 other nurses decided to go with them. They met Dr Dudley on the way out who now told them they could wear badges, but he refused to reinstate the rebel five. Their reply was adamant: 'All or none.' The strike had begun.

The strike caused a sensation in the town, and support was widespread. Refreshments were provided for pickets on the gate and accommodation for those who needed it. On Thursday the strikers paraded through the Cornish town, headed by their banner inscribed 'All or None'. As the week wore on, other workers joined the strike, and the previously more timid male staff at the asylum began to join the union. On Saturday the meeting of the Visiting Committee was attended by the five rebel nurses and addressed by Herbert Shaw, who claimed that their dismissal was an outright act of victimisation, and won reinstatement of all the strikers. Nurses could now be permitted to wear their union badges.

Work resumed the next day, but more was to happen later. The Visiting Committee set about revising staff pay and conditions. With the involvement, behind the scenes, of the Board of Control, tentative steps were made towards the establishment of a joint Advisory Committee between the staff and the Visiting Committee. Yet trouble continued to fester among the nurses and the Matron. Eventually, Miss Hiney was given a succession of periods of 'sick leave' and resigned in February 1919 'in view of medical opinion on the state of her heart'.[4]

The second dispute in the West Country in which women figured prominently was at Exeter City Asylum, which lasted for six months from the end of April 1919. Phillip Glanville, a carpenter with 28 years' service, and President of the local branch of the NAWU, had been dismissed from his post in December 1918, after presenting a petition to the Medical Superintendent for all-round wage increases, plus trade union rates for artisans. Dr Barlett is reported to have told Mr Glanville that he did not believe him to be worth trade union rates. The NAWU sought to achieve Glanville's reinstatement for four months before his appeal was finally turned down by the Visiting Committee on 29 April. The strike duly began the next day with 42 of the staff of 73 coming out in support of their dismissed colleague. A majority (26) of the strikers were women. According to Herbert Shaw the authorities claimed that 'flighty girls led the men out, but the steady-going conscientious men refused to embark on this escapade and stayed inside'. Whether women are militant or passive, their behaviour is accounted for by reference to supposedly 'feminine' personality traits. The authorities immediately advertised in the situations vacant column of the *Devon and Exeter Gazette* for replacements for the strikers. Most of the strike-breakers who offered their services on the male side were ex-servicemen. Many of the women strike-breakers were wives of male attendants who had not joined the strike. The women who did not originally join the strike tended to be older, more established nurses, the strikers often those who had been taken on during the war.[5] The authorities were prepared to take most of the men back (with the exception of Phillip Glanville), but not the women.

The strike enjoyed considerable support from the local labour movement, because it involved an important point of trade union principle. Transport unions sought to blockade the asylum and a local 'general strike' was even mooted, but the unions were not sufficiently strong in the Exeter area to mount such a venture. The dispute came to a head after the NAWU's Annual Conference voted in July 1919 to ballot all members on a national strike of asylum workers, in order to put pressure on the Board of Control and Ministry of Labour to intervene more actively in the dispute.

The local council was not, however, impressed, and turned down, for the second time, a proposal to go to arbitration. Perhaps they felt that the NAWU was bluffing. Certainly the leadership of the NAWU was reluctant to risk an all-out strike over one dispute, when trends generally seemed to be moving towards national recognition of the union. The strike ballot was largely a pressure tactic, rather than one that would be pursued in practice. The truth was that the members of the Exeter branch had gone on strike against the advice of the President, Ted Edmondson.

The strike ended after the municipal elections in November 1919 did not lead to a change in control of the council, and without the promised national or local strikes taking place. In August the Exeter branch had circularised and received some support among other branches for a motion 'strongly condemning the new Executive Council of endeavouring to settle the strike unfavourable to the Union'. All the same, it appeared that relations between the strikers and the leaders of the union terminated on an amicable note. At the final meeting of the strikers, a presentation of a case of pipes each was made to Herbert Shaw and Teddy Edmondson, the two officials in charge of the dispute, and, after tributes, 'the meeting closed with cheers and a mutual expression of all-round goodwill and comradeship'.

A Growing Membership

Despite Shaw's claim made to the NAWU Conference in July 1919 that 'if this union allows itself to be defeated on this fight you can consider the National Asylum Workers' Union smashed', the membership and influence of the NAWU contined to grow. Between December 1918 to 1919 membership rose from just under 12,000 to more than 15,000, and by the end of 1920 reached an inter-war peak of 18,000. Membership was becoming more evenly spread between the sexes, with women's membership reaching 46 per cent of the total. It was also becoming more dispersed geographically. The number of branches was increasing and the union becoming more representative of asylum workers as a whole.

The largest growth of membership was in Scotland. In September 1917 correspondents had written to the NAWU describing the 'trying conditions' under which they worked. There were no branches in Scotland at this time (though there had been some small pockets of membership in Aberdeen and Perth before the First World War), and the union offered to help. Some indication of the effects of these 'trying conditions' can be gathered from the Annual Report of the Board of Control (Scotland) for 1918. Out of an estimated total of 2,500 attendants and servants in Scottish asylums, 1,071 had resigned, 24 died, 52 left for health reasons and 133 been dismissed. The wages and conditions in Scotland were generally inferior to those of England and Wales. They were bad in the seventeen public district asylums, and worse still in the seven Royal or charitable hospitals.

By April 1918 membership of the NAWU was
spreading rapidly throughout the whole of Scotland.
Some asylum workers had individually been members of
the union's 'Central Branch' established either for senior
nurses who deemed it undiplomatic to join their local
branch, or, as in the case of Scotland, for those who had no
local branch to join. These now formed the nucleus of the
union in Scotland. Branches were set up at Montrose,
Hartwood (Lanarkshire) and Kirkwood (Aberdeen). In
Glasgow the union faced fierce competition from the
Municipal Employees' Association (MEA), which eventually became part of what is now the GMBATU. By
January 1919 the NAWU claimed to represent about half
of the 2,500 asylum workers in Scotland.

The NAWU also began to recruit more in the higher
echelons of the service throughout Britain. With the final
disappearance of the AWA in 1919 the way was now clear
to admit them formally into membership, and in 1920 a
special Officers and Sub Officers Section of the union was
formed. Not all rank-and-file members of the union were
happy at such a development, on the ground that it
introduced 'class distinctions'. The main base of support
was in Lancashire where the section was soon in the thick
of things, as Winwick Asylum sought to forbade its senior
personnel from joining the union on pain of dismissal.
Firm action from the NAWU was effective in dealing with
such opposition. By the end of September 1920, the
NAWU had succeeded in winning significant improvements in the pay and conditions of officers throughout
Lancashire.

The NAWU's National Programme

Central to the development of the NAWU during this
period was its adoption of a National Programme. This
had first been proposed in the correspondence columns of
the *NAWU Magazine*, and was taken up by the NEC. On 28
September 1918 a Special Delegates Meeting was called –
the first since before the war – to discuss and approve the
National Programme suggested by the NEC. It was
undoubtedly a sign of growing confidence within both the

ranks and the leadership of the NAWU. As if to underline
the new sense of commitment to trade unionism, the same
delegate conference decided,` finally, to seek affiliation to
the TUC.

The list of demands in the National Programme was
wide-ranging and impressive: a minimum wage of £3 5s a
week, a 48-hour week, universal recognition of the union
and establishment of collective bargaining machinery,
abolition of the emoluments system, equal pay for women,
improvements in the Asylum Officers' Superannuation
Act of 1909, and state registration for mental nurses (note
that the term 'attendant' is being dropped). The most
striking omission from the Programme, which caused
some resentment among those affected, was the failure to
demand trade union rates of wages for all artisan (craft)
employees.

The Programme was duly ratified by the branches and
presented to the Visiting Committees of Asylums in
England and Wales in January 1919. These activities, as
well as the mounting public pressure for reform of the
lunacy laws, led the asylum authorities to consider setting
up a national body to protect their interests. At central
government level, the Board of Control was also turning
attention, after long years of neglect, to the welfare of
staff. Could it be that a few months of trade union
militancy had achieved more than years of patient
petitioning?

In February 1919, the London County Council (LCC)
called together a Conference of Representatives of Public
Asylum Authorities, which was addressed at length by Ted
Edmondson, the NAWU President. The conference
agreed to ask the Ministry of Labour to help it set up an
'Industrial Council' along Whitley lines, fully aware that
they might otherwise have to face industrial action from
the NAWU.

There was just one snag. Despite concord among
employers on the need to set up an industrial council, the
Ministry of Labour disapproved of the idea of forming a
separate industrial council for the asylum service. Instead it
wanted asylum workers to be included within the scope of
the proposed National Joint Council for Local Authorities

Non-Trading Services, and talked the asylum authorities round to this position. The union was furious, not only because consideration of the National Programme was being delayed, but because other unions would have jurisdiction over a group of workers it regarded as its own 'special province'. It was prepared to make compromises with craft unions, whose misgivings about the NAWU's attempts to recruit craftsmen at asylums delayed the union's application to join the TUC until 1923. However it was uncompromisingly opposed to incursions from local government and manual workers' unions and walked out of meetings to which they had also been invited. It claimed this would allow the employers to 'divide and govern'.

To show the authorities that it meant business the NAWU issued ballot papers for strike action, to be returned by 28 March 1919. Nearly 8,000 members voted for a strike but the threat was sufficient to effect a settlement. It was agreed initially to set up a conciliation committee solely between the NAWU and the authorities to deal with indoor staffs, i.e. nurses and attendants. A committee covering artisans would, it was promised, be established later, but in fact it was never set up. The Joint Committee sat for the first time on 4 April 1919. Its first offer was for a 60-hour week for indoor staff *exclusive* of meal times, but after some hard bargaining this was amended to *inclusive* of meal times, to be determined locally. The important of this lay in the fact that LCC and Metropolitan Asylums Board staff needed to protect the 48-hour week which had practically been conceded to them.

The question of wages was referred to a sub-committee, with the subsequent award backdated to 1 April 1919. The union did not succeed in winning its full National Programme, but it had established its right to speak as the sole collective voice of asylum workers, and important concessions were won, including: abolition of payments in kind (emoluments); increments to be paid for up to five years of service and on being promoted to staff nurse and charge nurse; female nurses to receive 80 per cent of male rates, including increments; overtime pay of time-and-a-quarter for the first two hours, and time-and-a-half thereafter; cost-of-living increases; abolition of the term 'attendant' and use of the term 'nurse' for both sexes.

A more controversial feature of the agreement was the establishment of different rates of pay according to whether the local hospital was judged to be 'urban' or 'rural'! A male probationer nurse in an 'urban' mental hospital was to receive the princely minimum sum of at least £2 a week (exclusive of war bonus). In rural asylums it was much less – in some cases as little as £1 15s a week – because it was linked to the wages of agricultural workers in the district.

The award only applied to England and Wales. In Scotland many authorities were resisting recognition, especially the Royal asylums. In its refusal to recognise the NAWU, the House Committee at Montrose referred to it contemptuously as 'this English union'. In December 1918 a conference of Scottish branches threatened strike action if recognition was not conceded within one month, but a meeting of employers at the end of January 1919 voted narrowly against recognition. Eventually in June 1919 a Conciliation Committee of public asylums was formed, with some of the Royal asylums agreeing to observe its awards.

Not everyone was happy at the establishment of collective bargaining between the NAWU and the authorities. By the end of 1919, the Asylum Workers' Association, excluded from the new machinery, had finally been wound up and given a decent burial. Many medical superintendents were also more than a little peeved. Through their professional association, the Medico Psychological Association (MPA), they had pressed strongly from February 1919 to be represented in an advisory capacity on the new Joint Conciliation Committee (JCC) 'to indicate how any alterations proposed would affect the welfare of patients' (and, perhaps, themselves).

A subsequent meeting of the MPA in March 1919 unanimously declared that standard hours and overtime pay were 'contrary to the ethics of the nursing profession'. The MPA was unsuccessful in its bid to establish an Advisory Board to the JCC to veto any proposals it did not like. This was partly because the employing authorities –

lay members of visiting committees – saw the JCC to some extent as a means of strengthening their hand in relation to the medical superintendents. The Board of Control was also worried that its position and influence might be eroded, and indeed the NAWU called for it to be abolished and its powers transferred to the newly formed Ministry of Health, describing it as 'antiquated' and ineffective:

> They are the laughing stock of the asylum world. Their 'surprise visits' provide entertainment for thousands, and the things they don't see would fill a book.

The NAWU had thus, within just ten years of being launched, dispatched a rival and well entrenched professional association, fought off the challenge of other trade unions and compelled recognition and significant concessions from one of the most reactionary and authoritarian groups of employers in the country. It was no mean achievement. It now remained to be seen whether these gains could be defended and consolidated in the difficult years that lay ahead.

Notes

[1] For a more thorough account of these developments see J. Hinton, *Labour and Socialism* (1983), Ch. 6.

[2] For example, *Liverpool Post and Mercury* and *Manchester Guardian* for 6 September 1918.

[3] *NAWU Magazine*, September 1918.

[4] C.T. Andrews, *The Dark Awakening* (1978).

[5] *Devon and Exeter Gazette*, 25 July 1919.

Chapter 6
From Conflict to Accommodation, 1920-31

In 1920 a new era appeared to be dawning for asylum workers. On 20 February a permanent Joint Conciliation Committee (JCC) came into existence, with the newly formed Mental Hospitals Association (MHA) on the employers' side, and the NAWU on the workers'. Negotiations between them led to further wage increases. In 1919 the Nurses' Registration Act had been passed which provided for the setting up of a General Nursing Council (GNC) to govern this newest of professions. From now on nurses would qualify after three years' training, and mental nurses would be included in the new scheme. The new Ministry of Health agreed that the NAWU should be represented on the Mental Nurses' Committee of the GNC. The influence of the union was growing daily and its membership increased to 18,000.

From then on, however, the going got harder. For a start only about a dozen authorities observed the award of the JCC in full: the South-West Authorities, under the Chairmanship of Alderman Munro (who had played a leading part in the Exeter strike) deliberately flouted the award. In Scotland progress was also proving difficult. A new revised version of the National Programme had been rejected by the employers' side of the Conciliation Committee, as it was by the JCC for England and Wales in 1921.

The most important developments were those looming in the external political and economic sphere. The strides made by asylum workers at the end of the war were sustained by a buoyant labour market, which was maintained for the economic boom that immediately followed the Armstice. But by the end of 1920 the beginnings of an economic slump were becoming apparent, and by 1921 it had definitely arrived. Exports slumped and unemployment rose; wages fell, but so did prices. By March 1922, more than 2 million insured workers were unemployed., The coalition government responded with deflationary economic measures. From February 1922 the 'Geddes axe' began to fall and large amounts were chopped off public expenditure.

The Gathering Storm

In late 1920 and early 1921, however, the NAWU fought two determined battles against intransigent asylum authorities, with some degree of success, at Cheadle Royal and Stafford Asylums. There were to be precious few such victories to follow for the rest of the inter-war period. At the private Cheadle Royal Asylum in Cheshire a recently re-established branch of the NAWU had been pressing the Management Committee for official recognition, reductions in hours and improvements in pay. The committee pleaded poverty, claiming that many of the patients were 'unremunerative', and relatives of others would not be able to afford higher maintenance charges. The only alternative to closing the institution altogether would be to sack many of the staff. It therefore refused to recognise the union, and offered only minor concessions. But after a determined two day 'stay-in' strike on 19 and 20 November the union won full recognition, and has retained it to this day. The second dispute illustrated the ridiculous lengths to which some medical superintendents could go in issuing regulations to maintain discipline. In February 1921, Dr Shaw, the Superintendent of Stafford Asylum, issued an order forbidding the female staff from using the front drive on pain of instant dismissal, forcing them to go the back way to the town, which was a mile longer. In March after a protest meeting, the female staff marched as a body down the drive, and the prohibition was quietly forgotten.

The tide was, however, already turning in favour of the employers. Rumours were in the air that the Mental Hospitals Association would insist that wage reductions be negotiated through the JCC. In July 1921, the NAWU urged mental hospital workers to 'stand fast' but admitted that some wage reductions 'may be unavoidable'. This did not necessarily mean *real* cuts in living standards, as the top of the inflationary spiral had been reached in November 1920, and the cost of living was now falling. The employers' side of the JCC now wished to tie the periodically negotiated weekly war bonus to an automatic sliding scale, and the NAWU reluctantly agreed. The basic wage was not affected, but it did not bode well for the future.

The most direct evidence of the declining confidence of asylum workers in the face of this new assault was a clear decline in membership of the union, which fell several thousand by May 1921 to a little over 15,000. Some employing authorities began to believe that the JCC was pussyfooting around. The first to break ranks was the Visiting Committee of Bracebridge Mental Hospital, near Lincoln. It withdrew from the Mental Hospitals Association and then, on 5 September 1921, reduced the wages of male indoor staff by 6 shillings a week, and took 4s 11d from the wages of female staff, in line with the reductions being imposed on farmworkers in the locality. After a strike in October, the employers decided to make reductions in line with the JCC agreement, but did not pledge themselves to observe it in the future. More signs appeared that confirmed the worst fears that this was not to be an isolated outbreak of employer hostility. In Scotland, the workers' side of the Conciliation Committee were forced to accept the 'sliding scale' imposed in England and Wales, while the employers deferred discussion of the union's claim for the minimum basic wage that operated south of the Border.

Wages reductions continued into 1922, as the economic crisis deepened. At central government level, the Board of Control which had in 1919 strongly and (one must suppose) sincerely associated itself with demands for an 'improvement not only in pay, but in rest and recreation', on the grounds that 'the comfort and health of the patients are largely dependant on the existence of a well qualified and contented staff', now sang a very different tune. It argued in its Annual Report for 1921 that the very improvements it had previously called for were now not only too costly, but also had a damaging effect on standards of care. Complaining of the rapid increase in the costs of maintaining mental hospitals, it ominously now declared that 'the whole subject of the work and wages of the nursing staffs in the mental hospitals requires to be very carefully considered'.

In most cases staff felt they had little option but to accept wage cuts. In Carmarthen and Lancashire workers went along with them. There was some talk of industrial action in Glasgow, but nothing materialised. It was perhaps surprising that the focus of fierce, but sadly isolated, resistance should have been at Radcliffe Hospital near Nottingham. What was less surprising was that yet again the women nurses gave a lesson in militancy and collective determination to the men. In a period in history when extraordinary events were commonplace, the Radcliffe strike was described by the press as the 'most sensational strike of modern times'.

The Battle of Radcliffe

The Visiting Committee of Radcliffe-on-Trent Mental Hospital in Nottinghamshire was a member of the MHA and had previously generally unheld the agreements of the Joint Consultative Committee. In February 1922 however, it announced without warning that it proposed to cut wages for men by 4 shillings and for women by 3s 4d a week, from 5 March 1922. It also increased hours from 60 to 66 hours a week by cutting the staff's days off from two days a week to three days a fortnight. This was in clear breach of the national agreement of the JCC. The workers met inside the hospital on 3 March. They accepted the wage cuts, but not the increase in hours, declaring that they would continue to take two days off a week as usual. They were urged to make a stand on this issue by both George Gibson and Herbert Shaw, who addressed the branch meeting and called on them to resist in the interests of asylum workers generally.

Tension mounted and on Sunday 5 March the female night staff refused to go on duty when they discovered that the matron had placed a non-unionist on nights. They suspected she was being placed there to learn the ropes in preparation for a strike. When the next day saw male craftsmen being recruited for the same purpose, Gibson and Shaw urged the married men to stay overnight in the hospital in case negotiations were broken off. At the same time, however, Gibson and Shaw sought to extricate the union from the potentially explosive situation, by seeking an urgent meeting with the visiting committee. The committee's view was that the stff had committed an act of insubordination by refusing to work the new hours, and insisted that staff work normally. Anxious to avoid confrontation, this was resumed from seven o'clock on Wednesday 8 March.

It subsequently became clear that the authorities were simply buying extra time in order to lay more thorough strike-breaking plans between themselves and the Nottinghamshire police. According to press reports they regarded themselves as simply 'subscribing members' of the Mental Hospitals Association, and not bound by its agreements.[1] They refused to allow the union to hold meetings in the hospital unless Mr Gell, the Clerk to the Committee, was allowed to be present. Union members were forced to meet at the nearby Black Lion public house. There they found a plain-clothes policeman and placed pickets outside the room 'to keep away undesirable characters acting as amateur detectives'. The Visiting Committee held its meeting without notifying the union, which nevertheless got to know of it. George Gibson, Herbert Shaw and Mr Booth, the union's solicitor, arrived at the Shire Hall, Nottingham on 24 March and, together with six representatives of the staff at Radcliffe, they were allowed to make representations to the committee. It was apparent that the employers felt 'badly let down' by the staff, who were in their view guilty of gross insubordination. Nevertheless a decision on the crucial issue of hours was yet again 'postponed'.

The next the workers heard was on 27 March. They had all been sacked, and offered re-engagement only so long as they signed the following form:

> To the Clerk of the Committee
> Notts. County Mental Hospital,
> Radcliffe-on-Trent.
>
> I beg to make application for the post of ... ... and hereby undertake to faithfully carry out all instructions of the Committee of Visitors, and to loyally obey the Officers of the Mental hospital appointed by the committee to put their orders into operation.
>
> Signed ... ...

They were given until four o'clock on 6 April to sign the forms. The union instructed members not to sign the forms. All the women followed these instructions, but some of the men – especially married men living in tied accommodation on the estate, who had been given a month to quit – did sign. Others were worried about the prospect of losing their pension contributions. Herbert Hough, a young probationer nurse in his twenties who had recently taken over as NAWU branch secretary, set about trying to organise the crumbling resistance of the male staff. The women struck as a body on the morning of 11 April. They would not allow the matron or other officials, except medical officers, to enter the wards. In line with national union instructions, the kitchen staff prepared the patients' meals but would do nothing for those in authority. When this led to their suspension they joined the nurses on the wards.

The men were taken aback by the women's militancy. They met in the lane the same evening when, according to Herbert Hough, they were taunted by Herbert Shaw. As he told me:

> He apologised for the absence of the ladies who were fighting the men's battles. You know, he was a pretty good rabble-rouser. The upshot of it was that most of us, well, in

fact we all decided to strike, but one or two of the men
funked.[2]

It was decided that it was only practicacl for the men to
occupy three of the six male wards on the ground floor,
and the next morning non-unionists were evicted from
them while the men loyal to the union barricaded
themselves into wards 11, 12 and 14. They took with them
extra supplies of twist and packet tobacco, chocolate,
cigarettes, tea and other items for the male patients. By
mid-morning a 'large detachment' of pickets arrived from
the Netherfield and Colwick Unemployment Committee,
and put up posters appealing to the unemployed not to
apply for jobs at the institution.

The committee met and sacked the 17 men and 50
women strikers for 'insubordination'. A bus load of
women strike-breakers arrived and were billeted in the
recreation hall, entertained on the piano by an ex-member
of the union. Contact with the barricaded strikers and the
union officials outside the gates was improvised by means
of semaphore. George Gibson, it will be remembered, had
served at the front, and one of the strikers inside had also
learned semaphore in the army. George Gibson and
Herbert Shaw surveyed the subsequent events through
field-glasses, while Mr Booth, the union's solicitor, went
off to the nearby Nottingham race meeting.

Events reached their climax on the afternoon of
Thursday 12 April. Press descriptions of 'bedlam', 'scenes
of the wildest description', appear to have been only slight
exaggeration. At 1 pm Mr Gell, the Clerk to the
Committee, and Mr Jones, the medical superintendent,
arrived at the door of one of the male wards, accompanied
by strike-breaking artisans and a force of bailiffs and
plainclothes policemen. 67 uniformed police were posted
round the building, supposedly to keep order, but did not
take part in the events which followed. Mr Gell shouted to
George Gibson in the lane to call upon the strikers to leave,
who shouted back: 'No, the responsibility is yours, and you
must get them out!'[3] Dr Jones then stepped forward and
called on the staff to surrender. As Herbert Hough
explains:

The superintendent came to argue with us at the window of one of the wards and a patient – a miner – he picked up the nozzle of one of those huge brass things, and was going to take it off. So I said, 'let me have it Jack', and I took it and gave him a nod and he spun the wheel, you know, and we turned the fire hose on the Super. They promptly turned the water off the mains.

The attack then began in earnest. At first the artisans tried to unlock the doors but the staff had wedged home-made keys into them, to jam the locks. The bailiffs then took over and broke down the doors with heavy crowbars, pushed their way through the improvised barricades, and engaged in hand-to-hand fighting with the staff. The strength of staff resistance was such that they were not able to repossess the hospital for the authorities until 5 pm, or four hours later. According to the *Daily Sketch:*

After a fierce hand-to-hand struggle, the nurses on strike in Radcliffe Asylum were overpowered and ejected by the police, assisted by a newly appointed staff. Insane inmates joined in the struggle on the side of the strikers. Many people were injured, windows were smashed, and the furniture of three of the wards reduced to matchwood.[4]

More details were provided by the *Nottingham Journal*:

Never in the history of trade unionism in the Midlands have more amazing proceedings been witnessed. Doors were broken in; barricades of furniture overturned; lunatics got out of control and smashed windows, pictures and anything else within their reach, hand-to-hand struggles took place between officials and patients, in the course of which Superintendent Smith, of the Notts County Constabulary, was bitten on the hand, while others were scratched and buffeted. Finally, the asylum authorities gained, by these drastic means, complete control of their asylum.[5]

The strikers had fought a brave rearguard battle through each of the wards of the hospital, improvising barricades on the way, until they were finally cornered. The female wards held better than the male ones: they were upstairs, there were more strikers and more of the patients joined in on the side of the staff. The female staff had, like the men, trained fire hoses on the force of attacking bailiffs and it was reported that one nurse broke down and cried 'when she turned the handle and no water came'. In Herbert Hough's words:

> There was a battle of course, particularly on the female side. The patients were all sympathetic to us, and on the female side they fought the police. One policeman had his hand bit. When the policeman put his hand on the nurse, the patient went for him. They [the female staff] made the mistake of putting a table against the door, rather than sideways. They knocked in the panel of the door and the policeman, a plain clothes chappy, crept through, and as he was coming from under the table, just got his head nicely in a good position, and Louie Burley, the charge nurse, she weighed about 14 stone, and she gave him an uppercut and by remarkable timing, she knocked him out. He fell flat and Louie thought she'd killed him, but he was, you know, a boxer's K.O. Well Louie fainted and fell on him, and the patient rolled her over and the chap was able to get up, but there were various incidents like this. They smashed windows – the patients tore legs off chairs and attacked ... In some of the wards there was no glass at all left in the windows. So all the female wards were held. We only held three of the six male wards. You see we hadn't staff enough, being on the ground floor, we hadn't staff enough to man them.

The staff were taken prisoners and collected together in the nurses' sitting room at about 5 p.m. Their spirits still high, they sang songs, including 'Rule Brittania', according to the *Nottingham Journal*'s account, 'laying great emphasis on the passage "Britons never shall be slaves" '. The defeated strikers collected their belongings and left:

> The union officials who had remained at their points of vantage in the lane outside the main gates of the institution, had provided transport, two motor charabancs being in waiting. Piled up with bags, baskets, boxes and bicycles, and crowded with ex-employees of the asylum, they made their appearance in Radcliffe at about 7 o'clock, and were met by a crowd of several hundred people. There has never been so

much excitement in the town, for years, not even over an election, said an old inhabitant.[6]

They held a meeting at the Black Lion, posed for photographs, were billeted overnight by sympathetic villagers and subsequently dispersed. So ended what the union described grimly as 'one of the worst cases of official tyranny in the history of the union'.

Many of the dismissed strikers experienced severe difficulties in finding alternative employment. A number of nurses were sacked when it was discovered they had formerly worked at Radcliffe. Herbert Hough did not get another job until nearly a year later. But if the strikers fared badly, Herbert claimed that the impact on the hospital was devastating:

> They had all sorts of people brought in. You should've seen the ragged lot that came in on the male side. They were dregs … broken down school teachers and that sort of thing, you know. On the female side, of course, they had officials' wives. They managed to get a few ex-nurses to come back, but it was a long time before they really got a settled staff.

Herbert blamed the committee and portrayed the medical superintendent and the matron as people caught in the middle. The matron was 'ill for weeks' and Dr Jones was 'not the same afterwards'. All the certificated staff had gone, and he died within a year or two of the strike, 'it shook him so much'. The last words on the dispute itself are best left to Herbert Hough:

> The day they ejected us, the bailiff called me and he said that I'd been ejected from that hospital and if I went in again I would be arrested. 6 or 7 years ago [in 1972] on the [50th] anniversary of that day I thought 'I wonder what it looks like.' I got on a bus and got off at the hospital and I walked up to the front door. I walked the full length of the front drive and up to the front door, just to show that I could go back. It was a mad idea, but … then I walked down to the village, and tried to look up various people, but I didn't meet anyone who was

very involved in the strike. I did go back. It was a very late act of defiance but, there, I did it.

Setbacks and Survival

The defeat of the Radcliffe strike was the green light for employers to go further on the offensive against workers' living standards. The victory of 'stay-in' strikes at Cheadle Royal and Lincoln had lulled the union into a false sense of security. George Gibson had told Conference in 1921 that the occupation tactic

> is one that can only be used as a last resort, and when the case which the union proposes to fight is one which is certain to command public sympathy; given these conditions, there is little doubt that the stay-in strike will always succeed in its purpose.

Now he had been proved disastrously wrong. A meeting of the JCC was called at the behest of the employers on 16 June 1922, just two months after the Radcliffe strike. Union membership had fallen further by the end of May to 13,000. The employers now wanted to negotiate reductions in the basic wage, in addition to the automatic deductions being made in the war bonus. The authorities in the rural areas were especially militant, with many of them threatening to secede from the MHA and hence the JCC if large reductions were not made. A reduction of 3 shillings a week was therefore imposed in the overall basic minimum in rural districts, lowering it to 35 shillings and widening the gap between them and urban asylums. In addition annual leave was cut from four to three weeks, and maximum hours were increased from 60 to 66 hours a week, inclusive of meal times. These were the new benchmarks established with the help of crowbars, bailiffs and the Notts County constabulary two months earlier. The NEC balloted members, recommending acceptance of what it called 'these unsatisfactory proposals', since otherwise the employers would disband the JCC, and with it any semblance of national pay and conditions.

Between 1923 and 1924, the NAWU's position

deteriorated seriously in Scotland. It had appeared late on the scene and had never been fully accepted by the authorities. By September 1923 only five authorities remained on the employers' side of the Scottish Joint Consultative Committee: Dundee, Fife, Govan, Lanark and Kirklands. At a special meeting held in Glasgow on 11 September these five agreed to invite the absent authorities to a meeting called to secure the continuation of joint machinery with the NAWU. These efforts came to nothing. By January 1924 Dundee was reported to have flouted the JCC's recommendations. By February 1924 the Scottish JCC had been disbanded. The NAWU made efforts to revive it in subsequent years. In 1928, the NAWU launched a Scottish Organising Campaign, even appointing a temporary 'lady organiser – Mrs Beaton – to go round the asylums'. This yielded 'disappointing results'. Membership had 'fallen considerably' in Scotland, and there was not any immediate prospect of reviving the JCC. It was not to reappear until the Second World War.

The NAWU's only option – throughout Britain – was to seek local improvements wherever it could. In England and Wales it had to face the opposition of the Mental Hospitals Association to such a strategy. In February 1924 the MHA complained that local branches of the NAWU were seeking reductions in hours greater than those recommended by the JCC. The union's Executive, not surprisingly, saw nothing wrong in this, but agreed to discuss the matter with the MHA. Local pressure continued to be applied where it could be mustered. It was perhaps in the North-East of England, where the Labour Party was taking a firm grip on local government, that most gains were made in this period.

One response of the union, in circumstances where gains from collective bargaining were hard to achieve, was to develop the 'friendly society' side of its activities. This was vigorously pursued as the 1920s wore on. Many of the initiatives in this direction were first developed by branches. By 1923 the East Midland Federation of NAWU branches had set up a trading club, in which discounts were available on a wide range of goods. Claybury branch organised a savings club. Napsbury had 'thrift' and sick

clubs, as well as a 'tobacco co-operation'. The aim of such
schemes was to develop the social side of the branch and to
hold on to members in difficult times.

The union could have sought to deal with the increased
difficulties of recruiting and retaining members by
strengthening its full-time officer force. This was
exclusively situated in the head office in Manchester, the
North-West being the birth place of the union. Yet, while
Lancashire remained powerful in union affairs – it no
longer contained the largest concentration of members, as
the NAWU had become a genuinely national union. The
union's structure was creaking at the seams. The pressure
of militant action, the developments of national bargaining machinery, a growing membership that required
servicing – all these and other influences pointed to the
need for a thorough and speedy overhaul of the union's
structure. Yet the Executive Council showed signs of
hesitancy and, although it encouraged branches to form
themselves into regional Federations in order to relieve
some of the heavy burden of work on head office staff, it
was much less enthusiastic about developing a scheme of
area representation for the NEC, or appointing full-time
officers in the localities.

NAWU/PLWTU Federation

The London branches – now the biggest concentration of
membership in the NAWU – had been partially appeased
by other developments during 1921. The trend in the
trade union movement as a whole was towards the creation
of giant unions by amalgamation, most notably the
Transport and General Workers' Union in 1921, and the
National Union of Corporation Workers took the lead in
the public sector and convened a meeting in London on 6
December 1919, to see whether it was possible to form a
Federation of 'all unions catering for the public, health
and utility services'. The unions present, the National
Union of Corporation Workers (NUCW), the NAWU, the
Poor Law Workers Trade Union (PLWTU) and the
National Union of Waterworkers Employees agreed after
'an exhaustive discussion' to take the issue back to their

respective Executive Councils. The NUCW, under the leadership of Councillor Albin Taylor, was seeking to move too fast for the other unions and the idea of one union for health services and public utilities got no further. From June 1920, however, a Federation was established between the PLWTU and the NAWU, with the ultimate aim of creating a single union for the health services. An integral feature of the joint arrangements was the appointment by the NAWU of a London Organiser (to work from the PLWTU's head office) and a Northern Organiser by the PLWTU (to work from the NAWU's Manchester head-quarters). The PLWTU's members thus gained officer support in the north and the NAWU gained the same in London and the south.

At first it seemed that the joint arrangements between the NAWU and the PLWTU might indeed be a prelude to greater things to come. The recently formed Professional Union of Trained Nurses (PUTN) and a doctors' union, the Medico-Political Union (MPU) showed an interest in join-ing the Federation, but the NAWU/PLWTU Federation did not survive for long. From the NAWU's point of view, despite its loss of membership after 1921, it was a financially secure organisation and could survive without amalgamat-ing with another organisation. Tensions had also been emerging at local level. By 1 October 1921 the Federation had been wound up and the two unions had gone their different ways, but not – as we shall see later – for all time.

The services of the Revd Stanley Morgan were retained as London Organiser and his position was made per-manent. He was the only official of the NAWU or its successor, the Mental Hospitals and Institutional Workers Union (MHIWU) ever to have been appointed from out-side the asylum service. London therefore had the privilege unique within the NAWU of possessing its own organiser. The London District Council (LDC) was becoming virtually a union within a union, especially since the London County Council would not participate in the Mental Hospi-tals Association or follow the recommendations of the JCC. But it did accord the LDC recognition, and the LCC's Asylums and Mental Deficiency Committee met regularly with the NAWU's negotiating committee.

The organisational problems of London were therefore
eased, but other sections of Britain still had no local
full-time officers. Scotland was unsuccessful in its attempt
to get Conference to pass a resolution allowing them to
employ an organiser. Instead the Revd Morgan was sent
up as a roving emissary of the union for six months during
the summer of 1922. His 'organising tour' could, of
course, do nothing to solve the necessity of providing
day-to-day back-up to the branches. This situation was
leading to simmering discontent. Most localities had
neither full-time officer support, nor a geographical
system of NEC elections which ensured them a voice at
national level. However in 1924 such a scheme did finally
become operative, and the union's structure became better
adapted to changed conditions.

On the Defensive

The union survived the lean years following the defeat of
the Radcliffe strike. Membership fell from the high point
of around 18,000 at the end of 1920, to 10,600 in 1926.
The NAWU participated fully in the General Strike of that
year, called by the TUC in support of locked out miners. It
had in fact the honour of being the first union to be called
to vote in favour at the special Conference of Union
Executives held on 1 May 1926. When the 'asylum
workers' voted in favour of the proposed strike this caused
some ironic amusement among those delegates who
thought that the whole adventure had a faint touch of
madness. Though NAWU members were not called upon
to withdraw their labour, the union threw its weight
behind the strike. The strike was, of course, defeated, and
the miners ultimately starved back to work after six
months.

These circumstances were hardly ones in which the
NAWU could launch a major campaign for the
advancement of asylum workers. Yet 1926 was the
NAWU's lowest point. Membership began to pick up and
rose steadily for the remainder of the decade, and stood at
12,500 by the end of 1930 – hardly the dizzy heights of the
immediate post-war years but, in the context, quite an

achievement. Claude Bartlett, who had become President of the union, put his finger on it in his New Year Address for 1927. Reviewing the dismal general situation, he observed that

> Unemployment has very considerably increased, and drastic wage reductions in many of the large industries have not been uncommon. Altogether it has been a year of much concern and anxiety to the trade union catering for the interests of those affected ... However, as far as our conditions of employment are concerned, we are in a much more favoured position. Wages have not been drastically reduced, the hours of duty remain unaltered, and the general conditions unchanged. Furthermore we are free from the ever-increasing and menacing problem of unemployment and many of the other unhappy circumstances which are consequent upon economic and social instability.

This of course, did not mean that the NAWU was making great strides in its negotiations with the employers. On the contrary, very little visible progress was made. However, in the difficult climate of the times, relatively minor concessions were hailed as a 'success' and, following them, membership of the union began slowly to rise.

In describing the late 1920s, the first official history of the NAWU was hard put to say 'What the Union is Doing'.[7] It claimed small – if not insignificant – victories here and there. For example, in March 1927, the Prestwich branch succeeded in winning a gratuity of £203 for Mrs Stringer, the widow of a member, and prevented her being evicted with her daughter from tied accommodation. In such circumstances, the emphasis was bound to shift towards the conservation of existing advantages. Job security was the biggest of these, and was generally assured so long as the worker did not antagonise his or her superior and get 'sent down the drive'. In a period of falling prices, those in stable jobs enjoyed modest but real increases in wages, even if their money wages did not rise. The more representative structure of the Executive Council, through federated areas, which led to the election of more nurses from rural asylums, also reinforced trends towards caution, conservatism and co-operation with the employers. Claude Bartlett was himself a product and symbol of this new situation, as a young mental nurse from Plymouth at the time of his election to President. It was an office he was to occupy for more than thirty years. After George Gibson was elected to the General Council of the TUC in September 1928 (from the Public Employees Section) Bartlett began to exercise a growing influence over the national union.

Closely associated with the shift to caution and conservatism was a growing emphasis, within the union, upon questions of status and professionalism. How this occurred, and its consequences, is the subject of the next chapter.

Notes

[1] *Nottingham Journal*, 12 April 1922.
[2] Interview with Herbert Hough in 1979.
[3] *Nottingham Journal*, 15 April 1922.
[4] *Daily Sketch*, 15 April 1922.
[5] *Nottingham Journal*, 15 April 1922.
[6] Ibid.
[7] MHIWU (George Gibson), *21 Years: A History of the MHIWU* (1931).

Chapter 7
From Attendants to Mental Nurses

They are our waiters, head, house and parlour maids,
the nursemaids of our second childhood, our herdsmen
and gaolers, and our playfellows.

A 'certified patient's' view of mental nurses, *NAWU Magazine*
April 1923.

We have already seen how NAWU was created out of a
hard-headed opposition to the pretentions of professionalism and a disbelief in the sincerity of those, mainly in
authority, promoting it. In place of the intangible benefits
of status and prestige, the union had demanded better
pay, improved conditions, shorter hours and less irksome
discipline – and won them.

From the early 1920s, however, a subtle change of
emphasis began to take place. No longer were the two
methods of advance, 'trade unionism' and 'professionalism', always seen as antagonistic to each other. The idea
that they might be complementary began to gain ground,
and along with it the idea that improvements in staff
conditions might also lead to better care for patients. This
change in union strategy accelerated when the conditions
of the 1920s weakened the ability of the NAWU to make
progress by aggressive tactics against the employers. Thus
professionalism became associated with the new spirit of
co-operation between the union and asylum authorities.

Yet defensiveness was not the only reason for the
NAWU's new interest in professional issues. During the
inter-war period, cautious attempts were made to reform
the custodial 'asylums' and transform them into curative
'mental hospitals'. Although only very small moves were

taken in this direction, it resulted in limited material improvements for both patients and staff, while the slow shift away from penal methods began to create the potential for staff to exercise an enhanced treatment role, instead of simply watching over their charges or setting them to work at one of the asylum industries. Asylum workers had previously made the transition from being 'keepers' of the 'mad', to 'attendants' of the 'insane'. Now, during the inter-war period, they would become 'nurses' in 'hospitals' for the 'mentally ill'.

The Battle with the GNC

After 1919, the term 'mental nurse' was the official designation of both male and female staff in mental hospitals, more or less as a by-product of the movement that was finally carrying general hospital nursing towards state registration. As early as 1912 the Executive Council of the NAWU had supported the pre-war agitation in favour of state registration for nurses, and George Gibson in particular had been an enthusiastic supporter of such a change.

The Nurses Registration Act of 1919 established a register of trained nurses which was divided into a number of parts: general, mental, sick children and any other prescribed part (under which mental deficiency was later included as a separate nursing qualification). The Act also set up a new governing body for the profession, the General Nursing Council (GNC), consisting of a majority of nurses, appointed initially by the Minster, and charged with compiling a syllabus for future examinations and an initial register of nurses. Mental nursing was included in the scheme after a deputation from the MPA went to see the Prime Minister. While the Bill was going through Parliament, the NAWU pressed strongly for and was promised representation on the Council.

Maud Wiese, from the Claybury branch, was the first NAWU nominee to be elected to the Council in 1922. She proved to be something of a thorn in its flesh, often taking issue with the policies of a Council dominated by general hospital matrons and doctors. One of her first protests – to no avail – was against the expensive premises taken by the GNC in Portland Place, given the high fees charged to nurses for taking its examinations. She was worried that the fees would discourage mental nurses from transferring from the MPA to the GNC form of training. From the 1920s two alternative forms of training existed for mental nurses. The established certificate of the MPA and Registered Mental Nurse (RMN) training under the auspices of the GNC. GNC draft rules proposed that holders of the MPA certificate, or anyone else with three years' training would, as a transitional arrangement, be permitted to register as mental nurses. In return the MPA would in future cease to examine and award certificates to mental nurses. They were to be invited to appoint examiners for the RMN finals. When this provoked strong protests from certain quarters – the Matron's Council of Great Britain and Ireland passed a strongly worded resolution opposing what it saw as an incursion by psychiatrists into nursing territory – the GNC began to backpedal. It announced that after 1925 it would only recognise the RMN qualification. The MPA retaliated by declaring that it would continue to train nurses for the certificate.

This was not the only issue of dispute between mental nursing and the general nursing establishment. Advancement to senior positions in mental nursing was increasingly dependant on possession of SRN, even in the absence of any qualification in mental nursing. In order to compete against general trained nurses, mental nurses would have to obtain State Registered Nurse (SRN) status. It became clear that the prejudiced attitudes of general hospital matrons was a serious obstacle in their way. In 1924 when the GNC circularised matrons on its proposal to allow MPA certificate holders to undertake a shortened SRN training, many declared that they would not accept such candidates. Maud Wiese leaked the results – quoting replies which showed deep seated prejudices against mental nursing – in the *NAWU Magazine* and, at the instigation of the GNC's chair, received a rebuke from the Minister of Health.

The dispute over the future of mental nursing was not

easy to resolve. General and mental hospital nurses were deeply suspicious of each other, and when contact occurred, friction was often the result. Some of this surfaced in the *NAWU Magazine* from time to time, when, for example, in June 1920 'Scottie' complained that

> For years back we have helped considerably to swell the numbers of the inactive and the apathetic, we have sat down and viewed with a calm submissiveness the invasion of our territory by individuals who, due to the snobbish idea that they are the all-superior trained, invariably prove round pegs in square holes ... What fools we have been!

A female nurse wrote:

> Hospital Matrons and sisters have made life unbearable with their tyrannical rules and regulations, and I have seen more kindness in a week in a mental hospital than I have seen in a year in a general hospital.

These were recurrent and deeply felt themes, and in the conflict between the GNC and the MPA such feelings were to draw mental nurses back into closer alliance with the psychiatrists and their professional association. General nurses began to be seen as the enemy more than medical superintendents.

Maude Wiese resigned from the GNC in 1927 because she, at least, had obtained a place to train as a general nurse. She stayed on the NAWU Executive in the meanwhile as its solitary woman member, resigning in August 1927 when she was appointed an Assistant Matron at Bexley Mental Hospital. In December 1927 the two NAWU candidates, Miss Jean Brown, and Mr E.H. Blackman from Bexley, a former President of the union, won both of the nurses' seats on the Mental Nurses Committee of the GNC. In the years that followed, the crisis between the GNC and the (by now) Royal Medico-Psychological Association (RMPA) deepened and internal divisions opened up within NAWU about how to deal with it. Though the RMPA training was not quite as academically oriented, the two systems of training were very similar. The main difference was that the fees were much lower for the RMPA exam: 5 shillings to take the prelim and 10 shillings to take the finals. In May 1928 the GNC's Mental Nursing Committee passed a resolution calling for a conference between the GNC (and its associated bodies in Scotland and Northern Ireland), and the RMPA, in order to sort out the apparently absurd fact that two certificating bodies existed for mental nursing, both offering virtually identical qualifications. The RMPA's view was that the problems would be solved if the GNC would only allow RMPA certificate-holders to register automatically as RMNs under the GNC.

The conference between the two organisations was held on 23 May 1929. Dr Robertson of the RMPA declared that mental nurse training for the register was a 'fiasco'. Only 212 candidates had taken the GNC test in the previous five years, while in the same period 4,229 nurses had taken the RMPA exam. He hinted that prejudice against mental nurses might be a factor in the GNC's obstructiveness, pointing out that mental nurses were at that time not admitted as members of the College of Nursing. The RMPA was prepared to operate the same syllabus as the GNC and allow the GNC to inspect courses and refuse any individual nurse from admission on to its register. The GNC's chair, Edith Musson, replied that it could not in her view delegate to an outside body powers which had been granted to it from Parliament. Accordingly, a letter was sent out on 15 June 1929, rejecting the RMPA's proposals, on the grounds outlined by Miss Musson.

Within the NAWU there was considerable friction over the issue. While majority opinion was behind the RMPA – if only for the pragmatic reasons of its lower fees and the protection of those members who held its certificate – the two union sponsored members on the GNC took a rather different view. In 1929 when the GNC finally turned down the RMPA's proposals for working in co-operation with it, Mr Blackman and Miss Brown again defended the GNC's position to the NAWU Conference, saying that registration 'means a very great deal for the future', despite the higher fees, much to the annoyance of George Gibson. The dispute between the GNC and the RMPA rumbled on, with the two systems of training continuing side by side until after the Second World War, when, as we shall see later, the RMPA finally wound up its examinations.

The union had been caught between two devils, and most members had chosen the one they knew, primarily to defend their immediate interests. As far as wider issues were concerned, there was little to choose between the two systems of training. Neither really met the training needs of mental nurses, being modelled on general nursing and medicine.

A Few Steps Forward

The 1920s were a time when the system of lunacy administration which had survived intact since 1890, came under increasing attack. A head of steam for reform built up from inside and outside the service, which resulted in some limited reforms by the end of the 1920s. The NAWU quickly realised that the reform movement held opportunities but also posed dangers to the interests of its members. Although it did not initiate the campaign for reform, once it was under way it very quickly entered the fray.

There were a number of different participants in the campaign, not all of whom always saw eye to eye with each other: civil libertarians represented particularly by the National Council for Lunacy Reform (NCLR), who believed that large numbers of people were being incarcerated unnecessarily in asylums, suffering indignities, drab routines and, on occasions, rough treatment from staff; medical men who desired greater recognition from medicine as a whole, and were pushing the idea that insanity was a form of treatable illness like any other; and social reformers who argued that if more people could be treated effectively at an early stage, through voluntary admission, this might in the long run prove less expensive, though in the short run it required more investment in acute services.

The reform-minded political climate immediately following the First World War was one which encouraged all three groups to press their particular case. The creation of the Ministry of Health in 1919 and fleeting plans to abolish the hated Poor Law were products of this environment. This spirit of reform largely evaporated after the inter-war economic crisis began in 1921. Nevertheless, the fact that some reforms were initiated at all, indicates that traces of this reform spirit lived on. They were particularly associated with the short-lived Labour governments of 1924 and 1929-31, which took tentative steps towards reforming the mental health services.

The reform movement was boosted in 1921 by a sensational exposé of conditions in Prestwich Asylum during the war by Dr Montagu Lomax. His book detailed his two years' experience as an assistant medical officer. He claimed that patients were herded together in insanitary barrack-like conditions, without any thought of classifying them into different types, with the main aim being confinement rather than treatment. Although he suggested that attendants and nurses were responsible for cases of ill treatment of patients, Dr Lomax attacked the whole system: especially the legal framework and the fact that medical superintendents sought to control too many extraneous activities, rather than concentrating on patients' welfare.[1]

The book was a sensation. Here was a young doctor condemning his own superiors in the most forthright possible terms. Since he also advocated that the authorities should be compelled to recognise the NAWU, the union's initial reaction to his book was not an entirely hostile one, but his criticism of staff eventually led it into conflict with him, especially as the press subsequently concentrated on these aspects.

The government appointed a three-person Departmental Committee of Enquiry into the accusations concerning asylum administration contained in Dr Lomax's book. It consisted of Sir Cyril Cobb, chair of the LCC Asylums Committee, and Drs Bedford Pierce and R.P. Smith – all of whom were in some way associated with the system of administration as it stood at present. Dr Smith had even published an unfavourable review of Lomax's book.[2] Dr Lomax called instead for the

appointment of a Royal Commission, a call echoed by the
union. There were, of course, instances of cruelty to
patients. Some were verified, and in a spate of disciplinary
cases nurses were sacked and sometimes prosecuted. The
Board of Control now had powers to initiate enquiries into
individual hospitals, and this led to the glare of outside
publicity, even in cases where accusations were disproved.
But the attacks were on the whole sweeping and
unsubstantiated, by their nature difficult to prove. Often,
however, critics missed the main point: the whole system
of administration of mental hospitals needed to be
overhauled. Cases of abuse were inevitable in a service
which sought mainly to confine 'pauper lunatics' at the
lowest possible cost.

These and similar points were made in an anonymous
article in the *Nursing Times* in 1923, said to have been
written 'by a mental nurse', and expressing 'our point of
view'. Its author complained that 'for all that is bad in the
administration of our mental hospitals the nursing staff
appears to be blamed', and described the (now retitled)
National Society for Lunacy Reform (NSLR) as 'ever eager
to advertise any sensational criticism of mental nursing'. It
claimed that for all the publicity, the various official
enquiries had 'the usual result of leaving the man in the
street just as wise as he was before.' The article did not
deny that much was wrong with the administration of
mental hospitals, but it placed the ultimate responsibility
more widely:

> Many of those people who are agitating for a Royal
> Commission to enquire into the accusations made against the
> administration and staff would be amazed to hear that they
> are responsible to a great extent for any abuses. Do these
> people realise, when they elect men and women to sit on local
> councils on condition that they pledge themselves to practice
> economy, that they are causing insanity? It is impossible for
> men and women to lead healthy lives under present
> conditions ... The chief aim of most members of committees
> is to reduce expenditure, and the medical superintendent
> who does not do likewise is seldom popular.[3]

It pointed out that the NAWU had been responsible for

many improvements, such as the shortening of the working day, which had also been beneficial to patients. Despite this, the beneficial role of the union had not been given due recognition by critics. As we saw in the previous chapter, 1923 was a year in which mental hospital employers were seeking to regain the initiative and impose cuts in pay and an increase in hours. The implications of this for the service – which were once again totally ignored by the NSLR – were made explicit in the article:

> Happily pressure has brought about many improvements, but these are in danger now that it is in the minds of the authorities to force mental nurses back to prewar conditions while they pretend to be anxious to improve the status of the mental nurse, and to attract a better class of probationer nurse. How can they expect to do this by worsening the conditions?[4]

Thus the ultimate failure of the NSLR and the NAWU to work in tandem was largely due to the failure of the former to see that a close link existed between improving conditions for staff and patients alike. It did not recognise the role that the union had already played, and failed to see that it represented a line of defence against a future deterioration in conditions.

The Committee of Inquiry reported late in 1922. It declared that many of the conditions described by Lomax had been the result of wartime economies, and came to the conclusion that his main accusations were unfounded. The union described the findings as a 'whitewashing' exercise, and added its voice to the growing pressure for a full-scale Royal Commission. The Board of Control tried to fend off this pressure by instituting an Inquiry into Mental Nursing in March 1922. Out of its nine members, only one had a nursing background – a fact that did not go uncriticised by the NAWU. Given that the Board of Control, as we saw in the previous chapter, thought that the problems of the mental health services could be solved by increasing nurses' hours and cutting their pay, the NAWU decided to boycott the Inquiry.

Two years later, in 1924, the first ever Labour

government was elected. It did not have an overall majority, and was very short-lived. Before it disappeared, however, it appointed a Royal Commission into the operation of the lunacy laws.

The Board of Control Inquiry into Mental Nursing reported late in 1924, after the decision to set up a Royal Commission had been announced. It had therefore become largely superseded. This hardly mattered anyway, because its conclusions were extraordinarily timid. It argued that there ought to be a greater recognition of the value of training and that this ought also to be reflected in pay. But that was about all.

The proposals of the Royal Commission were not revolutionary, but they did advocate that where possible admission should be 'voluntary' or 'temporary', and certification used only as a last resort. It did not argue, therefore, that the lunacy laws be abolished. These proposals were broadly in line with the NAWU's own thinking. In its evidence to the Royal Commission it called for an end to 'pauper' status for mental hospital patients, an increased government grant for patient maintenance, and an increase in the proportion of trained mental nurses to be at least 50 per cent. The union wanted to see the development of out-patient facilities and the majority of patients to be treated informally without certification. They also suggested a broad range of improvements in social and recreational facilities for both staff and patients.[5]

The Royal Commission had reported in 1926. Yet despite its relatively modest proposals, legislation did not appear on the statute book until four years later, in 1930. Yet again, it was a Labour government which took action, through Arthur Greenwood, the Minister of Health. Thus, by the end of 1930 'asylums' had overnight become 'hospitals' and 'pauper lunatics' were transformed overnight into 'rate-aided patients'.

Mental Hospitals and Institutional Workers' Union

Alongside these changes, 'attendants' officially became 'nurses' and the National Asylum Workers' Union changed itself into the Mental Hospitals and Institutional

Workers' Union (MHIWU). Wages and conditions had been undoubtedly improved out of all recognition. The 48-hour week had been established in a quarter of the mental hospitals in England and Wales. Despite the allegations and scandals of the early 1920s the status of mental hospital staff was steadily, if slowly, rising. The union itself had weathered the storm of the early 1920s, and membership was growing. It had won significant improvements for its members and the service as a whole. A certain air of self-satisfaction was settling upon the union, symbolised perhaps by the increasingly stout figure of George Gibson now, as a result of his TUC activities, a leading figure in the trade union world. Both the Mental Hospitals and Institutional Workers' Union, and its rotund General Secretary, had come a long way from the fledgling organisation of aggrieved Lancashire asylum attendants which, at the end of its first year, had assets of just 1s 6d. Only one thing slightly disturbed the union's 21st anniversary celebrations of 1931, and that was the severe economic and political crisis that was affecting the country ...

Notes

[1] M. Lomax, *The Experiences of an Asylum Doctor* (1921).
[2] According to the *NAWU Magazine*, April 1923.
[3] 'Our Point of View', *Nursing Times*, 28 April 1923.
[4] Ibid.
[5] *21 Years*, pp.76-8.

Chapter 8
Surviving the Thirties

As we have seen, the union had by 1930 adopted a much more cautious approach, seeking above all to consolidate what had already been achieved. There were many small signs of this more 'softly, softly' approach. For example, the new badge issued as a result of the change of title from January 1931 to the Mental Hospitals and Institutional Workers' Union was much more discreet than its predecessor. As a promotional leaflet announced:

> Its neatness, beauty and unobtrusive appearance will commend it to all our members. There is no lettering on the front of the badge, but the initials 'M.H.I.W.U.' are on the reverse side.

The 'objects' of the new union were achieving 'reasonable hours of duty and a fair rate of wages.' The problems and grievances of members now received less attention in the union journal than they had previously. At a time when there was always someone worse off than oneself, those with a job were often simply grateful for the fact, and there seemed little point in ventilating unresolvable grievances.

Yet the process of adjustment was not *that* smooth. Despite its more cautious approach, the union still found itself in conflict with the employers at the beginning of the 1930s. On 22 January 1930, the JCC met at the Guildhall in the City of London to consider the union's latest set of applications. The MHA made some concessions. Staff were to be permitted to have the union represent them if they were summoned to appear before the Visiting Committee; staff with five years' service were to be allowed the option of living out 'where practicable'; married men were to be allowed to bring their own rations in with them; and 'acting up' pay was to be made after seven consecutive days' service in the higher rank. However, the MHA rejected the more substantial claims of the union: for the establishment of local consultative committees, attendance of a union representative at all meetings of Visiting Committees which were to discuss 'any matter concerning their staff ', the abolition of the lower 'rural' rate of pay in favour of the higher 'urban' rate, and a reduction in the maximum hours of 60 (exclusive of mealtimes) a week established after the Radcliffe Strike of 1922.

The union's demands were bold ones, seeking not just higher rewards for their members but also a much greater share in decision-making. A Labour government was in power and Arthur Greenwood, the Minister of Health steering the Mental Treatment Bill through Parliament, was said to be a 'friend' of asylum workers. There may have been a speculative element to the union's claim, but the leadership were particularly disappointed at the JCC's failure to recommend a reduction in hours. It therefore encouraged branches to mount pressure at local level to achieve a shortening of the working week.

The MHA was unhappy at this attempt to bypass the JCC, and protested to the union's NEC. The Executive Meeting of 13 March replied by declaring that it wanted to reopen the question of hours with the MHA, encouraged by growing membership figures – now nudging 12,000. Under pressure from the branches, Gibson continued to press the issue, writing also to the government urging an enquiry into mental hospital working conditions, as recommended by the International Labour Organisation. A compromise was reached in September 1930 when the union agreed to the MHA's suggestion of a Joint Committee of Enquiry into Hours of Duty.

When the Committee reported late in 1931, the two sides had predictably failed to agree. The MHA rejected MHIWU calls for a 48-hour week, offering only a reduction of two hours to 58 hours a week. Since

organisations were bound by decisions of their respective
Conferences, there was no room for negotiation. The issue
was not settled until November 1934 when the JCC, 'after
prolonged discussion', agreed to recommend maximum
hours of 54 hours provided that no further revision
should be made for less than five years. After a ballot of
branches, the MHA offer was reluctantly accepted.

The truth was that, after 1930, the union was in no
position to press the issue of hours with any vigour. Not
only had Fenner Brockway's Private Member's Bill in
Parliament to regulate hours of the nursing profession
failed, but the Labour government itself fell later in the
same year. In December 1930 unemployment rose to
2,500,000 and by July 1931 the May Committee Report
called for big reductions in public spending, much of it to
be achieved by reducing the level of unemployment
benefit. Ramsey MacDonald split with his party to form a
National government to implement the proposals. The
Labour government fell in the Autumn of 1931 and
remained out of office until the end of the Second World
War.

The most immediate impact in the mental hospital
service were temporary wage reductions of 2.5 per cent a
year, for two years. However, in some areas, particularly
the North-East, some Visiting Committees imposed no
reductions.

In succeeding years pay negotiations naturally proved
difficult. Union applications were routinely turned down.
By 1935 the only further progress made – except for the
long delayed reduction in hours – was the prevention of
further wage cuts. In March 1936, as a result of
Conference resolutions, the MHIWU put forward eleven
proposals to the JCC (including such long standing claims
as equal pay, abolition of the urban/rural distinction in
rates of pay, long service increments, etc.) All were
rejected by the MHA with the exception of two extremely
minor concessions. Rates of pay had not changed since
1927, when the basic wage and the war bonus had been
incorporated. The minimum weekly wage at an 'urban'
asylum was £2 for a male and £1 12 shillings for a female
nurse. At 'rural' asylums the minimum was £1 13 shillings

and £1 8 shillings for men and women respectively.
Qualified RMN/RMPA holders only received 6 shillings
(men) or 4 shillings (women) a week extra. Male charges
got a maximum per week of 4 shillings extra, and women
3s 2d. Night nurses were paid as charge nurses.

Not surprisingly, some critical voices were raised. For
example, D. Jones of the West Ham branch suggested in a
letter to the *MHIWU Journal* in December 1938, that the
JCC might be retitled 'the Non-Intervention Committee'
(an allusion to the international aspect of the Spanish Civil
War then raging) since

> ... the only useful purpose this Committee is now serving is
> to act at an Old Comrades' Association with periodical
> reunions, paid for by the Mental Hospitals Association and
> our Union.

In 1937 a motion came before the MHIWU Conference to
withdraw from the JCC, but it was decisively defeated. In
the debate one influential view was that the branches in
'backward areas' particularly needed it. The union was in
no position to take an aggressive stance. At this stage in its
existence, the JCC was a very fragile body. Many of its
so-called 'recommendations' were no more than tentative
suggestions, and by no means all authorities were
members of it.

Majority opinion in the union was in favour of keeping
the JCC, even if it was a largely ineffectual body. It at least
preserved some of the advantages won during the union's
more militant phase. By 1934, membership was rising,
wage cuts had been restored and some reductions in hours
had been achieved.

Mental Nursing in the 1930s

But beneath this apparent tranquility staff were grappling
with increasing difficulties. The mental hospitals were no
longer the centre of public attention. The Mental
Treatment Act had been passed and the law partially
liberalised. But immediately afterwards, the country's
economic crisis had obliterated all good intentions in its

path. The numbers of in-patients grew from 138,100 in 1914 to 150,300 in 1939, largely in line with the rise in population, and to accommodate them the average size of hospital had grown to over 1,000.[1]

The overcrowding caused pressure on already scarce resources, the effects of which were documented in a thorough journalistic investigation by Paul Winterton.[2] He found that nurses were working under great stress, and their health, as well as that of their patients, was threatened. Homeliness and individual treatment were impossible when beds were often only three feet apart. Patients often did not have locker space and could be seen carrying their possessions around in a bundle during the day. Occupations and recreations could not be properly organised. Yet at the same time, with only minimal resources, mental nurses were now expected to be skilled in treating the mentally ill. It all added up to an intensification of working conditions.

Despite the difficulties, some authorities made improvements: out-patient facilities were expanded, barbers introduced for men and hair-dressing salons for women, films shown, occupational therapy introduced and individual rather than institutional clothing permitted, especially for women patients. In some hospitals in the 1930s canteens and shops were opened. New forms of 'physical' – and often physically hazardous – treatments were pioneered, particularly the induction of malaria in patients suffering from the final stages of syphilis, prolonged narcosis for manic depression, insulin shock treatment in schizophrenia, and various other kinds of experimental treatment.

Thus, despite the apparent good relations between the union and the employers, working conditions had deteriorated without any compensatory improvement in pay. Winterton concluded that

> Mental nursing at the moment is no career for an ambitious man. It expects a high degree of ability and intelligence, but its rewards for capability are mean and miserable.

He asked one mental nurse why he continued to do it, who replied:

The trouble is that there doesn't seem anything else for me to do. Either I've got to leave the service and try for some better job or live all my life on £3 10s a week.

As Herbert Hough explained to me, in the 1930s

it was a common thing for some of the officials to say to you, 'If you don't like the job, there's plenty of folks queuing at Lucy Tower Street', which was the Labour Exchange, of course.

The chief attraction of the work was still the security and superannuation rather than the intrinsic satisfactions that might be gained from it. During the depression years, large numbers of men, particularly from the North of England and Scotland, uprooted themselves and started new lives as mental nurses. The competition was fierce, and many of those applying were expected to possess a skill useful to the hospital community, such as being able to play a musical instrument or being good at sports; one retired mental nurse I interviewed had been a pianist in the cinema in the 1920s before talkies came along and made him redundant.

Difficulties in Recruiting Women

Yet while mental hospitals could always fill their establishment of male staff, chronic shortages of female staff persisted throughout the 1930s. All branches of nursing were experiencing difficulties in recruiting women. The shortage was due to a combination of factors: increased demands for pairs of hands as the public health service expanded; the competition of alternative factory and office work; and the low pay, long hours, poor conditions and petty restrictions within nursing itself. Hospitals could never attract enough women, nor keep those they recruited for long. Mental nursing, as the most unpopular and low-status branch of nursing, suffered worst of all. One option might have been to improve pay and conditions but, as we have seen, the MHA turned

down an application from the MHIWU for equal pay for
men and women.

The MHIWU for its part was hardly in a position to
press in any concerted way for improvements, since many
women nurses did not join it. It is not easy to tell why more
women did not join the MHIWU and participate in its
affairs because, of course, they did not make their reasons
known. The separation of hospitals into male and female
sides, and the growing domination of female sides by
matrons who had started off their careers in general
nursing, may well have been a factor. The perennial
problem of many women nurses not regarding the job as a
career but as a fill-in between school and marriage, may
also have been influential. There appears to have been
surprisingly little discussion within the union at this time
about the problems of women mental nurses. A rare
exception was an article in the union's *Journal* of October
1935 which asked 'Are female nurses getting a square
deal?' and answered with a 'very big decided "NO" '. It
found that even hospitals which belonged to the MHA
regularly evaded JCC recommendations, as far as its
women nurses were concerned:

> It is not unusual to find concessions granted to the male staffs
> whilst the same concessions are withheld from female staffs.
> Days off are cancelled at short notice, irrespective of any
> personal inconvenience to the nurse. Hours of duty are split
> up in a most extraordinary way, devised, one would imagine,
> with the sole object of preventing the nurse from getting away
> from the Institution for any reasonable period of time!

Female nurses suffered greater restrictions on their
freedom than male nurses, and frequently did not receive
the two consecutive days off a week 'recommended' by the
JCC. Behind all this lay the growing power of the matron
in relation to the medical superintendent and the Visiting
Committee:

> In some places, Matron's word is absolute law, and appeals to
> the Medical Superintendent (should there be one) would be
> worse than useless.

In short:

> ... it is evident that the female nurse is not being treated on an equal footing with the male nurse. She is expected to be contented under conditions which the male nurse would never tolerate; she is denied concessions granted to the male nurse; she has to work for 20 per cent less wages; and in every way she is made to feel herself inferior to the male nurse.

The remedy to the problem facing the female nurse, according to the author of the article – Cliff Comer, the National Organiser of the union and later its General Secretary – 'lies in her own hands ... The female nurses must organise themselves as strongly as the male nurses have done'. That was all very well, but mere exhortation to join and be active was not enough. It has to be said that the union could have done more to help female nurses to organise, especially given the fact that men's relatively better pay and conditions had been largely established by the militancy of female members between 1917 and 1921.

The chance to do something positive came rather belatedly at the 1938 Portsmouth Conference when a resolution was put to appoint a Woman Officer, in line with the practice in other unions. Out of 122 delegates present, only three were women; and one of these (Miss G. M. Hall from Brentwood) put the resolution, while another (Miss H. Ackland from Portsmouth) seconded it. It seemed the motion would easily succeed, when Mr Flanagham rose to oppose it on behalf of the NEC, doubting whether it would be effective. After a debate, Conference defeated the proposition on a card vote by 228 votes to 164. It was put again in 1939 without success.

An opportunity had therefore been lost. While the MHIWU had, it is true, pressed the issue of equal pay at the JCC, there was little concerted effort to deal with the glaring gap in union membership and the problems that women as a result faced. By 1939, when nurses amounted to 16,000 out of a total of MHIWU 19,000 members, there were only 6,000 female nurse members. Since there were approximately 30,000 mental nurses in England and Wales alone, and female sides of mental hospitals were

larger than male sides, there was no doubt where the
largest shortfall in membership lay.

There were some improvements in the working
conditions of female mental nurses by the end of the
1930s. On the whole, however, it was mainly the pressure
of chronic staff shortages that led authorities to review
their policies. The most concerted attempts to deal with
the difficulties of recruiting women nurses were those
undertaken by the LCC which started employing married
women in 1937. The LCC issued a special booklet *A Career
for Women* subtitled 'An Explanation of how a Young
Woman may become a Mental Nurse and of the
opportunities offered in the Mental Health Services of the
London County Council'. LCC wages were well in excess
of JCC rates, and considerable effort was put into
improving residences and recreational facilities. But by
1939, on the eve of the Second World War, the female
short staffing problem had not generally been solved.

The MHIWU and the Mental Health Services

The continuing emphasis on professionalism in the 1930s
partly arose from the union's defensive stance, and when
in 1934 the union adopted, on the advice of the NEC, an
additional object:

> To consider any matters related to the care,
> treatment and general welfare of the patients

this did not meet with universal approval. A minority
agreed with the objection of Mr A.R. Farmer, from West
Park, that it was an attempt to 'look after the employers'
side of the question'.

The majority agreed, however, that this was a rather
narrow conception of the role of unions in the health and
welfare services. Quite apart from status considerations,
the 'scandals' of the 1920s and the battles with the GNC
had shown that the workers' side of the question might
also be affected by matters affecting the treatment and
welfare of patients. Changes were occurring in the mental
hospital service which held profound implications for

staff, and the union would have to enter into the realm of professional arguments if it was to respond effectively.

An example was readily at hand in the recent development of occupational therapy. The development of craft workshops as a form of therapeutic treatment for patients had been pioneered in Holland and spread to England in the early 1930s. While it varied considerably in different hospitals, occupational therapy commonly involved taking the most ambulant and treatable patients from the wards, farms and asylum industries, to work under the supervision of a specially appointed 'occupation officer'. By 1932 both the MHA and the Board of Control were recommending its adoption to Visiting Comittees.

Opinion in the union was divided on the value of 'occupation therapy'. There were fears that instructors and instructresses were taking over the role of nurses. George Gibson was even more scathing in an article contributed to the *MHIWU Journal* in February 1934. He claimed that there was a good deal of 'ballyhoo' and even 'codology' about the current craze, and felt that psychiatrists were covering up for the fact that they had not found a cure for insanity. Gibson's outspoken views naturally led to a lively debate within the union. Many supported him, but others favoured occupational therapy as an alternative to the asylum industries as long as nurses were involved.

The issue finally surfaced at Conference in 1935. As a result of pressure from the South Wales and South-West Federation, the NEC was instructed to set up a committee of enquiry into occupational therapy and report back to Conference the following year with recommendations. It was the first ever major enquiry by the union into a professional issue affecting members. The committee prepared a wide ranging questionnaire for branches, and achieved a good response rate. In addition its members visited three mental hospitals – Ryhope, York and Exminster – in order to see for themselves how occupational therapy operated in practice.

The results of the questionnaire were issued as an Interim Report to the 1936 Conference. The results showed that occupational therapy had resulted in more patients becoming active than before, those involved spending on average four and a half hours a day at various activities. Most branches thought its effect had been beneficial, though some female nurses were concerned that they were now being expected to do the sewing work on wards. The Final Report to the 1937 Conference pronounced in favour of occupational therapy, but argued that it should form part of a definite course of treatment, rather than merely being introduced to counteract idleness. While it was no panacea, wards had become quieter, even if at the expense of standards of cleanliness, since fewer patients were performing the work of unpaid skivvies. The Conference approved the committee's recommendations, though one or two delegates wondered if George Gibson, in signing the report, was going back on his previous opposition. The union had, despite some reservations, sided with progress.

The 'Mental Deficiency' Service

The other major issue in which the union intervened in the 1930s concerned the direction of the 'mental deficiency' services. In contrast to growing official optimism about prospects for treating the mentally ill, there was a profound pessimism regarding the mentally handicapped.[3] The Wood Committee's first report published in 1929, had estimated that there were something like 300,000 'mental defectives' in England and Wales, about double the previous official estimate of 1908. It increased pressure to expand services under existing legislation of 1913 and 1927. The report assumed that about one-third of the total urgently required institutional care, either because they were too severely ill, needed training, or were of 'incorrigible criminal tendencies'. The press joined in with sensational stories of crimes committed by male patients, and large families reproduced by female 'defectives'. The Board of Control itself described 'high grade defectives' as a 'menace' in its Annual Report for 1929.

Pressure mounted for the prohibition of marriage and for sterilisation of the 'unfit', as practised in many

American states. Britain's economic decline was said to be due to the fact that while the 'better classes' were having fewer children, the 'unfit' were continuing to breed. Even labour movement organisations like the Women Public Health Officers' Association, the Women's Co-operative Guild, and the National Council for Labour Women all supported the call for sterilisation at one time or another during the 1930s. In 1934 the official Brock Report urged legislation to permit voluntary sterilisation.

The MHIWU's initial response to these developments was cautious. It opened its pages to the debate, in which two contrary views tended to be put: one which thought that defectives were a major social problem, countered by another more left-wing view which claimed that population problems were largely economic in origin. The union became increasingly opposed to sterilisation, especially when George Gibson came out against it. In 1934 he successfully moved a resolution at the TUC opposing the Brock Report's advocacy of voluntary sterlisation 'until the social aspects of the problem have been examined by a Royal Commission'. The TUC's opposition helped to kill off plans by the Board of Control to get legislation introduced. Yet though 'defectives' may not have been sterilised, they were certainly segregated in increasing numbers. In many cases, old workhouses rather than new buildings formed the basis of provision. The scale of expansion was considerable: from 17,101 beds in 1924 to nearly 36,000 by 1934.[4]

During the inter-war period mental deficiency nursing developed as a distinct branch of nursing, with first the RMPA and subsequently the GNC organising examinations separately from those for mental nursing. However, by 1934 only 40 of the 67 'mental defective' institutions with more than 100 patients had training schools recognised by either the RMPA or the GNC. This was a much lower proportion than in mental hospitals, and a greater proportion of staff were in consequence untrained. Thus, the JCC's conditions did not apply since the administrative authorities were not members of the Mental Hospitals Association. The workers were also generally not so well organised in the MHIWU as mental hospital staffs. An article in the *Journal* for September 1938 pointed out that the authorities seemed to want to place

> the patients out of sight and out of the public mind. This applies equally to the staffs, whose conditions are as much in need of improvement as are the care and treatment of the patients. Very few of these institutions provide facilities for training of their staffs in nursing ... Nursing certificates being unobtainable, the staffs have to remain on a lower scale of pay with very little prospects for the future. Long hours of duty, with unnecessary restrictions are the common lot of the male and female staffs.

If the status and material conditions of mental nursing were gradually rising during the 1930s, in 'mental deficiency' nursing they remained abysmally low.

Union Organisation in the 1930s

Branch secretaries and branch collectors (often one and the same person) were the main props of the union throughout the 1930s. Without their unrelenting efforts, the union could not have survived. If by the end of 1937 membership exceeded 17,000, passing the figure of the previous peak year of 1920, it was largely due to their efforts. A number of secretaries and active union members shared their reminiscences of this period with me. According to their accounts, as well as making collective representations to the officials, there were two other key aspects to the secretary's role. The first was individual casework, such as recovering a member's superannuation contributions, representing a man discovered drunk on duty, and so on. The second, to which a massive amount of branch resources were devoted, involved keeping the membership lists intact: contacting new members of staff, trying also to get non-members into the union and, above all, chasing up members in arrears of contributions (for, of course, there was no deduction of dues at source in those days). Given that membership was split into male and female sides, and into different shifts during the day, as well as into day and night staff, keeping track of the members was not always an easy task. The new 'villa' system of mental hospitals also meant that staff were more scattered and fragmented than under the previous 'barrack' system of the asylums.

The biggest organisational problems lay in London and Scotland. Although London had the largest concentration of members in the union, it also had a high proportion of non-members, particularly among female nurses. Added to this, the Revd Stanley Morgan was due to retire as London Organiser at the end of 1936, on reaching 65 years of age, and the NEC had made it clear that it would insist on his retirement, in conformity with union rules. The London District Committee (LDC) was unhappy, and worried that any replacement would not be able to represent them before the various authorities handled by the Revd Morgan – many of whom were not party to JCC agreements. The LDC was also in the middle of complex negotiations over the regrading of staff transferred to the LCC from Poor Law mental deficiency institutions. Cliff Comer, previously National Organiser, took over from Morgan in 1937. Relations between him and sections of the LDC were not always amicable.

In Scotland, the union made great strides during the 1930s, recovering all the ground lost in the 1920s, and more. By the Second World War, Scotland had become the third largest area in the union – a remarkable achievement given that for all of the period there were no nationally negotiated pay and conditions. These were in consequence generally worse than in England and Wales, and MHIWU branches often simply had to strike as good a deal as they could with local management. For some time the Scottish Federation had been pressing for its own organiser. As the general wealth of the union increased, part of it due to the growing financial contributions of Scottish members, their case became an extremely strong one – even though Conference turned it down yet again in 1935. They got round the problem informally in March 1938 by appointing Councillor Alex White as a 'temporary' organiser, with the Scottish Federation footing the bill for the running of the office in Edinburgh.

One footnote to the development of union membership in the 1930s was its growing concentration among nurses, or 'indoor staff', as opposed to craftsmen, the 'artisan' or 'outdoor staffs'. The latter identified more often with their respective craft unions, especially since they had served an apprenticeship elsewhere before working in a mental hospital. In any case the MHA refused to set up a separate sub-committee of the JCC for craftsmen, simply recommending that they should be paid the current trade union rate in the locality. Craft unions themselves were not too happy at the MHIWU's recruiting activities and, as we saw, their displeasure had helped to delay the NAWU's affiliation to the TUC until 1923. In the 1930s the MHIWU again found itself in trouble with some outside unions and was forced to concede priority recruitment rights to the craft unions. In some respects the MHIWU faced similar problems in seeking recruitment of the relatively few 'ancillary' workers – mainly domestic and kitchen workers – in mental hospitals. There were no national pay scales before the Second World War, so many ancillary workers could see little reason for joining the union. Those who did sometimes found it less than congenial, and sometimes complained in the letters to the *Journal* that they were looked down upon by nurses.

While the overall stance of moderation was maintained, there were nevertheless signs of a revival in union activity towards the end of the 1930s, particularly in Scotland and London. The continuing shortage of female staff strengthened the union's bargaining arm. In Scotland, the impressive growth of MHIWU membership was bound to lead eventually not only to concerted pressure for improvements at particular mental hospitals, but also to renewed demands to re-establish the Scottish JCC. Successful pressure to obtain local improvements from 1936 onwards convinced some employers of the need for a unified response. A joint conference between the MHIWU and employers got things moving, but the problem, as ever, was the reluctance of the royal mental hospitals to participate.

The Scottish JCC itself was not re-established before the Second World War. The union continued to press, and win, concessions at local hospitals, the most notable victory being at Glengall (Ayr) in December 1938. In September, a majority of the female nurses, with the support of the MHIWU, collectively gave a month's notice of resignation in protest at the conditions of service at the hospital, including low wages, and as many as 70 hours a week. The Hospital Committee had consistently refused to meet union officials to discuss staff grievances. The struggle lasted two months, with the nurses concerned being financially supported by the union until they found other work. On 2 December the union won recognition, a large number of concessions (including increased pay and reduced hours) from the management and a promise to look at other complaints in the future.

The shortages of staff and the effects of the beds crisis in leading to an intensification of work for nurses were two of the main factors in the growing restiveness of LCC mental hospital nurses towards the end of the 1930s. The third was the rise in expectations that accompanied the election of Herbert Morrison's incoming Labour administration of 1934. Some of these were fulfilled. The LCC had generally progressive intentions. In 1935 it made clear its belief that 'all employees should be in unions'. It relaxed the disciplinary rules on nurses and increased staff leave to three weeks. It brought in improvements for patients such as holidays by the seaside, hairdressing and cafeteria facilities. But the pressure on beds continually outstretched its financial resources.

The result was at first growing staff disenchantment and, finally, open rebellion. Relations became particularly soured in 1938 when the MHIWU's application for a 10 per cent increase on pay rates of £3 12s a week was flatly turned down by the Mental Hospitals Committee. The union's case was that members' duties had become 'more onerous' in recent years due to pressure of work, new and improved methods of treatment, and the complexities of operating the 1930 Mental Treatment Act. The cost of living in the London area, and the lack of promotion opportunities – it apparently took an average of 15 years for a man to become a staff nurse – all added to the sense of grievance, as did the more favourable pay and conditions of adjacent counties such as Middlesex. The management accepted that the levels of skill exercised by staff had increased, but did not agree 'that this in itself constitutes grounds for an increase in remuneration'.

Athlone and the MHIWU

A central prop of the LCC's refusal to pay increases was the insistence that these should have to wait upon the report of the recently established government inquiry into nursing, the Athlone Committee. This had been set up in 1938 as a result of the continuing shortage of nurses in general, the pressure of Labour backbenchers for a reduction in nurses' hours, and the growing trade union organisation of nurses themselves. We shall be hearing more of such matters in Part Two of this history. The Athlone Committee issued an Interim Report early in 1939. It recommended a wide-ranging programme of reforms to deal with shortages and discontent among nurses, most notably a Salaries Committee on the lines of the teaching profession's Burnham Committee, a 96-hour fortnight, other improvements in holidays, pensions and catering, and a relaxation of 'unreasonable rules and restrictions.'

George Gibson told the NEC that he thought Athlone to be 'generally speaking, an enlightened and valuable document'. The report made no specific reference to mental nursing. However a Mental Nursing Sub-Committee had been set up, which included one representative each from the MHIWU (Gibson), the MHA (L.T. Feldon) and the RMPA (Dr Masefield). The bodies which gave evidence to the sub-committee all drew a sharp distinction between male and female nurses, emphasising that shortages and poor conditions of employment were to be found mainly among the latter. A résumé of the history of the JCC, presented by George Gibson and L.T. Feldon, expressed general satisfaction with the collective negotiating machinery, except that it believed all authorites should be compelled to join the MHA, and that its 'recommendations' should become mandatory upon participating authorities. They suggested that standards of nursing had risen, even though the problems of recruiting female nurses persisted.[5] Both the MHA and the MHIWU drew attention in their evidence to the high rates of wastage of female nurses compared to men. The MHIWU recommended a package of practical reforms, which included a 96-hour fortnight, a month's leave, more personal freedom, improved catering and facilities for recreation. They wanted to see a proper reception given to new recruits and their gradual 'breaking in' to 'the atmosphere of a mental hospital', with 'suitable preliminary lectures', all arranged by 'some suitable officer'.

The other major issue which surfaced at the sub-committee was the continuing rift between the GNC and the RMPA. Most mental nurses continued to take the RMPA exams, because the fees were lower, and they could take them in their own hospitals rather than having the expense of travelling to a distant centre. The union was less concerned to favour one system over the other than to protect the interests of RMPA qualified members.

In the event, the war interrupted the work of the sub-committee, and its report, which was in the process of being drafted when war broke out in the autumn of 1939, never appeared. The main Athlone Committee, which had commenced its work earlier was, as we have seen, able to publish an Interim Report in February 1939, putting forward proposals that were broadly in line with what the MHIWU and other trade unions had been calling for. But the war prevented it from moving to produce a final report. With the publication of the Interim Report, the LCC, as it had promised, agreed to negotiate over the MHIWU's claim for higher wages. The basic rates were not changed, but extra increments were granted, which for many nurses meant substantial increases.

The union thus departed the 1930s on a note of modest success. Membership had passed the 20,000 mark for the first time in its history. A policy of moderation, astute investment of the union's money and reliance upon branch secretaries in the localities meant that organisation was solid and finance secure. The influx of men from the depressed areas, often with previous trade union experience had reinforced the union's organising strength in the branches. The head office staff, on the other hand, were representatives of an older generation, who had trained or worked in mental hospitals at around the time of the First World War or before. Bartlett, Gibson, and Shaw remained at the helm, one of the most experienced triumvirates in the trade union movement. These two generations of men largely determined the character of the union in the 1930s – the older generation of men still in control, but with the younger beginning to assert itself.

Notes

[1] K. Jones, *A History of the Mental Health Services* (1971), Appendix I.
[2] P. Winterton, *Minding Minds* (1938).
[3] For the historical background, see J. Ryan and F. Thomas. *The Politics of Mental Handicap* (1980), Ch. 5.
[4] Source: Board of Control *Annual Reports*. Figures are for England and Wales only.
[5] COHSE Archive, loc. cit.

Chapter 9
The Road to Health Service Unionism

The war, which broke out in September 1939, had two contradictory effects on the union. On the one hand it strengthened the bargaining position of labour because it led to a drop in unemployment, and because the co-operation of the workers was necessary to the war effort. On the other hand, as far as the mental health services were concerned, it was likely that standards of care would fall yet again, as they did between 1914 and 1918, especially as provision this time would have to be made for large numbers of civilian casualties. George Gibson pledged the union's support for the war effort, but emphasised that 'We shall expect a square deal from our employers. We will neither exploit during the crisis, nor be exploited.'

To show it meant business, the MHIWU called an emergency meeting of the JCC in December 1939 to discuss the union's case for a war bonus to compensate for the rising cost of living. In January 1940, the JCC met again and nurses were given a 3 shillings a week increase on basic rates. In Scotland, things also appeared to be moving fast. Agreement was reached in December 1939 to re-establish the Scottish JCC separate from the bargaining machinery for other local authority workers. The MHIWU accepted (as it did not for England and Wales) the principle of proportional representation with other unions; in the mean time it was given all the workers' seats on the JCC 'until a claim for representation is made by any other association of employees'. By February the JCC had also recommended a 3 shillings cost-of-living increase, and had referred the question of standardisation of wages to a special sub-committee. However, the employers' side of the JCC insisted that the increase must be ratified by the Scottish NJIC and that the JCC should become a sub-committee of that body. By January 1941 the Scottish JCC had collapsed as a result of the MHIWU's refusal to collaborate with the NJIC, insisting as always on the 'special' character of the mental hospitals service and, more particularly, the union's sole right to represent mental nurses.

The union was also having its problems in England and Wales. The employers could not see their way to include domestic staff and officers and sub-officers within the scope of the JCC until after the war. Furthermore the compromise 54-hour agreement of the 1930s was coming to an end, but the employers were not prepared to reduce hours of work. Added to this, workers were being asked to put up with deteriorating standards of care and massive amounts of overtime. When war broke out many of the beds had been turned over to the military authorities as part of the government's Emergency Medical Service, leading to even worse overcrowding.

Shortages spread from female nurses to other grades of staff. Within the first year of the war 2,000 male nurses had left to join the forces and 600 women nurses for war work. Some of these were replaced, but in most instances by less experienced personnel. By the following year many hospitals were up to one-third under strength. The female sides suffered most, as the choice of alternative work for women had widened due to the war. Standards of care inevitably fell, and wartime regulations, like those governing blackout, placed restrictions on the institutions. At the very least the war led, as Kathleen Jones has suggested, to 'the return of the locked door, and inactivity, of isolation' [1] At the worst it was responsible for higher rates of sickness, particularly tuberculosis and dysentery, among patients, and to an extent among staff. As in the previous war death rates rose, but by no means to the same degree.[2]

Nurses were not the only grades to be affected by

shortages. The popularity of domestic work was already low as a result of the abysmally poor wages and bad conditions, and fell even further during the war. Yet as we saw, the MHA was still resisting union pressure for a national wages scale for domestic and other 'ancillary' workers. The shortages of domestic staffs, like management's neglect of their welfare, had deep roots. The shortfall could partly be met by the traditional and well tried method, of getting patients to do the work. The growing shortage of doctors, on the other hand, was a direct result of the war and could hardly be remedied in the same way. Many doctors went into the army and, as a result, staffing ratios deteriorated. From 1940 the Aliens War Service Department allowed doctors and nurses of Austrian, German and Italian origin to be employed in mental hospitals.

Things were getting so bad that early in 1941 the Mental Hospitals Association and the union issued a joint appeal to staff not to take sick leave if they could avoid it. Finally the Ministry of Health acted, and in August 1941 issued the Mental Nurses (Employment and Offences) Order, which became known as the 'Standstill'. It prohibited nurses with more than twelve months' service, working at institutions which observed the JCC pay-scales, from leaving without the permission of their Visiting Committee, on pain of a maximum fine of £10 or one month's imprisonment. Prosecutions were made under the Order, though only nominal fines were imposed.

The Standstill Order only applied at institutions which paid the union-negotiated rates. The coalition government was anxious to secure the co-operation of organised labour in the war effort, and any restrictions on workers' normal right to leave should not seem to give the employer an unfair advantage. This was why, a month before the Standstill Order, the JCC agreed in July 1941 to a new national scale of wages which abolished long-standing distinctions between 'urban' and 'rural' rates of pay that had been maintained since 1920, and granted a rise in basic rates to cover the cost of living. The minimum starting pay for men was now £2 10s a week, and for women £2, plus war bonuses. The vast majority of authorities adopted the new scales, including many of those not members of the employers' association, the MHA. Intervention from the Ministry of Labour in the light of the Standstill Order finally led, by December 1941, to the revival of the Scottish JCC. The employers now negotiated a war bonus of 11 shillings for men and 19 shillings for women, and a 48-hour week.

State intervention during wartime was therefore at long last prodding the employers into action. The state had effectively taken over the running of the hospitals, and become their paymaster. The General Secretary of the Transport and General Workers' Union (TGWU), Ernest Bevin, had also become Minister of Labour in the coalition government, which led to pressure for greater union recognition. Thus, in 1941 just two years after the Interim Report of the Athlone Committee, the government had also taken action to set up the Nurses' Salaries Committee under Lord Rushcliffe (and its counterpart in Scotland, the Taylor Committee) in order to settle national rates of pay and conditions of service for hospital nurses. Rushcliffe was divided into two sides with appointed representatives of nurses' organisations on the one side (with a majority granted to professional organisations by the Labour Minister) and representatives of employing bodies on the other. The participation of George Gibson in the Committee was in his capacity as one of five TUC representatives.

The MHIWU itself viewed the Rushcliffe Committee with profound suspicion, worried that its monopoly over representation for mental nurses might finally come to an end. Combining forces with the MHA, it pressed the Minister of Health not to extend the Rushcliffe Committee to cover mental nurses.

The Ministry agreed in May 1942, a decision which was strongly attacked by Lord Latham, a Labour peer who had long been associated with the LCC which, it will be remembered, had not participated in the MHA or observed JCC agreements. In a speech to the House of Lords he argued that it would be inconsistent to exclude mental nurses from the terms of reference of the Rushcliffe Committee as they formed one-third of the total of hospital nurses. Arthur Moyle, of NUPE, and also a TUC member of the Rushcliffe Committee, agreed with him. NUPE had a long standing objection to a separate Whitley Council for mental hospitals, having been excluded from the JCC when it was first set up in 1920. It saw Rushcliffe as a means by which NUPE might become a recognised union for mental nurses. Since the late 1930s it had succeeded in establishing some branches in mental hospitals, particularly in the London area.

Equally understandably, the MHIWU was implacably opposed and was concerned as much as anything to protect the relatively favourable pay and conditions of its members in comparison with general nurses, by remaining a separate bargaining unit.[3] Lord Latham had referred in his speech to the increased status and standing that would come as a result of mental nursing's closer association with the wider nursing community. Mental nurses were cynical about such vague promises. After all, more than 20 years of State Registration had not so far reaped many material benefits for general nurses. Nor had the contact with general nursing, through the GNC, been an entirely happy affair.

The Report of the Rushcliffe Committee for general nurses was considerably delayed and did not appear until February 1943, more than a year after the Committee had been set up. The key stumbling block was the old one: employer opposition to the expense of any worthwhile proposals. This was only overcome when the Treasury agreed to pay 50 per cent of the cost. Even then, the proposals were not to be made binding on employing authorities. A 96-hour fortnight was not to be introduced then or in the foreseeable future. Student nurses were to receive a paltry minimum salary of £40 a year plus emoluments, no more than they had previously been offered. Qualified staff nurses and sisters were, however, to receive substantial increases on the existing rates paid by most hospital authorities.

Meanwhile, the MHIWU was negotiating with the MHA over new pay scales. The MHA was keen to obtain the 50 per cent Treasury grant, but the Ministry was insisting on some formal link with Rushcliffe Committee. In June 1943 the MHIWU finally relented, and a sub-committee of Rushcliffe was established for mental nurses, consisting of six representatives from both the MHA and the MHIWU. The sub-committee's report was not presented to Parliament until August 1944. It recommended higher percentage rises for basic grades than Rushcliffe had given to other types of nurses, to maintain the relatively advantageous economic position of mental nurses. It also recommended that the two systems of training between the GNC and the RMPA should not continue and that for the purposes of remuneration, of the RMPA certificate and registration by the GNC should be regarded as equivalents. The sub-committee and the Rushcliffe Committee itself were eventually reconstituted as the Nurses and Midwives Whitley Council under the National Health Service in 1948.

Progress was eventually made towards nationally agreed rates of pay for domestic staffs. Fairly early in the war the MHA had put aside its long standing objections to the idea, and got down to discussing the practicalities with the MHIWU, but the negotiations proved slow. Not only were there enormous variations in pay and conditions between different hospitals, there was not even an agreed nomenclature, let alone anything resembling a common system of grades. In September 1942, however, after lengthy negotiations, a breakthrough was achieved and the first ever national wages scales for domestics staff in the health service came into existence. Minimum wages for male staff were set at £2 10s and £2 a week for women. In addition, a new system of grades was introduced. For male domestic staff the following grades were created: head cooks or chefs, deputy head cook or chefs, messmen and senior messmen, kitchenmen and youths (16-20 years); for female domestic staff: head cooks, senior assistant head cooks, sewing room maids, canteen charge hands and assistants, senior maids and grade I, II, and III maids.

In 1943 faltering steps towards a national rate of pay for 'domestic' grades in the health service as a whole were made with the appointment of the Hetherington Committee, at a time of acute shortage of both domestics and nurses. Wards were being closed up and down the country due to lack of staff to run them. The Ministry of Labour had spent a great deal of money advertising for women to come forward without a great deal of success. To cope with the shortages Belgian women refugees were drafted in and even prison labour was used. The rates that the Hetherington Committee recommended in November 1943 were far from adequate, but Ernest Bevin, as Minister of Labour, used them to justify direction of labour to those institutions which paid recognised rates. Shortages continued, and in 1945, the Minister of Health in the new Labour government, Aneurin Bevan, transformed the Hetherington Committee into a properly constituted National Joint Committee for Hospital and Institutional Domestic Staffs. As with Rushcliffe, a sub-committee comprising the MHIWU and the MHA was set up. The NJC eventually became the Ancillary Staffs Council in the NHS.

The State of the Union

A transitional stage had therefore been reached on the eve of the MHIWU's amalgamation with the Hospitals and Welfare Services Union to form COHSE. The MHIWU had not entirely surrendered the JCC. Through its participation in Rushcliffe and in the NJC for Hospital and Institutional Domestic Staffs, it had one foot in the future, but by insisting on its own sub-committees, the other was planted in the past. And with good reason: the union had negotiated wages and conditions for both nurses and domestic staffs which were considerably better than existed for any other section of health workers. There could be no more fitting tribute to the union's achievements since 1910, nor of the necessity for strong trade union organisation in the National Health Service that was in the process of being created.

All this new activity had severely tested the union's organisation, which was more adapted to the conditions of the 1930s than those of the 1940s. The bulk of organisation was carried by the branches, yet the emphasis was now shifting to the centre, as the government increasingly intervened in the regulation of health workers' pay and conditions of employment. The full-time organising staff in consequence became overstretched. In 1943, Alex White, the Scottish Organiser, resigned because he 'could not carry on any longer'. He was eventually replaced by Michael MacBride, from Larbert, who was given the status of a National Organiser. In Manchester much of the work, as in the First World War, fell on the shoulders of Herbert Shaw. He took over as Acting General Secretary when George Gibson was away for several months in 1940 on government business, including a secret mission to Norway. In 1941 Gibson became Chairman of the TUC, and was preoccupied with his work on the Rushcliffe Committee. In 1943, he was appointed Vice-Chairman of the National Savings Committee. In 1944, the union's problems were magnified when Gibson and his wife were hospitalised as the result of a serious road accident. To cope with these difficulties, Claud Bartlett sought temporary leave of absence from his employment, after Herbert Shaw had complained to the NEC that 'it had been a difficult time and work had to be done at night and during the weekend'. Bartlett subsequently deputised for Gibson on the Rushcliffe Committee.

The union survived these difficulties. After all, during the past 35 years of its existence it had overcome many problems. It had withstood attempts to victimise union activists, blazed a trail in the years after the First World War, survived the disappointments of the 1920s, clung tenaciously to its achievements in the 1930s, and inched its way forward during the Second World War. With nearly 25,000 members, it was stronger than ever before. Now in the dying days of the war it was faced with a new challenge: what role would it play in the new National Health Service? The White Paper on the NHS in 1944 had urged the integration of the mental health services with the rest of the health service. The next logical step was the creation of health service unionism, and the abandonment of the union's long held view that mental health workers were 'special' and must be catered for separately.

These were the considerations such that finally led to the amalgamation of the MHIWU with the Hospitals and

Welfare Services Union in 1946, to form the Confederation of Health Service Employees (COHSE). The amalgamation negotiations themselves were yet another pressure on the overstretched MHIWU organisation. How the merger between the two organisations finally went through, with not a few misgivings by the membership, is a complex story. It will be told in full when we have looked in more detail in Part Two at the chequered history of the Hospitals and Welfare Services Union.

Notes

[1] Jones, *Mental Health Services*, Ch. 10.
[2] A.S. MacNally (ed.), *The Civilian Health and Medical Services* (1953), Vol. 1.
[3] G. Gibson, *Lord Latham and the Mental Nurses* (1942), COHSE Archive, loc. cit.

Part Two

From Poor Law to Health Service Unionism

Chapter 10
Working for the Poor Law

The history of the Hospitals and Welfare Services Union (HWSU) has many parallels with that of the MHIWU. It, too, was formed as a result of growing dissatisfaction with a slumbering professional association and its espousal of industrial unionism also led it to compete with other trade unions. Yet this is where the comparisons end for the HWSU never established itself with the same degree of success as the MHIWU. It did not win the loyalty of a majority of the staff, nor did it achieve substantial recognition from the authorities.

Much of Part Two will try to explain the reasons for these difficulties, and their effect on the union's organisation. Not least among them was that the 'industry' which it sought to cover had been transformed several times by the time of the amalgamation with the MHIWU, forcing the union itself to go through several changes of identity. The HWSU had in fact started off life in 1918, as the Poor Law Workers' Trade Union (PLWTU), an organisation covering workers for the Poor Law services of England and Wales, of which health services formed only one part. The separation of the health services only really occurred with the 'break up' of the Poor Law at the end of the 1920s. It was merged with local government and its functions spread among various committees of local authorities. The PLWTU, whose name had already been changed to the Poor Law Officers' Union (PLOU), was now an industrial union for an industry which no longer existed. It sought unsuccessfully in the 1930s to become a union for the generality of local government workers, as the National Union of County Officers. It survived – but only just – by increasingly becoming a specialised health service union, recruiting the growing army of hospital and health staffs who had no established organisation. Thus the story of the emergence of health service unionism from Poor Law unionism closely parallels development of the health services out of the Poor Law.

By the time the PLWTU was set up in 1918, the nineteenth-century Poor Law was in deep crisis. Its nineteenth-century architects had originally designed it as a means of disciplining workers into accepting low wages by offering them incarceration in the workhouse as the only, unattractive alternative. However, the workhouse system could not deal with the effects of large numbers of workers thrown into poverty by booms and slumps of the capitalist market. Nor had it originally been framed to deal with the fact that ill health (rather than, as it was assumed, an unwillingness to work) was a major cause of people applying for relief. Perhaps the biggest strain of all came from the extension of the franchise, as the subjects of Poor Law administration themselves now had political power and began to expect more from society than the inadequate and stigmatised system of relief it offered.

The end of the Poor Law was signalled in Sidney and Beatrice Webb's Minority Report of the Royal Commission on the Poor Laws in 1909. Their main charge was that the system was inefficient as well as inhumane, and they called for its various functions to be distributed to agencies more competent to deal with them. Though their advice was not originally heeded, the historical irony was that by 1929 a Tory Minister of Health, Neville Chamberlain, had acted on the radical vision of the Webbs, abolishing the Poor Law very much on the lines they had advocated.[1] Thus whatever the justifications for trade unionism within the Poor Law – and there were many – to launch it at a time when the very future of the 'industry' was uncertain, did not augur well for its success.

The Poor Law and its Workers

Poor Law workers had long had sufficient material reasons for organising collectively on their own behalf.

The Poor Law, as M.A. Crowther has suggested, justly had the reputation among its staff of being a 'second class' service. The reason for this, a Poor Law official quoted by her claimed in 1920, was that the Guardians in charge of the service, 'were always torn between the interests of paupers and of rate payers, and the officers were generally forgotten.[2]

There was a general expansion in the numbers of staff at the end of the nineteenth-century, particularly among medical and nursing staff, as pressure mounted to improve the quality of service, but this did not generally lead to substantial improvements in the material position of staff themselves. Since most of the finance came from the local rates, central government would not act to standardise pay and conditions, which therefore varied enormously according to the attitudes of individual Boards of Guardians.

The basic division in the system, upon which all others were built, was between what was called 'indoor' and 'outdoor' relief, i.e. within or outside the workhouse. In all there were about 50,000 workers in the Poor Law service in 1918.[3] At the pinnacle of the hierarchy was the Clerk, the chief administrator and advisor to the Board of Guardians. He was responsible for such matters as appointing staff (including doctors) and organising contracts with local tradesmen. Corruption was by no means unknown.

The pivots of the whole system were the relieving officers, nicknamed 'destitution officers'. In 1909, according to the Webbs' Minority Report, there were just under 2,000 of them with wages said to vary between 30 shillings and £3 a week, yet they could make more by taking on other functions, such as collector of the poor rate. There appears to have been few formalities in the system of entry, and favouritism seems to have played an important part in gaining a position. It was a distinctly lower middle-class position which, unlike some other local government white collar occupations (for example sanitary inspectors), did not require professional qualifications. In an age of growing specialisation the relieving officer remained a generalist, often responsible for a bewildering variety of duties, as the Webbs were quick to point out.

By all accounts, the relieving officers, as first point of contact in their system, often seemed to have wielded considerable power. They visited peoples' homes, decided whether they should see the Poor Law medical officer, made decisions on whether cases should be treated at home or in the workhouse, and often made the key initial decisions in the determination of insanity. They were, therefore, extremely powerful figures in local communities, a means of access to resources people might desperately need. Yet theirs was a power that must often have been constrained by living in close contact and having to deal directly with those in greatest dependance on them.

Among 'indoor' staff, complex relationships existed. The backbone of the service were the masters and matrons of the workhouses, responsible to an overseer. Rates of pay varied according to the size of the workhouses, but they generally earned much less than relieving officers. They were, typically, husbands and wives, 'without encumbrances', that is childless couples. Norman Longmate has suggested that:

> Inevitably, superivising a workhouse tended to attract the rootless couple with no home of their own – the man often a badly educated bully, the wife a nagging shrew with pretentions to gentility, delighted to command an unlimited supply of free servants.[3]

This image is, of course, close to the fictional stereotype. It is difficult to say how far it fitted in reality, although certainly many masters and matrons seemed to have pursued their deterrent role with enthusiasm. The worst were certainly appalling, yet it was the conditions under which they worked, and not just the personal traits of those employed, which encouraged excesses. The mountains of paperwork, the inadequate salaries and lack (until the 1890s) of pension rights, the long hours in depressing surroundings and the expectation that the regime would serve to deter applicants either exerted pressure on officers to behave in repressive ways, or encouraged them to abuse their position. And, of course, the whole official philosophy of the Poor Law encouraged workhouse officials to treat those who came within its net with severity bordering on cruelty. It is therefore not surprising that this border line was often crossed. As Crowther suggests:

> In the conditions under which they worked the officers had little incentive to be kind to workhouse inmates. Their own lives offered little except the chance of power over these relatively helpless subjects. The institution took its toll of staff as well as inmates.[4]

Below the master and matron came an assortment of staffs: porters, industrial trainers and drillmasters, lunatic attendants, labour masters and mistresses, needlemistresses, lavatory maids, cooks and nurses. Sorting out the 'proper' relations between masters and matrons on the one hand, and nurses and doctors on the other, had become a source of difficulty by the beginning of the twentieth century.

Disputes over spheres of responsibility were common. Where, as in many workhouses, the doctor was only part-time, the master wielded greater power. The authorities appear to have initially regarded doctors as more or less on a par with other 'tradesmen', and this attitude was slow to change. Thus for much of the nineteenth century their services were secured by means of competitive tender, encouraging one doctor to undercut another. Even when this practice ended doctors were often required to pay for medicines out of their salaries.

It was not uncommon for the workhouse master to intervene to curtail what he regarded as doctors' extravagant expenditure, for example on patients' diets.[5] The chief aim was of course cheapness rather than good quality care. Medical assistance to the poor in their homes was also only provided when the authorities (and sometimes the doctors) were convinced they could not afford to pay for it.

The condition of the sick poor in the workhouse was the subject of considerable public criticism from the 1860s. Nursing reformers, Poor Law doctors and concerned lay people combined to demand improvements. Although humanitarian motives played a significant part, the reformers often justified their case with economic arguments that it would in the long run save ratepayers expense. The fact that the reformed voluntary hospitals were not providing a better standard of medical and nursing care reinforced these 'efficiency' arguments. They also helped doctors to press for higher rewards, greater status and professional autonomy within the Poor Law system. Nevertheless, Poor Law doctors remained the poor relations of the medical profession as a whole, treating an 'inferior' class of patients with few resources.

A similar story could be told concerning the growth and gradual improvement in standards of workhouse nursing. The matron was not originally a trained nurse at all, but, as we have seen, the master's wife, and most of the nursing care was given by other inmates. Some of these 'pauper nurses' were, it was said, so frail as to require care themselves.[6] Yet the growing employment of paid nurses appears also to have been influenced similarly by considerations of efficiency. Providing higher standards of skilled nursing care to return people to the community was an investment which was thought might in the long run save the ratepayers extra expense.

As a result, not only were increasing numbers of paid nurses employed, but training schools for nurses were set up on similar lines to those established by Florence Nightingale and others in the voluntary hospitals. The pace of change accelerated after 1897 when the Local Government Board finally issued an order formally to prohibit the employment of pauper nurses. Although this did not immediately end the practice, the first years of the twentieth century saw a considerable expansion in the number of 'probationer', i.e. student nurses, a development which was linked also to workhouse infirmaries taking on an increasing amount of acute work. In 1913 the Local Government Board laid down that workhouses with under 100 beds should appoint a trained head nurse, and those with more than 100 a superintendent nurse with responsibility for the supervision and discipline of nursing staff. Trained nurses were to be employed in all Poor Law institutions. The independence of nursing within the Poor Law was now finally in sight.

At the end of the war, the *Poor Law Officers Journal* published rates of pay scales, based on a survey of 514 hospitals, including 81 Poor Law infirmaries. These showed considerable variation for top posts but greater uniformity towards the base. For example a matron in a London General hospital could expect to earn £310 a year, while in a provincial Poor Law infirmary the average was only £156. A ward sister would earn £54 and £43 a year respectively. Salaries for first year probationers were universally low, between £13 to £15 a year.[7] The hours of Poor Law nurses were long, those working days averaged more than 70 hours a week and those on nights 84 hours a week. Like their medical colleagues, they were frequently looked down upon by their counterparts in the voluntary hospitals, as inferior people looking after an inferior class of patient more likely to be suffering from less interesting, chronic disorders. Workhouse nursing was therefore more likely to be carried out by women from a working-class background than in the voluntary hospitals, since fewer 'ladies' were prepared to come forward to train in the lower status Poor Law hospitals.

In short, while there had undoubtedly been improvements in the general conditions of nursing and medicine within the Poor Law, the staff in these institutions also knew how far these still fell short of what was considered the 'best'. As Crowther suggests:

> The ablest members of these professions (nursing and medicine) inevitably found the Poor Law service repellant. Fear of lay domination, poor pay and overwork played a part, but the staff also suffered because they felt isolated from the mainstream of their profession.[8]

A Divided Workforce?

From this brief survey of staff working conditions in the Poor Law, it can be seen that there were material reasons enough to form a union to fight for improvements. So why did trade unionism not establish itself until some eighty years after the service's inception? The main reason was that the social conditions of the work did not foster the sense of a common community of interest among workers themselves. When trade unionism appeared, it was largely favourable conditions in the wider environment *outside* the services that finally made the difference to tip the balance of advantage marginally in its favour.

A major obstacle to the formation of a collective awareness among staff had been the long standing practice of filling Poor Law positions by patronage. Guardians often employed people who might otherwise have become paupers themselves, such as widows, forcing them to work at sweated rates.

As Crowther suggests, this placed such workers in a vulnerable position from which they could hardly organise collectively to improve their lot. Any improvements within the patronage relationship were likely to be due to the 'generosity' of the local employer, which should be received with due gratitude. Consequently wages and conditions varied enormously from one area to the next. The 'better off' Poor Law workers were unlikely to risk the wrath of their employers, and the 'worse off' were too demoralised to fight on their own behalf. This fostered a sense of dependency upon the local employer, which worked against the formation of a national sense of unity among Poor Law workers.

The other major reason for the lack of unity among staff was due to the diversity of Poor Law functions and the consequent division of the labour force into many grades. By the twentieth century the system of patronage, which had previously hindered trade unionism, was in decline. The fragmentation of the workforce was continuing apace, however, and became more marked as health care became a separate service within the Poor Law, and the established divisions of medical and nursing hierarchies were imported from the voluntary hospitals. So while the decline of patronage and the emergence of more regular conditions of employment began to foster a sense of unity, other developments were working in the opposite direction, serving to fragment the loyalty of the workforce. As time went on, the service thus became even more prone to the petty jealousies which had characterised it from the outset. Porters resented and battled with

masters, who fought in turn with the doctors; the matron
was often in permanent conflict with the trained nurses,
who in turn were in conflict with the assistant nurses and
ward maids. Each group tended to view the others' powers
and privileges with extreme jealousy. Though these often
took the form of 'personality' clashes, such conflicts were in
fact built into the system.

Finally, the growth of workhouse infirmaries was creating a group of workers – doctors and trained nurses – who
tended to identify not with the Poor Law at all, but with
their wider professional groups. The fact that elite members of these outside professional groups tended to regard
Poor Law nurses and doctors as inferior or even doubtful
members of the professional community, did not, on the
whole, dissolve these wider loyalties. In fact, they probably
encouraged Poor Law nurses and doctors to mark out more
sharply the distinctions between themselves and the 'generality' of Poor Law employees.

Given all the problems that have been identified in this
chapter, it seems all the more remarkable that Poor Law
unionism emerged at all. That it should take the form of
industrial unionism, seeking to unite all workers, regardless
of local circumstances, hierarchical position, or specialised
function, was quite extraordinary. Although the ultimate
goal may not have been achieved, the ideal survived, due to
the tenacity of the minority of staff who clung to it. Let us
now turn to discover how such ambitions came about.

Notes

[1] For a more detailed account of the downfall of the Poor Law see D.
Fraser, *The Evolution of the British Welfare State* (2nd edition, 1984).
[2] M.A. Crowther, *The Workhouse System* (1981), Ch.6, on which this
section of the chapter leans heavily.
[3] N. Longmate, *The Workhouse* (1974), p.102
[4] Crowther, op.cit., p.133.
[5] B. Abel-Smith, *The Hospitals 1800-1948* (1964), Ch.13.
[6] R. White, *Social Change and the Development of the Nursing Profession*
(1978), Ch.6.
[7] B. Abel-Smith, *A History of the Nursing Profession* (1960), Appendices.
[8] Crowther, op. cit., p.140.

Chapter 11
Rebels with a Cause

The Poor Law Workers' Trade Union, like its counterpart in the asylums, was formed in response to widespread worker dissatisfaction with a sedate, status-conscious, professional organisation, dominated by high-ranking officials in the service. Faced with pressing material problems, lower-ranking workers and officials lost confidence in the organisation's ability to further their collective interests, and struck out on their own.

The organisation in question was the National Poor Law Officers' Association (NPLOA), or 'the National', as it was not always affectionately called. Found in 1885, it was eventually absorbed into the National Association of Local Government Officers (NALGO) in 1930. The cautious approach of the National was strongly influenced by the fact that its decision-making structure was dominated by higher officials in the Poor Law service, particularly Clerks to Boards of Guardians. Its only significant achievement in the first 45 years of its existence appears to have been the introduction of compulsory superannuation for Poor Law officers. Then, at the National's own insistence, the scheme was made a contributory one, due to its anxiety to prevent pensions from being a charge on the rates. This led to the Poor Law Officers' Superannuation Act of 1896, later to become the model for the much despised Asylum Officers Superannuation Act of 1909 – of which we have already heard. The similarities between the National and the Asylum Workers' Association are almost uncanny.

After the relatively successful accomplishment of

compulsory superannuation, the National tended to rest
on its laurels. After 1890 provision of friendly society
benefits became the main rationale for the organisation's
existence. By 1912 membership had grown to around
11,000 – still a minority of the eligible workforce, but
viable enough for the kind of organisation with the
National's aspirations.

The First World War sabotaged this apparently eternal
equilibrium between the National and its constituents,
particularly its effect upon the cost-of-living-index, which
rose dramatically and unremittingly from 1914 onwards,
at the rate of about 27 per cent each year.[1] Civil servants at
national level were compensated for this by means of war
bonuses, a supplement to their salary that rose in step with
movements in the cost-of-living index. Since they had a
common employer, the state, this applied across the board.
Poor Law workers were also employed by the state, but
they faced a diversity of employers, some of whom
granted war bonuses and others did not. Such anomalies
led to growing discontent, especially when combined with
the very real economic difficulties faced by workers who
did not receive any, or only inadequate compensation for
the rising cost of living.

The time was now ripe for this discontent to become
manifest in collective trade union action. The numbers of
union members were in general expanding phenomenally
– from 2.5 million in 1910 to 8.3 million by 1920 –
bringing into the ranks of the labour movement groups
who had formerly been outside its ranks. At the end of the
nineteenth century the trade union movement had spread
out from its relatively narrow craft basis to encompass the
growing army of semi-skilled manual workers. The new
wave of unionism prior to 1920 brought in yet more of
such workers – including many in the public sector – but
also brought in many 'white collar' workers, in both the
private and public sectors who had formerly stood aloof
from trade unions.[2]

Large numbers of women also joined unions for the first
time, partly because massive numbers of them became
asborbed into traditionally male jobs during the First
World War, but also because many were in occupations

(like teaching and clerical work) which were becoming unionised. Between 1914 and 1918 the total number of women in unions increased from 0.4 million to 1.2 million.[3] The growth of a mass labour force in both manual and white collar occupations created increasing obstacles to the personal and individual supervision upon which patronage was based. Both workers and employers were needing to organise themselves collectively to deal with modern conditions of employment.

Along with the swelling numbers and greater representativeness went increasing influence. The political confidence of labour was rising: in 1913 unions won protected status under the law. But it was the war that really enhanced the influence of the trade union movement. The coalition government was anxious to prevent the spread of labour unrest, particularly in the munitions industries. This led initially to the setting up of arbitration machinery. General unions managed to win awards from this machinery in order to compensate their members working in local government.[4] The biggest breakthrough in the public sector came in 1917 when the government set up an independent tribunal for all civil service grades earning less than £500 a year. The state was seeking to act as a 'model' employer by setting an example which it hoped would be followed generally.[5] After the Whitley Report of 1917 it took this one step further and encouraged employers to establish national bargaining machinery over pay and conditions. This advice was mainly intended to apply to more strongly organised groups in private industry, but it had obvious implications for the public sector.

Not surprisingly, given these developments, pressure mounted from within the NPLOA, urging it to transform itself into a trade union and adopt a more militant, active approach. The NPLOA's national leadership was forced to respond, but its reaction was not encouraging. In April 1918 its Executive stubbornly insisted that trade unionism was not necessary and criticised those who suggested it was. It did not wish to alienate its members who were senior clerks. If the National became a union, they might experience divided loyalties in a strike. However, it did

urge the Local Government Board (LGB) to order all local
Boards of Guardians to grant the civil service scale of war
bonuses. Sir Auckland Geddes, the President of the LGB,
would only circulate local authorities late in 1918 drawing
attention to the 'strong feelings' among officers in many
districts and including a copy of the bonuses for central
government employees, following recent arbitration
awards, but would not interfere with local authorities by
ordering them to act.

None of this was sufficient to quieten the growing
clamour for trade unionism. On 1 November 1918 Edwin
Ridley, an Assistant Clerk from Stockport, and President
of the Manchester and District NPLOA, led a delegation
of branches in favour of transforming the National into a
trade union. They arrived fresh from a conference in
Birmingham, held on 5 October 1918, which had
discussed plans to set up a breakaway organisation should
the National refuse to become a trade union. The
Manchester delegates, who had called the conference in
the first place, had put forward a well thought out, if
rather ambitious scheme for forming a union. A 6d a
week subscription would be levied to finance a General
Secretary in London and six provincial Assistant
Secretaries. Low paid probationer nurses could become
honorary members if they could not afford the
subscriptions. The union would become part of the TUC
but would not affiliate to the Labour Party. A strong
emphasis was placed upon friendly society benefits,
including an ambitious pension scheme.[6]

The NPLOA Council rejected the views of the
Birmingham delegates, and reaffirmed its decision not to
become a union. It sought to stall the growing movement
by declaring that it would reconsider the matter yet again
on 7 December. The dissident branches held off from
actually declaring the formation of a trade union to the
world. In a last ditch attempt to pressurise the National
into becoming a trade union, they called a final meeting on
the day before the NPLOA Council was due to meet.
Meanwhile they continued planning for the likely
eventuality of being forced to form a breakaway
organisation.

The Birth of the PLWTU

Despite these uncertain beginnings, there was, at the London meeting on 6 December, a high level of expectancy that the new infant would shortly see the light of day. The meeting was held in the board room of the Paddington Guardians' Offices, to consider the proposal, talked about throughout the service since October, to form a trade union for the Poor Law service for England and Wales. The *Poor Law Officers' Journal* described the meeting as 'a large, representative and enthusiastic gathering' of Poor Law officers, presided over by Mr A.D. Milne, an Assistant Relieving Officer for Paddington.

The most controversial issue facing the meeting was that of strike action. To the cheers of those present, Mr Ridley said that under the Manchester scheme 'a sufficiency of officers would carry on the statutory duties'.[7] Some wondered whether now was the time to form a union for the Poor Law service when talk of reorganisation was in the air, but such doubts were swept aside in an impressive speech by Vincent Evans, a 29-year-old Deputy Clerk from Paddington, who argued that only trade unionism would solve the problems faced by workers: indoor workers particularly were working under conditions of 'sweated labour'. The time for 'dilly dallying' was now past and workers should now 'unite for the common cause'. With only one vote against, a provisional committee was elected from those present and arrangements made for it to meet the next day if the NPLOA should decide against becoming a union.

The Executive Committee of the NPLOA met the same evening at the Connaught Rooms in Great Queen Street, and yet again reaffirmed the decision not to become a trade union. Major John Simonds, the National's Secretary, told the Council Meeting held the next day, 7 December, that the general feeling within the organisation was against it. He also advised against 'drastic action' pending the possible reorganisation of the Poor Law. At the end of the debate the vote was decisive: 74 to 24 against becoming a union.

So the nativity of the union took place when the

provisional commitee met in the appropriately humble surroundings of a basement in Holborn on 7 December 1918 to draw up an initial scheme for a union. A provisional Grand Council was established consisting of 24 members, 12 each from the indoor and outdoor staffs. It was emphasised that 'ladies may be on this Council'. A union was finally being launched, and its birth was announced to the world by means of an advertisement in the *Poor Law Officers' Journal* on 13 December 1918. Its first President, Wilfred Hardman, was an office storekeeper from Manchester, and its first temporary General Secretary, Archibald ('Archie') Milne, an Assistant General Relieving Officer and Collector of the Poor Rates in Willesden.

The rules of the Poor Law Workers' Trade Union were approved and confirmed at a special meeting in Holborn Hall on 15 February 1919, and the union was registered shortly afterwards. The PLWTU was open to Poor Law workers of all ranks, unlike the NPLOA, which was a white collar union. All men and women below the position of clerk could join the union and participate fully in its affairs. Clerks, and members of Boards of Guardians, could become honorary members, which entitled them to attend meetings but not to vote. (Later, in the 1930s, an ex-honorary member, Mrs Beatrice Drapper, an erstwhile member of a Board of Guardians and union sympathiser, became the union's first woman official.) The union's major objects were, as one might expect, modest ones: to 'regulate' relations between Boards of Guardians and their officers and servants, to settle disputes by 'negotiation, arbitration or other lawful means', to protect members against victimisation, and to obtain 'reasonable' pay and conditions. The union did not at that stage seek to affiliate to the TUC, but the rules allowed for it to join any other federation or association of workers. No wider political objectives were stated, and the union, prior to forming its amalgamation with the MHIWU, never affiliated to the Labour Party. Supreme government of the union was vested in the Central Executive Committee (CEC), elected by a secret ballot of the whole membership. Branches of the union were grouped into counties or provinces with their own executive committees, composed of representatives from the branches.

There was an extremely strong emphasis upon friendly society benefits. The union calculated that, given the low levels of trade union consciousness among its potential membership, it was necessary to lure people in with material incentives. Membership of the union's Provident Fund was compulsory, and a wide range of benefits w re offered, including sick pay, funeral benefit and dowry benefit for women leaving to get married. Most ambitious of all was the union's pension scheme, and generous arrangements were also made to superannuate the permanent staff of the union. With the benefit of hindsight, the union ought perhaps to have established itself first before committing itself to such a high degree of friendly society expenditure for years to come.

The diversity of the membership was – unlike the NPLOA – reflected on the Central Executive Committee. The President of the union was now Mr J. Heaton, described as a 'man of strong and vigorous personality, a splendid speaker and organiser'. He was a poor rates assessor from Manchester. He presided over the first Provisional Council of PLWTU, which met on 1 February 1919, and assembled together an assortment of indoor and outdoor staffs ranging from porters, labour masters and one chaplain, to a hairdresser and dispenser. Almost one-third were relieving officers.

The vast majority came from the London area, some from Manchester, as well as solitary representatives from Birmingham, Bristol and Merthyr Tydfil. The first meeting simply dealt with the rules of the union.

When proper elections were held shortly afterwards this wide spread of membership was maintained, but distributed among the regions. Sadly, however, no women were elected on to the CEC, despite forming a substantial proportion of the membership. Vincent Evans, formerly the London Organiser, was elected unopposed as General Secretary, a position he was to occupy for more than a quarter of a century. He had occupied a succession of junior clerical positions in the Poor Law service, and worked his way up by his twenties to become Deputy Clerk to the Paddington Board of Guardians. He was a deeply religious man, and 'well known in certain quarters as an accomplished organist and composer'. He had convened the meeting of 6 December 1918, which finally propelled the PLWTU into the world. He took over as General Secretary when Archibald Milne, a fellow Paddington branch activist, resigned 'after two months' nerve-racking effort'. Mr Heaton served only a short spell as President. He was succeeded by Dr William Wiggins, MRCS, LRCP, DPH, Medical Superintendent of Greenwich Infirmary since 1911, described in the union's newspaper, *Monthly Notes* as 'quiet in manner, somewhat reserved'.

These efforts seemed at first to be yielding dividends. By May 1919 the union had already enlisted 5,602 members, and during 1920 reached a peak membership of 14,000. It was able to take advantage of the favourable employment situation, and the surge among workers generally in favour of trade unionism. The PLWTU's main recruiting cry was its newly agreed national charter, which included demands for a 44-hour week with overtime pay for excess hours, war bonuses to be made compulsory and consolidated into permanent wages, a minimum wage for all grades, improvement of living-in conditions, extended holidays and trade union recognition.

The national charter developed out of the conviction that it was necessary to centralise efforts within the union. From time to time new demands were added, for example for equal treatment for women officers. Yet although the PLWTU possessed a national charter, it could not pursue it nationally because it did not enjoy national recognition from employers. Neither did it have sufficient membership strength to take on the employers at national level as the NAWU had threatened over its national charter. The nearest thing to national bargaining was the Conciliation Council established between the NPLOA and the employers' Association of Poor Law Unions. This met from April 1919 to February 1920. It made some concessions to workers in its short existence, recommending implementation of civil service war bonuses and a maximum working week of 56 hours. It collapsed when the employers refused to implement a further war bonus

(Award 101) of the Civil Service Arbitration Board, and the NPLOA was forced to withdraw.[8]

The PLWTU thus had little choice except to seek improvements through local negotiations. The chief obstacle, according to Vincent Evans in his Report for 1920, was the familiar one that the Ministry of Health (which had replaced the Local Government Board) 'will not interfere with local autonomy, especially when the local rates bear the upkeep of the expense of the service'.

The only alternative was to seek to mount pressure locally to 'educate' Boards of Guardians on their duties as 'employers of labour' as well as to the ratepayers. The PLWTU could point to improvements that had come about as the result of its intervention. By 1921 it had won awards of bonuses, sometimes without recourse to arbitration, in such places as Paddington, Edmonton, Exeter, Newton Abbot, Great Yarmouth and Stepney. The greatest success, however, was in London, with the Paddington scale of salaries serving as the model, won, according to Vincent Evans, 'owing to the fact that the branch is stable and united'.

The union's other major campaign was over the impending reform of the Poor Law. Whatever the problems, the union knew where it stood with Boards of Guardians. Any merger of the Poor Law into local government might threaten any advantages enjoyed by transferred officers, as well as the identity and recruiting base of the union itself. The PLWTU therefore had a vested interest in seeking to obstruct moves to disband the Poor Law. It also wanted to show it was quicker off the mark than the NPLOA. Aware of the general state of uncertainty among Poor Law workers, it moved to seek better co-ordination among the workers' organisations. From 1919 it actively sought to convene a Conference of Poor Law Officers' Organisations (CPLOO), initially to press for generous rates of compensation for officers displaced in any reorganisation. The PLWTU persuaded some of the small sectional associations, such as the Metropolitan Relieving Officers' Association, to affiliate with the CPLOO, but the NPLOA stayed aloof, weakening the position of Poor Law officers in their dealings with central government.

The Faltering Challenge

By the end of 1920 it was becoming apparent that the PLWTU was not going to emulate the success of the NAWU in driving the NPLOA out of existence. The PLWTU was an alternative to the National, but not its replacement. Furthermore, numbers of staff joined existing trade unions which, unlike the PLWTU, seemed to some to be more genuine unions, because they were affiliated to the TUC. The main hope for unity lay with a merger between the PLWTU and the NPLOA. There was strange love-hate relationship between the two organisations. Many PLWTU activists had been long-standing National members, and it seems likely that there was a good deal of dual membership between the two organisations.

The National took the challenge of the union very seriously, reforming its structure and approach to industrial relations. The worsening economic situation after 1920 adversely affected both organisations, but there is no doubt that the union was hit hardest. Membership fell to under 5,000 by mid-1923. At this stage the union was virtually insolvent, and was lucky to survive at all. Membership of the union began to pick up slowly, but never exceeded the peak figures of 1920 until the late 1930s. In the new, defensive conditions the balance of advantage shifted back to the NPLOA, as the *Poor Law Gazette* − as the union journal was now called − readily conceded in December 1923:

> The National has the advantage of the sympathy of the majority of the responsible officials. Its entrance in any union [i.e. area] is not barred. Adhesion to its cause is encouraged, in fact in some places insisted upon. Its claims are pressed with all the powers of assistance that chief responsible officers can give. Those who support it are not victimised, and every facility is offered its branch agents to effectively discharge the duties of the office.

This forced a recognition by the PLWTU of its relatively

FEDERATION *of the*

NATIONAL ASYLUM-WORKERS' UNION
———————— WITH THE ————————
POOR LAW WORKERS' TRADE UNION

Present Membership of the N.A.-W.U. - 18,000
Present Membership of the P.L.W.T.U. - 15,000

Combined Total - - - 33,000

Wherever there is an Asylum—there is also a Workhouse in the District.

E VERY Branch of the National Asylum-Workers' Union should endeavour to assist our Colleagues of the Poor Law Workers' Trade Union, by bringing its Aims, Objects, and Literature to the notice of the Staff of any Poor Law Institution in their vicinity ; by offering to assist Poor Law Officers to establish a local Branch of their Union, and by helping them in such other directions as may suggest themselves to our local Branches.

Full particulars of the Poor Law Workers' Trade Union and supplies of Organising Pamphlets, etc., can be obtained from Mr. G. Vincent Evans, General Secretary, Poor Law Workers' Trade Union, Room 7, 90, Charing Cross Road, London, W.C.2.; or from Mr. L. Wilkinson, Organiser, c/o National Asylum-Workers' Union, 27, Corporation Street, Manchester.

Printed and Published by the Co-operative Wholesale Society's Printing Works, Reddish.

Announcement in *NAWU Magazine*, November 1920

weaker position – an abandonment of its former goal of replacing the NPLOA altogether. Initially the PLWTU had in 1921 pinned its hopes upon the NAWU, and the possible unification of trade unions in the public sector. Yet, as we have seen, that uneasy alliance only lasted a year. The failure of the Federation, and falling membership, led the PLWTU to reconsider its uncompromising stance towards the National.

It soon became clear that the National would strike a very hard bargain from its position of relative strength. The Memorandum of Agreement that was eventually put to ballot in the two organisations conceded virtually all the demands of the NPLOA's negotiating committee: Clerks to Guardians were to be admitted as ordinary members, and the PLWTU's strike clause would be deleted from the rule book. But despite this the proposed new organisation never saw the light of day. When the terms of fusion were put to ballot in September 1922, PLWTU members voted massively in favour. National members, however, voted against, by a wafer thin majority, but with a large number of its members not even bothering to vote. The 'fusion fiasco' was extremely embarrassing to the PLWTU, especially since it had bent over backwards to meet the National's conditions. The union believed that the clerks 'killed' the fusion proposals, but it seems that doubts about the Provident Fund's financial soundness was a major source of NPLOA misgivings.

During the following eight years, the PLWTU regularly attempted to revive the issue of fusion, but with little success. Nearly all the overtures came from the union, although it sometimes seemed to be given encouragement by the National. Eventually the issue was resolved in 1929 by NALGO, long interested in the National, which offered amalgamation to both the union and the NPLOA on the eve of the Poor Law system's absorption into local government. The union turned the offer down because it would have meant sacrificing its manual worker membership in order to become part of a 'white collar' union. The National went ahead, striking a tough bargain as a result of which Major Simonds, the National's leading official and a trained barrister, became NALGO's Deputy General

Secretary in charge of its legal department.[9] NALGO's emergence as a significant health service union was very much assisted by its link-up with the NPLOA.

With the failure of fusion proposals the union was reorganised anyway, largely along the lines that had been anticipated by them. The term 'worker' was diplomatically dropped from the title of the organisation, and in November 1922 the Poor Law Officers' Union (PLOU) was born. Clerks to Guardians were henceforth admitted as ordinary members, and the withdrawal of labour clause was deleted from the constitution. The union was divided into eight Provincial Councils and the officer force strengthened considerably. Before reorganisation, the union had two paid organisers in addition to the General Secretary: Reg Crook who was appointed London Organiser in November 1920 and worked from head office; and John Deasy, the Northern Organiser, a former member of Batley Board of Guardians, President of the local Trades Council and Chairman of the National Union of General and Municipal Workers. In addition, Mr H. Hubert was appointed as the union's Assistant Secretary, and four more Provincial Secretaries were appointed, despite falling membership and uncertain finances.

Rumours were spreading that the PLOU was on the verge of collapse. They were taken sufficiently seriously to warrant an article by Vincent Evans to counter suggestions that the union was 'breaking up' after the failure of fusion. He admitted, however, that 'certain of our members appeared to be losing heart'. Evans admitted a loss of members, as had been suffered by all other unions in this period of high unemployment, but claimed, correctly as it turned out, that the union had reached its lowest point and would now gradually increase in strength.[10]

Yet nothing could disguise the fact that the challenge of the union had lost a great deal of its impetus. The failure of the PLWTU either to supersede or merge with the National had dealt a serious blow to the hopes for industrial unionism in the Poor Law service. The divisions of interest among workers had proved to be simply too powerful. And the union of 'officers' formed out of these disappointments in 1922 was inevitably a much more

cautious and conservative organisation than the uncompromising union of 'workers' established in the heady days
of 1918. In these latter more difficult days attention was
inevitably focussed on the need to survive, while at the
same time keeping the spark of industrial unionism alive.
It is to the credit of the activists and members at this time
that 'the little barque' – as Vincent Evans called the union
– was kept afloat.

The Union at Work

Given such problems, the union's power to improve
conditions of service for its members was limited, but small
victories were won here and there. The union records
contain numerous examples of the kind of treatment
meted out to 'subordinate' officials, and the efforts it made
to defend them. Many concerned 'dual appointments', like
the case in 1919 of Mr and Mrs Park, Superintendents of
Casual Wards at Brentford since 1906. When they came
back from extended sick leave they found their jobs taken
by others; Mr Park refused to take charge instead of
'mentally deficient' children, and both he and his wife
were given the sack. After representations from the union,
the guardians refused to implement this decision of the
House Committee.[11]

The records also show the difficulties experienced by
full-time organisers. John Deasy in his periodic reports
often spoke of the obstacles in his way. In April 1923 he
went to Doncaster:

> Visited the four members we have here with a view to trying
> to increase our membership. I found however that they are so
> afraid of Mr Long, the Master, that they do not do anything
> to help me.

But he did not give up, and sought an interview with the
Master who simply 'glared' at him, and then contacted
Labour Guardians and the town's Labour MP, Tom
Williams. He did not get very far.

The changing economic situation was the main reason
for the flagging fortunes of the union. However, it also

suffered from being neither 'fish nor fowl'. It was neither respectable enough for reactionary authorities in comparison to the National, nor sufficiently like a 'proper' union for many Labour authorities. It did seek periodically in the 1920s to affiliate to the TUC, which turned a Nelson's eye to its approaches, as other unions, already affiliated, were seeking to recruit in this area. Often the union favoured by Labour Guardians was the one to which they themselves belonged. For example, at Poplar in East London, of the rebel Guardians who refused to implement central government policies restricting the amount of relief payable to the unemployed, a number had either been members or officials of the Transport and General Workers' Union or the National Union of General and Municipal Workers.[12] The PLOU had an active branch at Poplar but was not regarded as an 'appropriate' union by the Guardians because of its non-affiliation to the TUC.

The union had sought to remedy its industrial weakness through political action. It had liaised over various issues with Frank Briant, the Liberal MP for Lambeth North, the radical socialist MP Dan Irving (a former associate of William Morris) and Charles Edwards, an ex-miner and Labour MP for Bedwelty in South Wales. Its most concerned campaign was to sponsor a Private Member's Bill to establish an Appeal Tribunal to which aggrieved workers could take their cases. However it did not succeed, since the tide in the early 1920s was turning against the labour movement. In the local government and Poor Law sector no permanent national bargaining machinery was set up, largely because the employers could see that workers were both divided between different organisations and unlikely to mount a campaign of industrial action. The exception in the public sector was the asylums. There, as we have seen, recognition was a direct consequence of a threatened national strike.

The PLOU could therefore do little more than soldier on as best it could. Its two most notable campaigns were at Stepney and its legal action on behalf of Joseph Dewhurst. In 1925 the Stepney Board of Guardians in effect tore up the existing contracts of its relieving officers. Instead the clerk asked them to fill in forms so that they could re-apply for their jobs on pay scales lower than their existing salaries. The Minister of Health was apparently 'sympathetic', but, as usual, would not intervene. Instead he simply advised the officers to re-apply for their jobs. All the union could do in the end was to seek return of superannuation contributions for those officers who had lost their positions, because they had refused to re-apply. Even so, they were not successful since, in the view of the Minister of Health, they had left voluntarily!

Joseph Dewhurst was the subject of a famous test case against his employers, the Salford Board of Guardians, which almost broke the union financially. It originated in 1922 when Dewhurst retired, and was not finally settled in his favour until 1926. By this time it had gone through a long legal process, reached as far as the House of Lords, and Mr Dewhurst himself had died. The issue to be settled was whether cost-of-living bonuses paid during the war should count for superannuation under the Poor Law Officers' Superannuation Act 1896. The union eventually won the case – even though counsel at one stage advised against proceeding further – and a sum of £508 19s 9d, equal to his entitlements, was paid to Joseph Dewhurst's widow. The case was important in helping to consolidate the PLOU's recovery from its precarious position in the early 1920s. It was one risk, at least, that paid off for the union.

The union survived the disappointments and setbacks of the 1920s and membership stabilised at around the 6,300 mark during the closing years of the decade, which made it just about viable. In seeking to explan its survival, perhaps some credit should go to the spirit of camaraderie that appears to have existed among the union's core of loyal supporters. The social side of union acitivities had always been strongly emphasised. Partly this perhaps derived from the union's projection of an ideal of a community of interest among all Poor Law workers. It was also partly to escape from the drabness of institution life. The Brentford branch explained its reasons for holding a dance in February 1922 in the following terms:

Life for the staff of any hospital or institution can never be very bright. Wherever you go there is always suffering and evidence of suffering so a Committee has been formed of the above Branch to promote these pleasant evenings whenever possible. The dance music was rendered by the Carlyle Orchestra and Jazz Band. Conductor, C. F. Preston, M.C. for the evening, Bert Hitchens.

Many branches organised such activities. For example, the Greenwich branch in 1920 organised a sports day which included tug-of-war, track races and swimming competitions. The highpoint was 'a thirty minutes display of ornamental and scientific swimming by Miss Eva Johnson, gold medallist'. In the evening there was dancing in the gymnasium.

In the face of all these setbacks, perhaps the strength of these social bonds helped to hold the union together through its period of adversity. If this was so, then it serves to remind us that there must be deeper bonds within trade union solidarity than simply the instrumental desire to achieve some collective material advantage. For when that ceases to be an immediate possibility, how else do we explain its continued survival?

Notes

[1] Hinton, op. cit., p.98.
[2] G.S. Bain, *The Growth of White Collar Unionism* (1970), p.142.
[3] S. Lewenhak, *Women and Trade Unions* (1977), p.161.
[4] See H.A. Clegg, *General Unions in a Changing Society* (1964) Chapter 3.
[5] S. and B. Webb *The History of Trade Unionism* (1920 edition), pp.508-9.
[6] 'Poor Law Officers and Trade Unionism', *NAWU Magazine*, October-November-December 1918.
[7] *Poor Law Officers' Journal*, 13 December 1918, which contains a full account of the meeting.
[8] Minute Book of the Poor Law Council, NALGO Archive, Modern Records Centre, University of Warwick.
[9] A. Bloor, *White Collar Union* (1967), pp.102-3.
[10] 'Gossip and Gossipers', *Monthly Notes*, December 1922.
[11] Central Executive Committee (CEC) Minutes, 1919, COHSE Archive, loc. cit.
[12] See N. Branson, *Poplarism 1919-25* (1979).

Chapter 12
Wake up, Nurses!

Of all the disappointments suffered by the union during the 1920s, perhaps the most disheartening was its ultimate failure to recruit and retain significant numbers of Poor Law nurses. This was a field in which the union had confidently expected to do well, especially after a respectable medical man such as Dr Wiggins had been elected as President of the PLWTU early in 1919. He himself had boldly predicted that, through his election, the 'snobocracy' which prevented nurses from joining trade unions could now be overcome, as 'false pride must give way to a spirit of co-operation'. But when Dr Wiggins was defeated by David Priestly in the December 1923 Presidential elections, it was admitted in a post-mortem to have been influenced by the fact that the hoped for influx of nurses into the union had not occurred, 'and, as a body, the nurses remain outside the union's ranks'. Priestly was from much humbler origins, being described at the time of his elections as 'a barber, etc, at Epsom' and chairman of the local PLOU branch. He served as President from 1924 to 1926, steering the union through its three most difficult years.

The roots of the moves to organise unions among general nurses extended back to the years before the First World War, when the reforms in the workhouse nursing services were bringing its staffing and administration closer in line with the pattern established in the voluntary hospitals by reformers such as Florence Nightingale. This process in part originated from imperialistic ambitions of the voluntary-hospital trained elite of nurses to extend their control and influence into another sector. Chris Maggs has described how, in order to do this, they had to create 'new nurses' out of rather unpromising material, for unlike the voluntary hospitals many more of the recruits were working-class rather than 'ladies'. He has amply documented how the new control structures sought to fashion the new nurses: managerial strategies were developed to routinise the working day and closely define the tasks expected of nurses; training schools through strict discipline helped to 'weed out' those who were regarded as unsuitable. Finally he shows how official ideology sought to instil a sense of superiority, and manipulate aspirations for social mobility – the promise of travel, position and, perhaps, a successful marriage.[1]

But was the elite as all-powerful as this description might imply? Were all recruits as successfully 'socialised' into compliance with their role as 'new nurses' as was intended? The general lack of success of the campaign in organising trade unionism among nurses would perhaps suggest that this was largely the case. However there are at least some countervailing signs of resistance against the new control structures in Poor Law nursing. If the elite appeared to have won a tactical victory by the mid-1920s it was not secured without a struggle, in which the worsening employment situation came to the assistance of the beleaguered elite to dampen nurses' spirit of resistance.

Nurses' Discontent

In the years running up to the First World War, the widespread industrial militancy began to spread into some unexpected quarters. In 1910, for example, there were spontaneous strikes of school-children. The suffragette movement was also resorting to ever more militant methods in order to win the vote. It is hardly surprising, therefore, that unrest also spread to nurses late in 1911. One of the most publicised instances was at Carlisle Workhouse Hospital, where the reprimand of two probationers by the Superintendent Nurse led to a protest among probationers when, according to the nursing press, they 'left the hospital in a body'. They presented a long list of complaints to the Board of Guardians including accusations that Superintendent Nurse Kirwen had deliberately delayed leave passes, locked away the butter and hidden someone's false teeth, all of which she denied. Five probationers subsequently resigned. The Guardians sought the resignation of the Superintendent Nurse, but it was not allowed by the LGB Inspector.[2]

Nor was this an isolated incident. In Aberdare in South Wales, two nurses walked off duty, went to the Medical Officer of Health and submitted charges against the matron. At York Union Workhouse nurses refused the sausages offered them for breakfast. According to the nursing press:

> Two links of sausages were subsequently found suspended from a gas bracket in one of the wards bearing the inscription 'No further use for you', which was certainly not the right way to give expression to their grievance.[3]

Those disputes were the subject of widespread comment in the nursing press. An editorial in the *British Journal of Nursing*, claimed that:

> The lack of discipline in many of the infirmaries and sick wards of workhouses – as revealed in constant reports in the public press – point to the conclusion that the nursing staffs are out of hand in these institutions.[4]

It concluded that 'further action is needed ... for where discipline is lax, the sick are the invariable sufferers'. The *Nursing Mirror* was more thoughtful and linked the discontent with the new structure of nursing management in Poor Law hospitals. 'The aggrieved nurse is a far more common figure in the present day,' it mused. Although it argued that though conditions were generally improving, this was a rather patchy process, and there was 'some dislocation of the system now established in well-governed institutions for the sick – of the matron's role'.[5]

The editor of the *Nursing Mirror* did not, however, approve of the growing tendency for nurses in such situations to walk off the job, let alone collectively to resign their positions. Patients would suffer and nurses lose their careers. Instead she suggested that an appeal to the matron couched in temperate language, confined purely to facts, and signed by all the staff ought to be met with fair consideration. But if this did not succeed, she could only recommend,

> that courageous acceptance of disagreeable conditions which makes up half the philosophy of life for those who succeed in their careers ... A little patience, a little laughter, and the hard years are gone by.[6]

The nursing press could not contemplate the possibility that trade unionism might help nurses in such situations, even though one nurse wrote to it asking if it knew of 'any society or union which pledges itself to safeguard the general interests of nurses'. She went on to make a classic statement of the case for trade unionism.

> Many people talk of nursing as a heavenly calling, and they will think that such a thing as a Union is desecration. But we feel that we could fulfil our heavenly calling better if our earthly welfare were better looked after. How can we play the role of 'ministering angels' to the best of our ability when our minds and bodies are wearied out by too long hours, the swallowing of half-masticated food, lack of change and pleasure, and last, but by no means least, the petty tyranny of hospital life?
>
> Surely, we do not need such treatment in order to become good nurses. Is it not time that nurses rebelled openly, and so made it easier for nurses in the future? We need shorter hours, longer mealtimes, larger salaries, and more freedom in our off duty. Nurses would fulfil their calling of healing and uplifting much better if their own lives were made brighter.[7]

An editorial in the same issue described the idea as 'distasteful', but many nurses wrote to the journal in support of the idea.[8] Such 'deviant' viewpoints indicate that there was already a rather different voice in nursing to the official one, already clear and confident in tone. Perhaps, in the light of its message, we need to revise our image of the typical nurse as totally devoted and self-effacing. There were obviously divisions in the ranks.

Subterranean rumblings, spontaneous collective action, even vocal expressions of support for trade unions were one thing, but permanent collective organisation was quite another. Though nurses had no lack of grievances – poor pay and conditions, long hours, irksome and often petty forms of tyranny – remedying them was another matter. The first obstacle was often the nurses themselves. As we have seen, official ideology often taught them to make a virtue of bad conditions, and impressed upon them the necessity of absolute obedience – influenced by the fusion of religious masochism, military discipline and feminine perfection in the origins of modern nursing. In the voluntary hospitals adherence to this ideology was greatest, but reinforced by other factors: the class background of the recruits, the acute and 'glamorous' nature of the work. The voluntary hospitals were both avenues to the higher posts in the nursing world, and marriage markets for the middle class. They were also financed from voluntary subscriptions and hence could plead insufficient resources to make substantial improvements.

Nursing After the First World War

The greatest possibilities for trade unionism existed in local government: among district, public health, school and Poor Law nurses. In these sectors the nurses were much less likely to be so starry-eyed about the dominant nursing traditions, and were more likely to be from a working-class background. Perhaps most important of all was the fact that being part of local government created the possibility of harnessing external political pressure, both for improvements to be financed through the rates, and to curtail the absolute power of the matrons. It was not until the end of the First World War that a concerted and successful attempt to recruit nurses into unions took place. Largely as a result of the war a new much more self-assertive notion of womanhood came to the fore which spread to nurses. For example, a Sheffield newspaper in 1919 described nurses who had 'served their country in the war' as not being 'disposed any longer to suffer the pettifogging methods by which their coming and going has been regulated'. There was said to be 'growing resentment of the old-style rule of matrons', and a desire for 'wages more in keeping with those paid to them in the war hospitals'. It was also said that:

> At one of the hospitals in the city the officials have been practically sitting on a volcano for two or three months. The maids in a mass joined a general workers' trade union, and immediately provoked anxiety. Their outspoken talk of revolt infected the nurses, and it was thought that anything was possible. Matters came to a crisis some days ago on the hours question, and the powers that be in the hospital were glad to make a prompt concession to both maids and nurses in face of a virtual ultimatum.[9]

There were reports of trouble elsewhere. At Bermondsey in December 1918, for example, there occurred what the *Nursing Mirror* described as 'a disgraceful incident'. After the nurses' rest day had been reduced to a half day off, due to the influenza epidemic then ravaging the country: 'at nine o'clock one morning a deputation appeared in the matron's office armed with threats'.[10] But what incensed the *Nursing Mirror* more was the fact that, due to the intervention of the Labour guardians, the nurses' rest day was restored, thus undermining the authority of the matron.

A profound shift of political power was taking place in the localities. Although the Liberal-dominated coalition had won the general election, Labour had swept to power in many working-class municipalities. This was a boost to the campaign to extend trade unionism to local government sevices, though, as we have seen, it did not benefit all unions equally. Long overdue reforms were also brought in elsewhere, in Lambeth for example under the influence of its chair, the Liberal MP Frank Briant who was closely linked to the PLWTU. Briant encouraged

Lambeth to lead the way in reforming conditions of employment for hospital nurses. The main impetus was the introduction of the eight-hour day which also required them to deal with the resulting staff shortage by trying to make nursing a more attractive occupation. Probationer nurses would henceforth start at £2 2s a week and have a choice of living in or out. *Nursing Times* commented:

> Two guineas a week, living at home or in 'digs', and learning a 'profession'. What would our nursing pioneers of fifty years ago have said to anything half so revolutionary?[11]

It was not entirely happy as 'students ought, strictly speaking, to pay for their training' and would only countenance it provided the salaries of trained staff were also raised.

The climate after the war therefore seemed in principle favourable for those who might seek to transform nursing's periodic discontents into permanent organisation. By late 1919 it was also suggested in the nursing press that some 2,500 or so general nurses had also joined the newly formed PLWTU, making up 25 per cent of the union's membership. For this reason *Nursing Times* felt moved to give some attention to the growth of trade unions even though it was sure that 'such a society [as the PLWTU] will attract very few of the best nurses'.[12] The union's journal chronicled the attempts to involve its nurses in the life of the union. It gave the pages of *Monthy Notes* over to Maude MacCallum, the tub-thumping leader of the newly formed Professional Union of Trained Nurses with whom the PLWTU had close links. She urged nurses not to join the NPLOA, because that organisation was controlled by a barrister-at-law, Major Simonds, and not a nurse. The NPLOA's nursing section had been formed in 1917 in the hope that it would be allowed direct representation on the College of Nursing's Council – which the latter organisation refused. It had recruited about 1,000 Poor Law nurses, most of them from the senior grades, by the early 1920s.[13]

Instead, Mrs MacCallum urged nurses in *Monthly Notes* of October 1920 to join organisations run by the workers themselves ('wake up: and be free women instead of slaves'). She admitted that the long hours made it difficult for nurses to participate in unions:

> I know what we all say: we are overworked and overtired, in the short time we are off duty we want to go to the theatre, or see the shops and have a little relaxation. That is all true, but what is also just as true, unless we take the management of our own affairs into our own hands, we shall go on being tired and overworked. 'Wake up Nurses', and take a little interest in your own business.

Such calls were not always heeded and it was admitted that nurses were not always easy to involve in the union. Dedication, snobbery and apathy may have played their part, but fear of victimisation was also influential. Nurses' superiors were doing everything in their power to encourage membership of professional associations, particularly the College of Nursing, and discourage membership of trade unions. And their power was considerable. Nurses were extremely vulnerable as probationers, and if they were to obtain a post afterwards they needed good references.

Matrons and the College

There is documentary evidence that the matrons did not sit idly by while the campaign to unionise nurses gathered pace. *Nursing Times* gave considerable space and approval to those matrons who were opposed to the PLWTU. London matrons of Poor Law infirmaries, who tended to be trained in the voluntary hospitals were, it was suggested, implacably opposed. One is quoted as saying:

> The fact that the power behind a trade union was the strike weapon should in itself be enough to make nurses think twice about joining. Furthermore nurses should remember, above all, that their calling was not a trade. Probationers, especially young ones, should (she thought) consult their parents before 'joining any such organisation'.[14]

Yet apparently not all matrons were opposed to trade unions. The *Nursing Times* article, while not reporting their views, admitted that some matrons in the provinces, who were not steeped in the traditions of voluntary hospitals, had joined the PLWTU. The most clearly stated view was one of fierce opposition to probationers joining. Unlike trained staff, they were not to be permitted a free choice in the matter. As another London matron declared: 'For apprentices to become trade unionists is an unheard state of affairs.'

But did this mean that probationer nurses would be victimised for joining unions? The claims of an unnamed PLWTU official were reported, who claimed that nurses were threatened with loss of promotion if they joined a union. *Nursing Times* could not believe this was the case:

> It may be contrary to discipline for a probationer, who is an apprentice, to belong to any such organisation, but a trained nurse has the right to join what society she likes. The most a wise matron would do would be to *advise* her nurses, *never to 'threaten'*.[15]

Along with the repression or discouragement of trade unions went the encouragement of professional associations, particularly the College (later Royal College) of Nursing as an alternative organisation. This was said to 'look after' the interests of all nurses even though matrons dominated its affairs. The College had been set up in 1916 on the initiative of Dame Sarah Swift – a former matron of Guy's Hospital who had been put in charge of the British Red Cross Society – and the Hon. Arthur Stanley, the Treasurer of St Thomas's Hospital and himself Chairman of the British Red Cross. It therefore possessed most of the characteristics it needed from the outset to guarantee success: links with the British establishment, and with the senior nursing and lay managers of the voluntary hospitals. All it now required was the loyalty of rank-and-file staff.

The original aims of the College were to rationalise the chaotic system of training, by setting up a register of nurses and a system for recognising training schools. In the longer term it sought also to win state registration of nursing. Membership was only open in the first instance to nurses who had completed training in a civilian hospital with 250 beds and a resident doctor.[16] The official connections it enjoyed undoubtedly helped it not only against trade unions but rival professional associations, such as the Royal British Nurses' Association (RBNA). It was portrayed in the nursing press as a more 'moderate' organisation, which it was hoped would 'accomplish its mission without creating bitterness and ill-feeling', in contrast to RBNA- and Committee for State Registration-inspired attempts before the war to secure registration.[17] There is no doubt also that the encouragement of the College by matrons and administrators in the hospitals was a prime factor in its growth. By 1918 it claimed 11,000 members, already probably four times as many as the RBNA, which had been established since 1896.[18] When these more subtle and respectable methods of political pressure appeared to pay off in 1919, with the achievement of state registration for nurses, the College consolidated its position in relation to all its rivals. By 1925 in its Annual Report, the College claimed approximately 25,000 members.

That does not mean that no doubts were voiced about the purported advantages of state registration. As always, the letters columns of the nursing press provide evidence of opinions other than the officially sanctioned ones. 'Registration for nurses is all right,' wrote one probationer from a London fever hospital, but we want more than that.' She went to detail her long hours, poor food and little free social time in the evening because of compulsory prayers and bible readings. No wonder, she thought, that nursing was facing a recruitment crisis:

> In these enlightened days, the modern girl expects comfort, good food, and a certain amount of social life. If these are not offered her in hospitals she will go elsewhere.[19]

This generational conflict was a potential Achilles' heel for the College. The dominant ideology still held that a nurse's dedication must be total. However the practical consequence of that view was that nursing was beginning to lose its popularity, not least among middle-class girls, in favour of such occupations as teaching and clerical work. The gap between the 'modern girl' and the rigidity of traditional nursing institutions was a contradiction which unions might exploit, especially since probationers (along with men, mental nurses, and assitant and other untrained nurses) were excluded from College membership. In London, where the PLWTU was strongest, the gap was at its widest. The hospitals were steeped in tradition, while the metropolis offered many attractions to the 'modern girl' who, though she was not necessarily less committed to nursing, was also committed to other things. She therefore began to rebel against the fussier aspects of nursing discipline, sought higher income and fewer hours, and more independence to pursue her own leisure interests.

The Brentford Dispute

Such factors lay behind the most significant trade union stuggle on behalf of nurses during the 1920s: the Brentford dispute of 1921, which the PLWTU described as 'one of the finest fights in the history of the Poor Law service'. According to the union's account the night nurses at the Brentford (subsequently the West Middlesex) Hospital committed the heinous crime of skipping their usual breakfast at 7.30 pm on the evening of 28 March to prepare the hall for the Easter dance.[20] The following day all the night staff were summoned before the matron for engaging in such an audacious act of insubordination. She suspended their 'privileges', including the right to get off early on Saturday afternoon at 4 pm and be allowed 'out' until 8 pm. As a result one Irish probationer would have missed seeing her sister 'who she had not seen for years'. She disobeyed this rule, was taken before the committee, sacked on 21 April 1921 for 'wilful disobedience', and ordered to leave by 9 am the next day.

Immediately 39 out of 52 nurses petitioned the Guardians for her reinstatement and were summoned to the Assembly Hall at 5 pm where the chairman of the board addressed them: his address consisted more or less of a 'jacketing' and, looking at the petition, he asked whether a Nurse Slatter was present. She answered – and was therefore summarily discharged and told to be out of the institution by 9 am the following day – no reason whatever being given. All the nurses considered taking strike action but were persuaded that it would be better to send a delegation to the chairman led by the union. He refused to see them. The next day two more nurses were dismissed by the matron, backed up by the medical superintendent and the Clerk to the Guardians. For a while even the assistant medical officer was suspended from duty for showing sympathy with the nurses. Other nurses who signed the petition were threatened with the sack. Miss Cumberbatch, who chaired the Hospital Committee of the Brentford Board of Guardians, was reported to have defended the dismissal of the nurses by arguing in uncompromising terms that:

> Those who are not prepared to give up EVERYTHING in the sacred cause of fighting disease should not be nurses at all.

The PLWTU took the case to the wider labour movement in Brentford, and on Sunday 8 May 1921 a meeting was convened by Reg Crook, Provincial Secretary of the PLWTU, attended by representatives of 172 branches of unions in the area, said to be 'representative of 85,000 men and women of the world of unionism'. Brother Crook informed the meeting of the events leading to the dismissal of the nurses, and was promised full support in his campaign to have the nurses' cases re-opened. A deputation to the guardians was elected which consisted of 17 trade unionists and 12 representatives of ratepayers, and on 21 May it arrived at the Guardians' office at Isleworth to ask for admission. The deputation was invited up to the vestibule on the first flight of stairs by the deputy clerk and asked to wait peacefully.

> Five minutes – eight minutes passed – and then to the complete astonishment of all concerned, there rushed up to the door on bicycles, a superintendent of police supported by

constables. Then the Deputy Clerk made known the unjust treatment of the Board. 'Officer', he said 'I am instructed to request you to remove these men and women who *have forced their way* into the Guardians' offices'. Protests were advanced by the three leaders of the deputation but without avail. The police had formed up around the stairs – it was a case of go at once or come into conflict with the police.

So they withdrew: but matters did not end there. The eviction of a representative delegation of working-class people in the area angered the local electorate. The next elections were to be held the following April, in 1922. Meanwhile the union's solictor had advised against pressing the Ministry of Health for an enquiry into the dispute, but instead to issue writs against the Brentford Guardians. To finance this course of action the Executive set up a Brentford Dispute Fund, and began paying the four nurses 25 shillings a week victimisation pay. So that the case should not be forgotten, union members wore artificial forget-me-nots in their lapels.

When the time for elections for the Board of Guardians came round, the Brentford branch of the PLWTU had unanimously adopted Mrs Councillor Cowell, the leader of the ratepayers' delegation to the guardians in the previous May. They worked assiduously for her and Reg Crook addressed two meetings in support of her candidature at the local picture palace. By one vote, Mrs Cowell topped the poll and subsequently chaired the Brentford Board of Guardians. The previous Chairman of the Board, Mr Greville-Smith, who had played such a central role in victimising the nurses, was not elected. The legal case was not settled until May 1923, when it came before Mr Justice Darling in the High Court. Counsel for Miss Florence Slatter made a moving speech on her behalf, in which he referred to her dismissal as

... the ill-considered action of those who, clothed in a little brief authority, seem to think that everybody is entirely at their disposal, that their word is law, that what they do is absolutely right, and that they are supreme.

Eventually the case was withdrawn by the union after the Board – by now very different in composition from that which had dismissed her – agreed to furnish Miss Slatter with 'a testimonial to her capacity and character', in order that she might find another position. In the light of this, the cases of the remaining three victimised nurses were also withdrawn. This was victory of a sort, but there was no question of reinstating the nurses.

The Late 1920s

The conclusion to the dispute marked the end of the union's campaigning efforts on behalf of nurses during the 1920s, by which time it was fighting for its very survival as an organisation. It had hoped to use the dispute as a means of recruiting many more nurses. By this time, however, trade unionism was generally in retreat in the Poor Law service, as elsewhere. Thus the College, with the help of the nursing press, hospital administrations, and the declining force of the wider trade union movement, recovered the initiative. But at a price: although it had sworn to oppose anything which smacked of trade unionism, it had in fact established a Salaries Committee in 1919, which published recommended pay scales. After 1926, when *Nursing Times* became the College's official organ, it refused to accept advertisements if pay and conditions fell below the College's minimum. In order to establish a hold over potentially rebellious probationer nurses, it also in 1926, relaxed its exclusive attitude, and set up a Student Nurses Association within the College. It had seen the writing on the wall. *Nursing Times* had warned the College in 1919:

> It is obvious that if professional societies work too slowly, the more impatient spirits will join something that will secure them benefits.[21]

The College, despite its natural inclinations, shifted ground just far enough to head such a movement off.

By the latter half of the 1920s the union's challenge to the College was therefore fading. One of the most significant triumphs for professional associations in their battle with unions came when the Labour Party itself accorded them honoured status in its 1927 conference on 'The Nursing Profession'. The conference had been called to consider the Draft Report prepared by the Standing Joint Committee of Industrial Women's Organisations, and the party's Advisory Committee on Public Health. The Draft Report, as Brian Abel-Smith has suggested,

> in many respects ... was close to the policy actually implemented under the National Health Service many years later. It advocated a 48-hour week, the separation of nurse training schools from hospitals, and student status for probationers with proper time for study. But one paragraph read 'the only way in which nurses can deal effectively with their conditions, and exercise any sort of equality in bargaining power, is for the profession to be organised on trade union lines.' This was anathema to the professional organisations.[22]

Unfortunately, the Labour Party had invited all and sundry, including the professional associations, to its conference when, given the Report's suggestions, one might have expected attendance to have been restricted to labour movement organisations. According to Abel-Smith's account of the Conference:

> Mrs Sidney Webb, who took the chair sensed the feeling of the meeting and proposed that the words 'purely vocational' should be substituted for 'trade union' in the offending paragraph. According to Mrs Fenwick (of the RBNA) this was a 'touch of genius'.

But there was another, though perhaps by now rather subdued feeling present at the meeting, which regarded the Labour Party's capitulation to the professional associations as a betrayal of the interests of rank-and-file nurses. It was expressed by Vincent Evans in an article in the *Gazette*, after he had attended the conference for the union. It was reported that:

he felt ... like a member of a fishing party. All appeared to be fishing for something, and what it was he had so far failed to discover ... Generally speaking it was all wasted effort. It appeared as if the Labour Party were out to make a good impression upon the nurses, and its chief speakers were hopelessly afraid of advocating the principles of trade unionism.[23]

Thus, by the late 1920s, the PLWTU's campaign to unionise nurses had not yet yielded much in the form of permanent organisation. Some nurses had been intimidated, others had probably been convinced that the College and the matrons had their best interests at heart. There could also have been some truth in the claim of Miss Seymour Yapp, the Matron of Lake Hospital, Ashton-under-Lyme, that nurses were poor union members, who would pay their subscriptions 'while enthusiasm burns', but would eventually become irritated with the weekly payments, 'especially if they do not see any return for them'.[24]

It does appear that the first fires of enthusiasm for trades unionism among nurses had largely burnt themselves out by the mid-1920s, but that did not mean that they had been extinguished for ever. In June 1921, John Dillon, the Branch Secretary of the Bolton branch of PLWTU, had drawn attention in 'Monthly Notes' to an inescapable contradiction:

The long hours of duty, the inadequate remuneration, the petty tyrannies which she smarts under, in the guise of the maintenance of discipline, are some of the evils which eclipse the brilliance of the nursing profession. They are defects which must be obliterated before the profession can make any claim to having raised its status, for if the conditions of employment are derogatory, the status can only be so in comparison.

It was not a contradiciton that would go away, or one which 'snobocracy' or the College of Nursing could entirely smother by cosmetic changes in structure and policy. In the 1930s, a fresh generation of nurses would rekindle the torch of trade unionism, handed down to them from the 1920s. The PLWTU and PLOU had, for the first time, established a tradition of trade unionism in general nursing, which future generations would enrich and renew.

Notes

[1] C. Maggs, *The Origins of General Nursing* (1983).
[2] *Nursing Mirror*, 27 January 1912.
[3] *British Journal of Nursing*, 10 February 1912.
[4] Ibid.
[5] 'Nurses with a Grievance', *Nursing Mirror*, 3 March 1912.
[6] Ibid.
[7] 'Everybody's Opinion', ibid., 9 September 1911.
[8] Ibid., 9 September, 7 October, 28 October and 4 November 1911. All correspondents gave themselves fictitious names, for reasons which should be obvious.
[9] Press cutting kindly given to me by Jane Salvage.
[10] 'A Disgraceful Incident', *Nursing Mirror*, 7 December 1918.
[11] 'Some Changes in the Nursing World', *Nursing Times*, 27 March 1920.
[12] Ibid., 18 October 1919.
[13] NPLOA Records, NALGO Archive, loc. cit.
[14] 'The Trade Union Movement Among Poor Law Nurses', *Nursing Times*, 18 October 1919.
[15] Ibid.
[16] G. Bowman, *The Lamp and the Book* (1967), Ch. 6 (the official history of the Royal College of Nursing).
[17] 'The College of Nursing', *Nursing Times*, 16 December 1916.
[18] Bowman, ibid., p.56.
[19] *Nursing Times*, 7 February 1920.
[20] Compiled from editions of *Monthly Notes*, and its successor, *Poor Law Gazette*, 1921-23.
[21] *Nursing Times*, 18 October 1919.
[22] Abel-Smith, *Nursing Profession*, pp.133-4.
[23] *Poor Law Gazette*, 7 February 1927.
[24] 'Trade Unionism versus Professional Union', *Nursing Mirror*, 22 November 1919.

Chapter 13
Going it Alone in the Thirties

In 1929 the Poor Law was finally abolished, although its spirit was to live on. The following year the PLOU was transformed into the National Union of County Officers (NUCO). Its membership was thrown open to all employees of county, county borough and metropolitan borough councils. Subscriptions were 6d a week, including funeral benefit, after an entrance fee of 1 shilling had been paid. Overnight the specialist union for Poor Law officers had been transformed into a union for the whole of the local government service.

The grand ambitions that lay behind this reorganisation were, however, never realised. Not for the first time, the tendency became manifest for the union's ambitions far to exceed its resources. The NUCO was lucky to survive its first two years of life, as it yet again sailed perilously close to the rocks of bankruptcy. Once more, the union defied the expectations of most of its critics and survived, growing moderately in strength throughout the rest of the 1930s.

The Local Government Act 1929 abolished the elected Boards of Guardians and redistributed their powers among various committees of county and county borough councils. As a result approximately 78,000 Poor Law employees, about one-third of them in London, were absorbed into the mainstream of the local government service. The Act allowed for hospital services to be transferred to Public Health Committees of Councils, to be financed partly out of the rates and partly by means of a block grant from central government. Relief was to be administered by Public Assistance Committees of Councils. In theory the basis had been laid for the complete separation of medical services from the administration of poor relief, apparently very much along the lines advocated by the Webbs, but this impression is misleading.

Sidney Webb himself believed that the 1929 Act was part of the Tory government's attempts to press home its undoubted advantages after the defeat of the General Strike.[1] The government had been incensed at the continued refusal of certain Labour-controlled Boards, particularly in mining areas, to restrict relief to be unemployed. Its hope was that the counties and county boroughs would be more remote bodies, less susceptible to politcal pressures from below that came from direct elections to Boards of Guardians. In any case, the government was not making sufficient central finance available to make the abolition of the Poor Law a reality. Indoor relief became 'institutional relief' and out-relief became 'domiciliary relief', workhouses became institutions and 'infirmaries' hospitals. The wording changed, but much remained the same.

The PLOU had fought against these changes, not primarily for political reasons, but because of fears of 'displacement', that their pay and conditions would worsen with the break-up of the Poor Law, or even that they would be made redundant. One effect of this was to bring the NPLOA and the PLOU closer together. The NPLOA had joined the Conference of 'Poor Law Officers' Organisations in 1925, under pressure of the Dewhurst case judgement, which at that stage had been lost by the union in the High Court. Now the National joined forces with the union at the end of the 1920s in the campaign to protect transferred Poor Law workers' conditions, particularly their more favourable superannuation rights. The pressure was successful in getting a clause inserted in the 1929 Local Government Act, protecting the employment conditions of 'transferred officers'.

The PLOU now had to consider its own future. It was being courted by a number of unions, but the most likely merger was one which brought the NPLOA, NALGO and the PLOU into one organisation. The NPLOA struck a favourable deal with NALGO, and although NALGO would accept all existing manual and non-manual members of the PLOU, it insisted that in future only white collar workers should be admitted. The PLOU felt this was a policy which 'fosters class interests' and does not develop 'recognition of a duty to each other irrespective of class or grade', and ran counter to the union's dominant philosophy since its formation in 1918.

These and other issues were finally resolved at a 'Future of the Union' delegate conference held in London on 7 December 1929 – eleven years to the day since the birth of the PLWTU. The 200 delegates present decisively rejected the NALGO proposals. The union would again 'go it alone', but in an even more uncertain and unfamiliar environment. After some argument, the name of the union was changed to the National Union of County Officers. The officer force of the union was to be strengthened and the union now divided into eleven (later twelve) areas or zones. Subsequently George Esther was appointed to organise the North-East, and the services of Alderman E.A. Hardy, a Labour Councillor from Salford, were enlisted to look after the North- West. John Deasy's activities now became restricted to Yorkshire and the East Midlands, while Councillor Mrs Beatrice Drapper, a former Guardian and now Labour member of Lewisham Council, was appointed to assist Mr Hubert in London and the South-East.

Guilds and an Industrial Union

Perhaps the most controversial feature of the reorganisation was the plan to reduce the importance of the branch by dividing the membership into specialist 'guilds'. The splitting up of the Poor Law system and its redistribution to different committees of county and county boroughs was one influence behind the idea; so also was a growing emphasis on 'status' and 'professionalism'. Guilds had been the monopolistic organisations of crafts and trades during the middle ages which were superseded by trade unions. Their adoption in principle by the 'Future of the Union' conference underlined the conservatism and professionalism ethos of the NUCO. The system was approved against the opposition of those who saw guilds as fostering within the union the very 'class divisions' that had led to rejection of NALGO's merger proposals. In practice the guild system was never adopted in entirety, as it was unwieldy in practical terms. By 1935, however, sectional meetings were being held for doctors and nurses, residential schools' staffs, relief and clerical staffs, female laundry and domestic staffs and engineering and maintenance staffs. Other sections were formed as demand arose, for example, among ambulance staffs.

The NUCO thus came into existence on 11 January 1930, with a structure and government largely resembling that of the PLOU, and with Vincent Evans still firmly at the helm. Early in its life the new union applied for affiliation to the TUC and was again turned down. Yet although there was considerable continuity between the PLOU and the NUCO, the world of local government into which the NUCO was entering was very different from the Poor Law service. The NUCO which had in theory become an industrial (although it preferred the term 'specialist') union for the whole of the local government service, had entered a cut-throat world of inter-union competition between a great variety of organisations. The most immediate threat was NALGO, already claiming 100,000 members, and with its rate of growth continuing to accelerate. Its merger with the NPLOA had given it a very useful presence in ex-Poor Law services, especially in London. The NUCO was also now exposed in London, still its strongest area, to competition from the London County Council Staffs Association (LCCSA), an organisation fostered by management, who accorded it special privileges. On the manual side the two big general unions (the TGWU and NUGMW) had considerable numbers, but they, too, had become increasingly concerned by the end of the 1930s, with the phenomenal growth of NUPE and its aggressive recruiting policies initiated under Bryn Roberts's leadership.

The NUCO sought to develop its appeal by reviving its friendly society activities, offering members an arrangement with the Whitehall Building Society at enhanced rates of interests. In 1931 it developed a 'safeguard' policy which, in return for contributions, provided a member's widow with a pension of £1 a week. Later, a motor insurance scheme was developed, as well as trading schemes and even 'special facilities' to use the libraries provided by Boots the chemists. The development of these sidelines was almost certainly the result of competition from NALGO, which for many years had been known as the 'goose club' on account of the enticements offered to conservative- minded local government officers.

The NUCO was lucky to survive the early 1930s. It was swimming against the tide, promoting unionism for all grades at a time when the trend in local government was towards separate organisations for manual and non-manual workers. Its new provident activities and the cost of extra organisers were causing a drain on finances and only drastic economies prevented the union from going bankrupt. Then in 1934, in a highly controversial measure, the responsibility for all unemployment relief was transferred to central government.[2] Some 6,000 ex-relieving officers – the group who had formerly been the mainstay of the union – were absorbed in the new Unemployment Assistance Board.

Despite these problems, the union pulled back from the edge of the precipice. In 1935 its long-standing application to join the TUC was finally successful. It was finding a growing base among health workers (especially in London) whose numbers were expanding rapidly in 1930s. By 1939 its membership had increased modestly to 13,000. In the process it changed from being a rather staid organisation of ex-Poor Law workers, into a campaigning, even militant union of health workers, yet with a strong professional ethos.

The 1930s saw a substantial, if uneven expansion of general hospitals. The counties hardly developed any, the boroughs only a few, but in London there was growth in London County Council (LCC) hospitals, particularly after Labour came to power in 1934. It had inherited a large number in 1930 with the transfer of Metropolitan Asylum Board (MAB) Poor Law hospitals. The opportunity was also taken to weld the MAB and LCC ambulance services together into a single unified service of 153 vehicles and 400 personnel, making it by far the biggest authority in the country. Its municipal hospitals grew rapidly in the 1930s, helped by the general prosperity of the area in comparison to the rest of Britain. By the end of the 1930s the LCC provided 60 per cent of all municipal hospitals, and a total staff excluding mental hospitals of 21,560.[3] This growth provided a solid recruitment base for the NUCO, which was able to harness the growing discontent of health staffs.

As the 1930s progressed the union's motto 'Unitate Fortior – Stronger United' – took on a more vital meaning. The first signs of impending trouble came in 1933 when the district auditor in London sought reductions in the wages of transferred officers who had previously worked for high paying Boards of Guardians, such as Poplar, Greenwich, Bethnal Green, Stepney and Bermondsey. It was the first sign that the guarantee in the 1929 Act to protect the conditions of transferred officers was by no means absolute. A NUCO delegation on 23 March 1933 to the Central Public Health Committee of the LCC, led by Vincent Evans, only brought the reply that individual cases would be dealt with by appeal against the auditors' decision, which in some cases involved considerable sums of money.

The London County Council Dispute

The first collective protests involving large numbers of health staffs occurred in May 1934 against the new system of 'rations' brought in by the LCC. It was the foundation for all the union's subsequent campaigns in the 1930s. The Labour Party had just arrived in power and was not blamed for the situation, which was regarded as one of the 'relics' of the old 'municipal reform' regime. The system was a centralised means of standardising staff diets throughout the LCC's hospitals and institutions, based on 'scientific' calorific calculations, but staff suspected that the main aim was to restrict the quality and quantity of food available to them.

A vociferous protest meeting was held by the NUCO at the Memorial Hall in Farringdon Street. Resident staff, especially those who had formerly been employed by the MAB, were particularly incensed. Since part of their salary was received in the form of 'emoluments' they experienced the new scheme as a real cut in the value of their wages. Nurses were very active participants in the protests made at the meeting. One was allowed to put a resolution to the meeting, protesting against the appointment of voluntary hospital trained nurses as matrons of LCC hospitals. Clearly the meeting was beginning to tap much deeper discontents.

A deputation was got up to go to the council to protest at the changes in the rationing system, and included rank-and-file workers as well as union officials. When received by the council on 21 June 1934, the delegation did not find the new Labour administration to be as sympathetic to its complaints as it had expected. The council's officials defended the new system as fair and rejected many of the claims of the union as wild exaggerations. One member of the deputation was the late Doris Westmacott, a young trained nurse and midwife sister at Mile End Hospital, who joined the union in 1933 after being persuaded to do so by male nurses. As she told me, she found herself on the deputation after she was 'pushed forward' by Vincent Evans. She could not afford to live out because of the poor pay. Apparently the council refused to believe her complaints about the quality of the soused herrings, but she spoke up for herself all the same.

This was the earliest experience of disappointment with the Labour LCC. It was not to be the last. Later that year there were accusations, particularly from ex-Poor Law staff, that the LCC was seeking to erode the preferential conditions of transferred officers. Among their complaints was that the LCC was asking them to work a 54-hour week as opposed to their established 48 hours. The MAB's relatively protected conditions were due to the pressure brought upon it by the National Asylum Workers' Union after 1918. The MAB also employed numbers of unqualified male nurses who were being regraded as ward orderlies as part of the council's innovative policy of relieving the trained staff of routine domestic duties. The male nurses – who became an

The Mental Hospital and Institutional Workers' Union

ORGANISATION OF NURSES

An Appeal

Following the Lancet Commission of Inquiry and the exposures of nursing conditions contained in the Report of that body, considerable dissatisfaction has been expressed by all sections of Nurses at the lack of professional organisation and facilities for mutual assistance.

The Mental Hospital and Institutional Workers' Union, with the approval of the Trades Union Congress General Council, and with the support of large numbers of Nurses, male and female, engaged in district nursing, private nursing, and other special branches of the profession, offers its services for the purpose of initiating a professional organisation on Trade Union lines.

Our ultimate conception is that of a self-governing federation of all sections of the Nursing Profession. We shall endeavour to raise still higher the status of nursing; we will strive to secure economic freedom for all engaged in the profession, and greater security of tenure for those engaged in district nursing; we shall try to protect Nurses from the exploitation now so common; we shall seek to obtain statutory provision for Nurses in sickness and old age, and to provide machinery that will enable Nurses to take part in the development and government of the profession to which they have dedicated themselves. We shall do nothing detrimental to the dignity of nursing, but shall do everything which the collective wisdom of Nurses themselves deems to be desirable for the greater efficiency of the profession and for the best interests of those engaged therein.

All who are interested in the development of an organisation on these lines are invited to communicate with:

GEO. GIBSON (General Secretary),
The Mental Hospital and Institutional Workers' Union,
1, Rushford Avenue,
Levenshulme,
MANCHESTER.

The Socialist Medical Association

At the Annual General Meeting of the Socialist Medical Association, held in London, on May 28th and 29th, the following Emergency Resolution was unanimously carried:-

Resolved—That we welcome the formation of an organisation representing all sections of the Nursing Profession on Trade Union lines and wish it success.

Appeal in *Mental Hospital Workers' Journal*, July 1932

increasingly important ginger group within the union –
felt aggrieved that they were now being asked to
undertake such 'degrading' work as scrubbing floors. On
16 October 1934 a crowded meeting was told by one of
them that

> We were transferred on All Fools Day 1930 and apparently
> the Council intends to make 'all fools of us'.

The 500-strong meeting then passed a resolution
detailing other deteriorations in the terms and conditions
of their service, and sought an early meeting between the
NUCO and the LCC.

This did not achieve anything, so the next stage was a
massive protest rally, the biggest in the history of the
union, held in the Central Hall, Westminster on 8 January
1935, and attended by 1,800 members. It was presided
over by Lionel Lunn, a public assistance officer in
Burton-on-Trent and the union's President throughout
the 1930s and beyond. The meeting was called in the spirit
of resistance to 'any encroachments on transferred
rights and conditions of employment ... What we have we
hold.' There appears to have been a highly charged
emotional atmosphere at the meeting. It began at 6.30 pm
with an organ recital by the General Secretary, followed by
the Wood Green Male Voice Choir, who sang such stirring
items as the 'Pilgrims Chorus' and the 'Comrades' Song of
Hope'. Finally Mr Ruttledge, the London Organiser, led
the meeting in community singing, before the meeting
even got down to the business of the evening. Speeches
were made by union leaders and representatives of
different grades of staff. Nurse Iris Brook, who, as she
told me, had recently been recruited to the union's staff
after contributing an article to the *Daily Herald* on 'How
Nurses Suffer', addressed the meeting. She was married to
Dr Charles Brook, who had helped to found the Socialist
Medical Association and also became a NUCO activist. 'If
Florence Nightingale were alive today,' she said,

> she would be ashamed of the profession, particularly
> comparing the scanty and inadequate recognition meted out

to highly trained nurses for years of self-sacrifice as compared to other professions. Florence Nightingale if alive today, would undoubtedly be the General Secretary of a nurses' union to see that nurses were not exploited.

The formal business of the meeting ended with a resolution in favour of 'one union for all grades'. It also called on the Minister of Health to instruct local authorities to maintain the status quo for transferred staffs. The rally then closed with the singing of the NUCO song, composed in 1933 by Vincent Evans, the refrain of which went:

> Sing aloud the message,
> Bringing hope and cheer
> For NUCO stands for comradeship
> And drives away all fear.

Feelings were running very high, and did not die down. The protest movement was unearthing some deep-seated anxieties which were linked to more than simply a deterioration in material conditions of employment. Many transferred officers seemed to have felt a loss of a sense of community with the break-up of the Poor Law system, and the abolition of the Guardians, and had not yet found a new sense of identity in a rapidly changing service. With the shift to a modern hospital system, new demands were being made on the staff, but without any major uplift in their pay, status and conditions of employment. At the same time, with the growth in size of hospitals, authority was becoming more remote and impersonal, increasing workers' sense of alienation. Nor should it be forgotten that the wider world outside the hospital, with the rise of fascism and the drift to another global war in the space of a generation, was also riven with anxiety. The NUCO, with its emphasis on 'friendship' and the solidarity of all grades, perhaps provided its membership with that sense of belonging that was disintegrating in their daily lives. Perhaps that was the way in which it drove away the non-specified 'fear' alluded to in the NUCO song, which led others to say that the NUCO had 'quaint ways of its own'.[4]

This sense of growing alienation lay behind union complaints of the LCC's increasing adoption of industrial methods. In November 1935, the *Gazette* published an open letter from a NUCO member to Herbert Morrison, Labour leader of the LCC, which, as well as listing many of the now familiar grievances of transferred staffs, also declared:

> What I fail to understand is your condemnation of capitalism, and all that it entails, and for the Council, the majority of whom condemn such a system, to apply it in a socialised service.

The writer in this particular instance was referring to the process of 'speed up' that was being introduced among LCC laundry staffs. Its laundries had originally been run by the MAB, which had, by 1910, granted laundry workers stable conditions of employment, including super-annuation.[5]

Their transfer in 1930 to the LCC was said by the union's *Gazette* in 1935 to have caused 'a rising tide of discontent' among their ranks. A meeting of London laundry workers held on Tuesday 26 November 1935 displayed this publicly. The discontent was focused upon the LCC's plan to 'centralise' the service. Alderman Miss E. Kellet, a leading NEC member from the London area, addressed the meeting and said whether it was called that or 'rationalisation', it

> meant the same thing to the workers, speeding up intensification of working conditions, and as such should be fought to the bitter end by the workers.

Revelations regarding the 'scandalous' conditions in the laundry were given to the meeting, such as the lack of facilities for staff to eat, or anywhere to hang their clothes. Vincent Evans later addressed the meeting and had few kind works for Herbert Morrison. At the close of the meeting a resolution was passed condemning the introduction of 'industrialism' within the public services. The LCC was planning to introduce a 'Bedaux' system, based on time-and-motion study, into its laundries. Such schemes had been introduced in private industry from the early 1930s and been the subject of a number of bitter disputes.

NUCO ambulance workers had also been in dispute with the LCC, especially after the introduction of a new grading structure in 1935. Ambulance workers came under the London District Joint Industrial Council (JIC), from which the NUCO was excluded, and the union's ambulance section campaigned vigorously for the ambulance service to be part of the council's Public Health Department rather than the General Purposes Committee. This issue too showed that ambulance workers were concerned with their status. The first London ambulances had been those of the MAB, transferring fever cases into isolation hospitals. By the 1930s the LCC service was more concerned with maternity cases, and accident and emergency work, but many ambulance workers believed that their status, training, pay and conditions had not improved in line with the demands now made of them. To be part of the JIC meant they were classed as manual workers.

In July 1936 an unsigned article in the *Gazette* listed a variety of grievances, including insufficient annual leave and the postponement of days off because of lack of relief staff, under the title 'The Grouse of an Ambulance Attendant'. The article also displayed a strong sense of alienation from senior officials in County Hall. There were certainly enormous variations in the pay and conditions of ambulance workers nationally. Sometimes ambulance work was attached to the Local Watch Committee, sometimes to the local fire brigade, which workers were sometimes expected to help out in an emergency. By September 1935 the NUCO was pressing for a nationalised service with uniform pay scales and shift system, overtime payments, sick pay and holidays.

Porters were another group actively discontented from the late 1930s. In 1938 the NUCO pressed the case of LCC porters who wished to end the practice of compulsory sleeping in at a number of hospitals, as a condition of allowing them to be non-resident. Pressure on their behalf to the Medical Officer of Health for the LCC did not succeed in changing his mind. In early 1939 the NUCO took up cudgels on behalf of temporary adult porters in the LCC who, after two years, were dismissed in favour of 18-year-old 'juveniles' at a lower rate of pay. The NUCO circulated a leaflet addressed to 'Ratepayers of London', detailing all kinds of unpleasant or difficult activities associated with portering, and asked them 'Do you, as an intelligent person, believe this to be a job for a boy?' The union subsequently organised a protest rally at the Memorial Hall on 10 January 1939. The council, for its part, claimed that the policy was a progressive one, providing permanent careers in the place of temporary ones, but it admitted that temporary workers themselves would be displaced. In *London News*, the official organ of the London Labour Party, it described the union as

> a rather quaint union organisation known as the National Union of County Officers ... Ever since the Labour Party has been in power on the London County Council the organisation has gone out of its way to make itself a nuisance in ways it did not when the Tories were in power.[6]

It called the union's leaflet 'grossly misleading'.

The union did not succeed with this protest, but it again illustrated the extent to which the NUCO would pursue the grievances of staff, even though a Labour authority was in power. It was one of the paradoxes of the NUCO that, though a 'non- political' union, it should be constantly reminding the LCC of its socialist duties. It even won itself the reputation of being an 'extreme left' union in some quarters, presumably because criticisms of the LCC were associated with the Communist Party, and because the *Gazette*, under Pat O'Gorman, had a 'distinctly left' flavour. Certainly Alderman Hardy, the organiser in the North-West felt that this was why he had faired so badly in 1937 elections on to the TUC General Council. Yet such a reputation may well have been exagerrated, at least, according to Pat O'Gorman, the most militant NUCO official working in the London area. He resigned in 1938 in protest, among other things, at the union's lack of concern about political issues, particularly the Spanish

Civil War. He felt that the established leadership of the
union was the obstacle, and only represented high ranking
grades in the service.[7]

The NUCO's militancy was therefore limited in scope – it
did not embrace wider political issues outside the employment sphere, or even industrial action within it. Nevertheless, it was real enough, and grounded in the discontent that
affected nearly every grade of health worker employed by
the LCC, including those far removed from contact with
the patients – stokers, for example, appear to have been one
of the most aggrieved groups in the 1930s. LCC staff were
not the only group with grievances, but they were bound to
be prominent in the campaign to unionise staff since they
represented the largest concentration of health workers in
the country. The LCC was also pioneering methods of
administration – dubbed 'industrialism' by the NUCO –
which were likely to dislocate traditional relationships.

The most significant dispute outside London was in
Canterbury in 1938. Its immediate cause was the resignation or dismissal of eight members of staff, following the
appointment of a new master and matron. But the most
contentious issue of all was the refusal of the town's Public
Assistance Committee to negotiate, or even see a NUCO
representative about the dispute. It became a local, even
national, *cause célèbre*. A massive meeting which crowded
out the town's biggest hall and appears to have generated
more excitement than the residents of Canterbury had seen
for years, was held on 15 March 1938. The workers drew
messages of support from the local and national labour
movement, and the meeting was addressed by a TUC
official, Victor Feather. This and other disputes did not
always yield results satisfactory to the members, but they
did show that health workers had the confidence to stand
up for themselves in a way that had never been seen before.

The Three Guilds

The development of the guild system within the NUCO
was central to its attempt to harness the specific grievances
of an increasingly diverse and specialist workforce. It was
also an attempt to marry trade union and professional

concerns. Guild members were separate from local branches, so would not have to associate with 'inferiors'. By 1939 three guilds were functioning for ambulance services, medical services and nurses. The Ambulance Services Guild was established in 1938 and issued its charter in 1939. It wanted a nationalised ambulance service which would be recognised as an essential part of the health services. A primary object was the establishment of a state register which 'shall operate similar to that applied to the nursing profession', and a three year course of training. The moves to obtain state registration did not get very far, but in 1946 the guild (then part of COHSE) sponsored an Institute of Certified Ambulance Personnel, with Vincent Evans as its first President. The Medical Services Guild grew out of the medical services section, set up in 1933, which originally included nurses as well as doctors. Membership of the guild was open to doctors and dentists, as well as pharmacists and qualified laboratory technicians. It specialised in 'service protection', usually on an individual basis, in contrast to the 'professional protection' already provided by the Medical Defence Union. Other staff groups were organised in sections rather than guilds. The Engineering and Maintenance Section had well defined objectives, including a 40-hour week, better holidays and sick leave, the abolition of industrial conditions and the establishment of a conciliation committee to deal with promotion 'as opposed to secret reports'. Institution and hospital employees, i.e. excluding nurses and doctors, also had their charter, including abolition of compulsory residence, better and more 'hygienic' conditions of employment, and more freedom for staff, with 'institutions and hospitals to be regarded as public necessities rather than "Labour Concentration Camps" ' (a play on the initials LCC).

But the Guild of Nurses was by far the most active and successful group within the NUCO by the late 1930s. How supposedly deferential nurses became transformed into militant trades unionists, and the vanguard of the NUCO, is a story worth telling in some detail, and is the subject of the next chapter.

Notes

[1] B. Gilbert, *British Social Policy 1914-39* (1920), p.219.

[2] For a full account see A. Deacon and J. Bradshaw, *Reserved for the Poor* (1983) Ch. 2.

[3] G. Gibbon and R. Bell *The History of the London County Council 1889-1939* (1939), p.204.

[4] Tory London Municipal Society, quoted in *County Officers Gazette*, the NUCO's official newspaper, 12 July 1935.

[5] For one matron's unfavourable opinion of such a system see *British Journal of Nursing*, 19 February 1910.

[6] 'Real Facts About Hospital Porters', *London News*, January 1939.

[7] Letter of resignation, 17 November 1938 in NUPE Archive, National Museum of Labour History.

Chapter 14
Nurses Must Organise

Throughout the 1930s public attention was focused almost continuously upon the plight of nurses. At the beginning of the decade it was largely as a result of agitation on behalf of nurses by others, whether the press, members of the medical profession or sympathetic Members of Parliament. As these well meaning efforts came to nought, nurses started to take matters into their own hands. As an article in *Labour Woman* in January 1937 declared: 'nurses must organise', for the alternative was 'no organisation – no progress'. Nurses began to learn the lesson in growing numbers, so that by the end of the 1930s a significant change had taken place: nurses themselves were agitating and organising in defence of their interests.

Throughout the nineteenth and most of the twentieth centuries, hospitals have been explicitly excluded from the protective legislation that began in the nineteenth century with the passing of the first Factory Act. Only those workers who would have been covered outside – such as those in workshops – have been included within their scope. Those on the wards have been largely unprotected by laws that were being extended, if not always applied, to increasing numbers of workers in outside employment. Periodic attempts were made to remedy this neglect by bringing in special legislation to cover health workers. We have already heard of one such unsuccessful attempt, by the NAWU in 1911, to place a statutory limit upon the number of hours worked by asylum workers. The reason why this, and all other subsequent attempts failed is a simple one: no government ever adopted the responsibility for such legislation, or when it did, as briefly in 1919, it subsequently dropped it. Almost invariably such Bills have been introduced on the initiative of individual MPs sympathetic to such a cause.

Fenner Brockway's Bill

This was the case with the Bill introduced in Parliament in December 1930 by Fenner Brockway, then the young member for Leyton, for a minimum wage of £40 a year and a maximum working week of 44 hours. Not only did the Labour Prime Minister refuse to give the Bill facilities, but it was bitterly opposed by professional organisations such as the College of Nursing, whose Council proclaimed in February 1931:

> That it is not in the interest of the nursing profession or of the public that standards of hours of duty and a salary should be enforced by legislation, since experience has shown that these questions can best be settled by the nurses themselves acting through their organisations.[1]

The reasons for opposition were various. In the first place the Bill was regarded as an insult to the dignity of the profession – 'Would doctors, artists, professors or university students call in the law to regulate their hours of study and service?' Also, private nurses were worried that their employment prospects might suffer. Above all, the matrons of the voluntary hospitals who dominated College affairs would have experienced extreme staffing and financial difficulties as managers in implementing the Bill.

The nursing press universally condemned the Bill and declared that nurses as a body were 'overwhelmingly' against it. Yet there is some evidence to the contrary, as the nursing press itself was inundated with letters in favour of the Bill, many of them from College members. The Bill failed. The Labour government fell in 1931 and Fenner Brockway was not returned to Parliament in the elections. But the Bill was a watershed because, more than anything, it raised the question of the limited effectiveness of the College for many working nurses. It appears to have

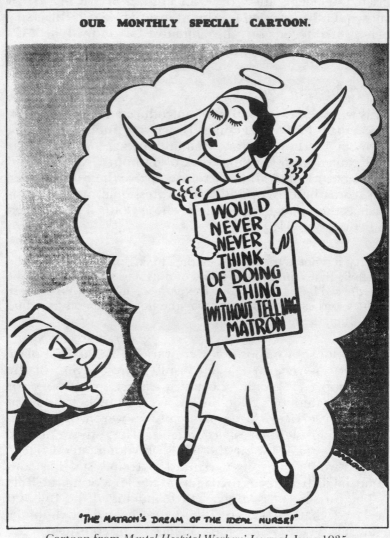

Cartoon from *Mental Hospital Workers' Journal*, June 1935

stirred the College into making a more energetic effort to secure reductions in hours for nurses. It also led to the renewal of the movement to unionise nurses which had lain dormant since the 1920s. The Bill therefore announced the beginning of an intense competitive struggle between the College and trade unions during the 1930s.

In the absence of immediate improvements in nurses' pay and conditions, the nursing press offered the consolation to be found in products such as Ovaltine and Bournevita. 'Nervous exhaustion' was not caused by short-staffing, long hours and financial worry but 'nerve starvation' which, of course, Ovaltine could easily remedy. Whatever the problem, the nurse had only to drink Bournevita to feel 'on top of the world'. Meanwhile the *Nursing Times* ran helpful articles advising readers on 'How to Live on £80 a Year', the average salary of a ward sister in the voluntary hospitals (though municipal hospitals paid more). Never mind if she

> considers herself very badly off, has no wardrobe to speak of and by the end of the month is reduced to borrowing. One is compelled to admit the justice of the criticism which considers her unbusiness-like and economically ignorant.[2]

Others felt that perhaps trade unionism might be a more effective solution to such problems, especially those who had come together in support of Fenner Brockway's Bill at a conference held at the House of Commons on Friday 19 June 1931, which Beatrice Drapper attended for the NUCO. One student nurse told the meeting that she had got up a petition in favour of the Bill at a London hospital which had been signed by the majority of students. The meeting concluded with a call to the TUC to develop a plan for organising nurses along trade union lines.

This call coincided with the TUC's growing desire to assist in the recruitment of more women workers into the movement, especially among poorly organised trades. In the same year, 1931, it established the National Women's Advisory Committee. The next year the TUC took its first hesitant steps towards organising the two most notoriously unorganised women's occupations, domestic service and nursing. As far as the domestic servants were concerned, however, the TGWU and the NUGMW both refused to help because 'the difficulties in the way of organising these workers are too great'.[3] Eventually the TUC was pushed into launching its own National Domestic Workers' Union in 1937. As far as nurses were concerned, neither of the two most likely organisations – the NUCO and NALGO – were affiliated to the TUC. The job on this occasion was therefore delegated to the MHIWU, whose General Secretary, George Gibson, was a member of the TUC's General Council. With the approval of Congress, the MHIWU offered its services to help general nurses to get up what it called 'a professional organisation on trade union lines', to improve pay and conditions.[4] The College recognised the implications of the MHIWU's move: 'We must stand together under the aegis of the trade union or strengthen our professional organisation to take its place.'[5] The College had only recently introduced a system of area organisers, partly in response to growing competition from trade unions.

The Lancet *Commission*

The campaign to organise nurses had recently received a boost with the revelations of the *Lancet* Commission on Nursing in 1932. It was researched and written by a group of doctors and educationalists concerned at the growing shortage of nurses, despite the professional recognition that nursing had supposedly achieved with state registration in 1919. As Abel-Smith has pointed out, the problem was not due to fewer nursing recruits, but a growth in demand for their services. The number of women coming forward to nurse had increased, but not in line with requirements.[6] During the inter-war period a shift in social attitudes occurred alongside developments in medical practice, which led to many more people being treated for acute illness in hospital. Hospitals, of course, needed nurses, and, increasingly, trained nurses, to undertake skilled technical duties delegated to them by doctors.

The *Lancet* Commission members were not being entirely altruistic. The modern doctor wanted a modern nurse, equipped with a degree of initiative, rather than the 'handmaiden' produced by the traditional system. Unfortunately the traditional system was increasingly deterring middle-class girls who, it was hoped, might adapt to these new requirements. The report went into great detail about how training sought to inculcate habits of 'uncritical obedience', serving to dampen rather than arouse curiosity. The first duty of the nurse was simply 'to get the job done', much of which consisted of back-breaking domestic duties. Outside the wards her life was subject to a multitude of petty regulations which were resented by women 'accustomed to modern standards of liberty in their own homes'. Her food and accommodation were poor. A first-year student nurse received £20 in voluntary hospitals or £29 in municipal hospitals in 1930, and her long-term material prospects on completing training were for the most part rather dismal; staff nurses received between £60 and £65 per year, ward sisters between £70 and £76 per year, while assistant matrons earned anything between £75 and £200 and matrons between £70 and £310 a year.[7]

These were some of the discoveries of the report and it made a large number of recommendations on the basis of its analysis, including the introduction of an eight-hour day, the appointment of more ward maids to relieve nurses of domestic duties, the relaxation of discipline in off duty hours, extension of superannuation to all hospitals, improvements to accommodation, and so on. It did not, however, advocate any definite salary scales, nor did it advocate any general improvement in student nurses' salaries. It even advocated that some 'voluntary' hospitals with 'good' training schools should experiment by advertising for students 'without offering remuneration'!

But it was its description of nurses' conditions of existence which received most publicity, rather than its prescriptions. For those anxious to organise nurses in unions, it implicitly indicated the neglect and complacent attitudes of the College of Nursing which, until that time, and even after, insisted that its methods were achieving great improvements for nurses. The College largely represented the leaders of the profession, the matrons who were responsible for defending the very traditional institutions of nursing that had been so much the target of the *Lancet*'s criticisms. If what the *Lancet* report was also arguing was true, and traditional nursing institutions were not necessarily appropriate to standards of care demanded by 'medical progress', then perhaps trade unionism might be more beneficial for nurses and patients alike. Both might benefit from resulting improvements in pay, hours and conditions, and the formation of more self-possessed and better balanced persons, less prepared to accept uncritically the edicts of higher authority, or have their lives entirely limited by the boundaries of hospital walls.

It is hardly surprising also that the report was interpreted in some quarters as an implicitly feminist statement of faith in the new freedoms and independence won by women, and an indictment of the failure of nursing institutions to adjust to them. Evelyn Sharp writing in *Labour Woman* in April 1932, argued as much. However, though the report argued that the hospital authorities must recognise and reconcile the 'basic differences between the traditional and modern outlook on women's work and aspirations', this change had still left women in an inferior position in a male-dominated society. Their role in the labour force was still regarded as a secondary one, just as the *Lancet* report's recommendations still left the nurse in a secondary role to doctors in the division of labour. She might be accorded more trust and responsibility, but she was still firmly subordinated to the doctor.

The revelations of the *Lancet* report also induced the press to expose the conditions under which nurses lived and worked. But newspaper revelations were one thing, results another. With the failure of the College of Nursing to take effective steps, an organisation which, in any case, excluded many from its ranks, including male nurses, fever nurses, children's nurses, mental nurses and assistant nurses – trade unions were increasingly able to harness the growing discontent. An article in the NUCO *Gazette* in May 1932 dismissed the efforts of others on behalf of nurses and drew an important lesson:

> Let nurses get this firmly fixed into their heads: that only by organised effort will they achieve reasonable working conditions and fair salaries.

Public sympathy, argued the article, no matter how widespread, never by itself won a penny for nurses, unless nurses themselves were prepared to utilise it by organising on their own behalf. From the mid-1930s they made the most concerted effort yet seen to obtain their just deserts, aided and (it must also be admitted) partly hindered by the wider labour movement. There were simply too many organisations competing to admit nurses into the ranks of the trade union movement. In addition to the NUCO, the TGWU, the NUGMW, and NUPE were the main TUC unions seeking to recruit nurses, at a time when the NUCO had only recently in 1935 been accepted as a bona fide union and allowed into the fold. But these difficulties were compounded by the activities of NALGO, then outside the TUC, which also made concerted efforts to recruit nurses. Nurses were therefore confused by the lack of unified opposition to the College of Nursing, which blunted the edge of the unions' thrust against them.

Nevertheless the NUCO made some headway in the early 1930s in its efforts to recruit more nurses, forming, in 1933, a medical and nursing section of the union, particularly in the North-East of England, South Wales and London. In London the NUCO faced the additional problems of competing against the management approved LCC Staffs Association, which in May 1933 sought to set up what the NUCO described as a 'dumb organisation' of nurses. The NUCO went ahead with its own campaign, organising a meeting at the Friends' House in April addressed by both Beatrice Drapper, as National Women's Organiser, and Vincent Evans, at which a debate ensued between the platform and some College of Nursing members who had come to defend their organisation.[8]

The NUCO crossed swords with the College again in

1935. In May Cardiff City Council decided, against vigorous protests from the NUCO and Labour members, to reduce student nurses' starting salaries from £35 to £20 a year. During the discussion at the Health Committee, it had been clear that such a move enjoyed the warm approval of the College which had a policy of an £18 minimum, while the NUCO was clear that such a move should be resisted. Throughout the 1930s the College opposed improvements in the pay of student nurses.

Between 1933 and 1936 the NUCO's medical and nursing section was consolidated, but there was no spectacular increase in membership. In 1936, when the medical and nursing sections split and Iris Brook became a 'temporary' paid organiser for nurses, its total membership was still less than 1,000, some 500 of them in London. The chair of the NUCO's section for nurses was the left-wing Pat O'Gorman. Two other registered nurse members of the section, Mr T.O. Morgan from Cardiff, and Doris Westmacott from London, were NEC members.

The report of the section to the February 1936 NEC talks frankly of 'the manifold difficulties we have encountered' in recruiting nurses. However, the three years between 1936 and the outbreak of war saw a dramatic improvement in the union's standing among nurses. The foundations for it had been laid in 1935 by Alderman Hardy who, on behalf of the NUCO, successfully put a resolution to the TUC's Annual Conference in favour of a statutory 48-hour week, with one clear day off in seven, for all hospital and institutional employees. This led to a TUC deputation to the Ministry of Health on 23 July 1936. The subsequent Annual Report of the Chief Medical Officer of Health gave prominence to the working hours of nurses. It urged local authorities to make improvements, on the grounds that it improved nurses' efficiency, and assisted recruitment, but it was against legislative enforcement.

TUC Initiative

In 1937 the TUC seized the initiative. It formed a National Advisory Committee for the Nursing Profession, consisting of unions organising nurses with the object of promoting trade unionism among nurses. These were the MHIWU, the NUCO, the TGWU, the NUGMW and the Women's Public Health Officers Association. In late April Mr Kirkby, the Labour MP for Everton, successfully moved the second reading of a Bill drafted by the TUC, from a NUCO resolution. This would have provided all workers in municipal hospitals and institutions with a statutory 96-hour fortnight or 48-hour week, overtime payments for all hours worked in excess, abolition of the 'spread-over' (split shifts) and one full day's rest a week. Although it would not have applied to voluntary hospitals, informed opinion suggested that they would have been compelled to follow suit or run into considerable difficulties in recruiting staff. True to form, the College of Nursing attacked the Bill, making the rather extra-ordinary assertion in an article in *Nursing Times* that the Bill 'will not be popular with the majority of nurses', but it candidly admitted that 'this goes to show that if we do not put our house in order there are others who will'.

The Limitation of Hours Bill was reintroduced into Parliament during the next session by Fred Messer, a member of the NUCO and Labour MP for Tottenham (South). The Bill fell as it did not enjoy the support of the National government, but only by the slim margin of 122 votes to 111, after the Minister had committed the government to legislation after the publication of the Report of the Athlone Committee that had just been set up to examine and make recommendations regarding the 'recruitment, training and registration and terms and conditions of service of persons engaged in nursing the sick'. Its appointment had been the result of the College's intervention to head off the growing movement for trade unionism among nurses.[9]

The College was particularly worried about the development of the Guild of Nurses, which the nursing section of the NUCO had now become. On 26 November 1937, a week before the Commons debate, the inaugural meeting of the guild had been held before an eager audience of more than 500 nurses at St Pancras Town Hall. George Lansbury, veteran leader of the Labour Party, presided over a procession of speakers, including rank-and-file nurses. The TUC sent 'good wishes' to the new organisation. At the end of the proceedings the meeting passed resolutions in support of the new Nurses' Charter published by the TUC, the Limitation of Hours Bill and an attack on the composition of the newly appointed Athlone Committee for including only one 'working nurse'. It had two members of the nursing establishment and no less than seven doctors. Doris Westmacott said later of the meeting, 'I do not think I have ever seen such enthusiasm,' and there was a 'rush for membership forms at the close of it'.

The publication of the TUC's Nurses' Charter had undoubtedly provided a strong focus for the campaign to establish the guild. It was the product of the TUC's recently established Nursing Advisory Committee, and had eleven points:

1 96-hour fortnight and abolition of 'spread-over' system [split shifts].
2 Enhanced overtime rates and discouragement of time off in lieu.
3 Minimum month's holiday with pay.
4 Minimum sick leave with 13 weeks' full and 13 weeks' half pay.
5 Sickness and disability compensation.
6 Trained nurses to have freedom to choose place of residence, and nurses' home conditions to be fully adequate.
7 Superannuation for all nurses, transferable throughout the service.
8 Abolition of unnecessary restrictions.
9 The creation of a National Council setting standard pay, hours and other conditions, and local consultative committees at hospital level.
10 All probationers to go through preliminary Training Schools before working on the wards.
11 Facilities for higher training in midwifery, massage [physiotherapy], etc.

The union's view of the charter was that:

it was put forward with real concern for the sick, the ailing, the afflicted and in the interests of the nation and the nurses ... It is hoped that it will arouse nurses to organise for these

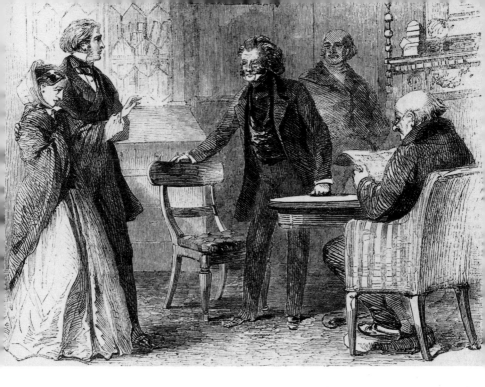

Before the Welfare State: *above* the image: a female asylum patient is gently but firmly introduced; *below* the reality: uniformed warders with a work-gang of patients at Horton Asylum, Epsom, 1907

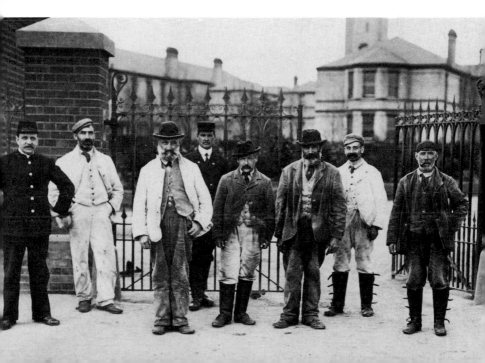

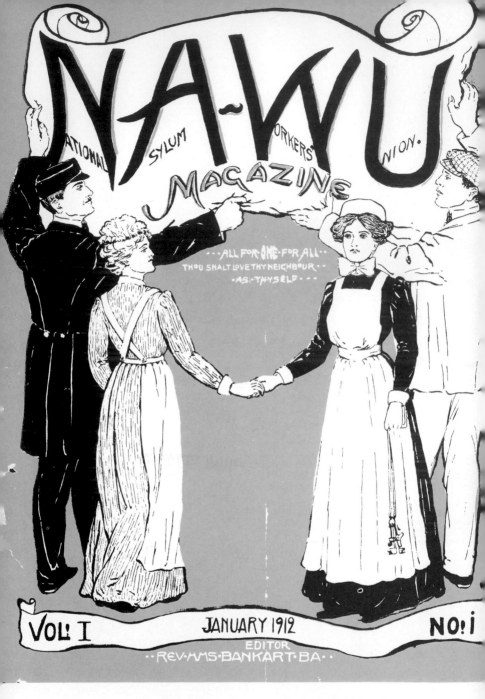

The Union Makes Us Strong: cover of the first issue of the *NAWU Magazine* emphasising the need for unity among all grades of staff, men and women, nurses and non-nurses

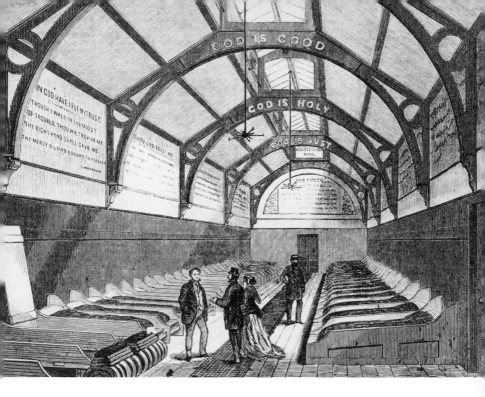

Religion and bare furnishing at the Marylebone workhouse (*above*), and mealtime at the St Pancras Workhouse in 1900 (*below*)

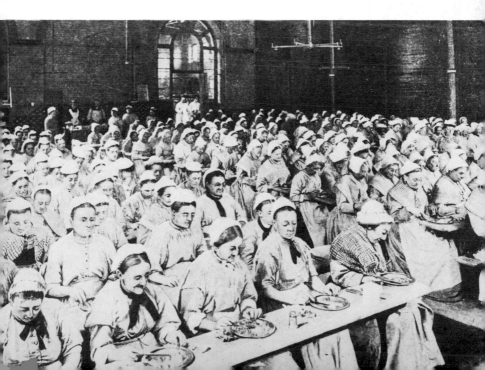

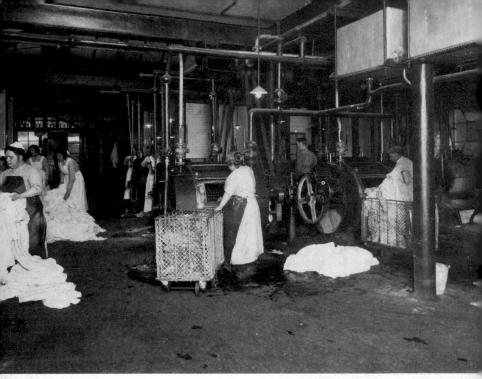

Across the Divide: unlike the professional associations, the National Union of County Officers, like its predecessors, sought to organise all grades of health workers, to improve the gruelling conditions in many laundries (*above*) and to enhance the position of nurses (*below*)

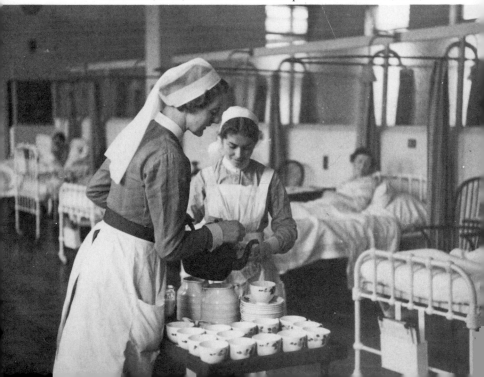

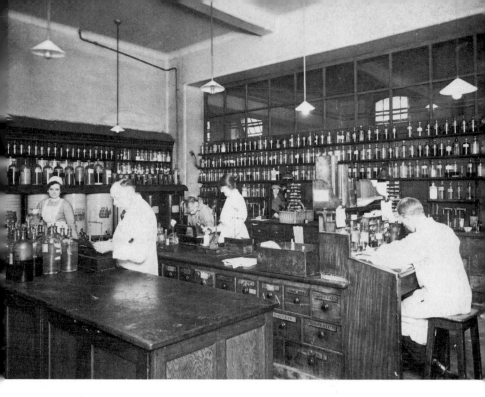

The NUCO also recruited among the new hospital occupations which emerged between the wars, such as those employed in pharmacies (*above*) and the ambulance service (*below*)

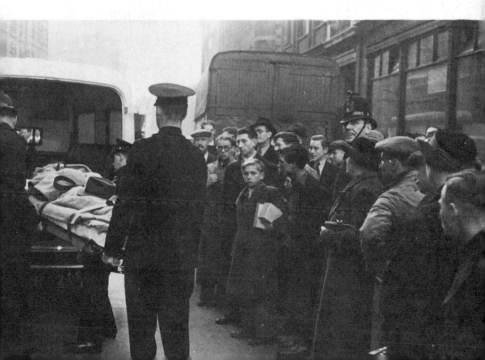

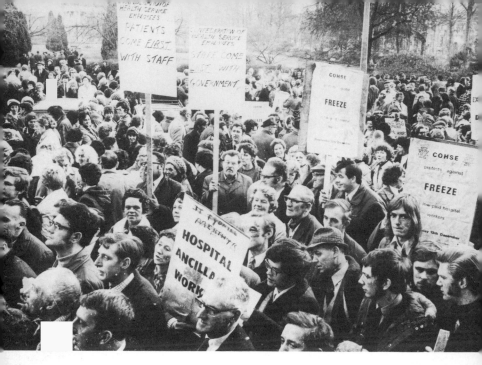

Health Service industrial relations at the crossroads: (*above*) ancilliary workers protest in Cardiff against the 1972 wages freeze and, (*below*), nurses campaign for better wages during the 1974 Halsbury campaign

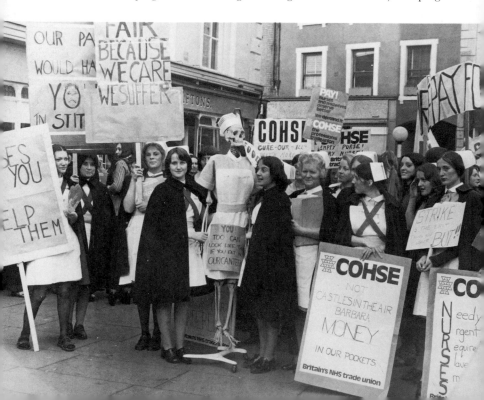

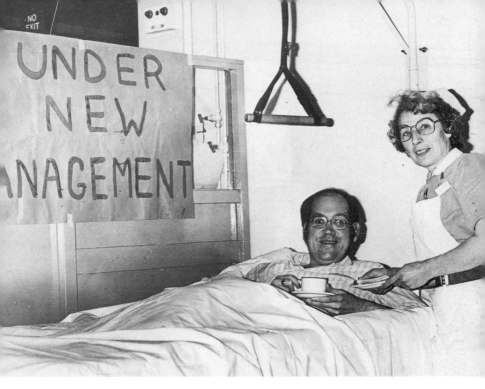

Hospital work-ins, like that at Etwall in Derbyshire (*above*) have helped to defend an increasingly threatened health service; *(below)*, COHSE members in the balcony at the 1982 TUC conference return the ovation they received in support of their 1982 pay campaign

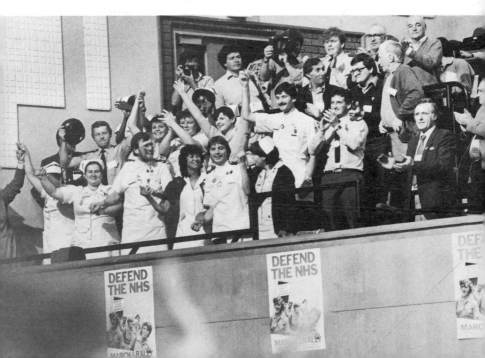

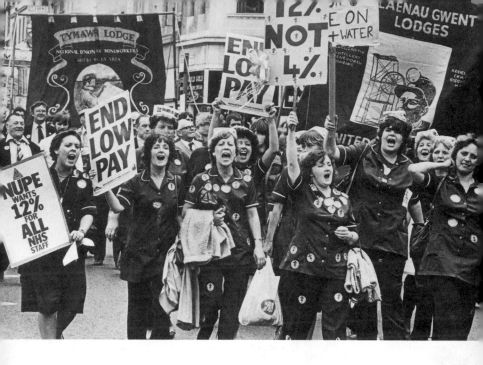

Demonstrating: *above*, during the 1982 low pay campaign and, (*below*), against the Prime Minister's visit to the East Surrey Hospital in 1984

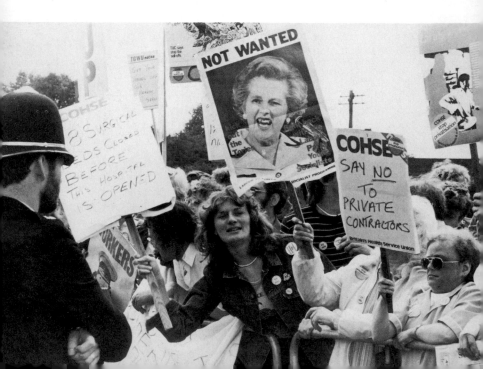

improvements in salary and general conditions of service which alone can make the profession efficient and attractive.

Certainly many of its demands were well ahead of their time. Bold in conception, the charter combined demands for the development of training and education, with traditional trade union demands for improved material conditions and greater democracy in the workplace. On a number of important issues, however, it said nothing, for example on the vexed questions of the relation between State Registered and assistant nurses, and between nurses and doctors. The charter was the occasion for a massive publicity campaign among nurses including the issue of a special booklet entitled *Off-duty*.

The other factor which served to crystalise the growing sense of grievances among nurses was a series of exposé articles in the *Daily Mirror* in November 1937. They were initiated by Dr A. J. Cronin, author of *The Citadel*, which had earlier exposed corruption among Harley Street doctors. He now turned his attention to nursing, which he uncompromisingly described as 'the worst job in the world'. He related the now familiar trials of students and the poor prospects of trained nurses. He declared:

> We must do something about it! ... The myth of Florence Nightingale is dead. It has haunted the nursing profession too long. And to invoke it now in the cause of sweated labour is sheer hypocrisy.[10]

Nursing Times was horrified. Its stated view of the problems faced by nurses was that 'the College is doing all that can be done'. It thought that nurses' grievances were exaggerated. For example:

> Lights out at 10.30 is not really so cruel when one remembers that the probationer must rise at 6.15 at the latest. It is really a kindness to the probationer to pack her off to bed (and incidentally it accounts for her nice complexion).[11]

So it is hardly surprising that it had little sympathy for Dr Cronin's views. Nursing was 'the best job in the world' and 'the work is constant joy in spite of irritations and difficulties'.[12]

But the hundreds of nurses who wrote in at the *Daily Mirror*'s invitation to tell 'nothing but the truth', had in the main rather different stories to tell. One probationer nurse told how she was put in charge of a babies' ward at night, which was put into quarantine when diptheria broke out:

> For 36 nights without a break I was isolated with the babies, and getting very tired. One morning I came off duty and went out for some fresh air – strictly against the rules. I was seen leaving the hospital and reported. As I went on duty that night I was hauled into Matron's office. She was green with fury and I was terrified.[13]

Complaints of restrictions on personal liberty figured highly, especially among trained nurses:

> We women who have reached the age of discretion, and are trusted during the day time with the lives of 30-40 patients and a staff of probationers to train are not allowed to use our own discretion as to what time we come in at night. Even now at my hospital we trained and untrained people have to be in by 10.30 pm. Admittedly we may have a late key, which extends the time to 11 pm. If we are later than that we have to apologise to Matron – SISTER.[14]

The daily grind:

> For breakfast fifteen minutes is allowed. This meal begins at 7 am. If we are five minutes late the door is locked ... For dinner twenty minutes is allowed. We average twelve working hours a day; we have lectures in our off-duty. The commencing salary is £18 for the first year – and reaches £40 in the fourth year! These days of sweated labour leave one with very little desire for social interests – THREE NURSES.[15]

One of the most moving letters of all:

> We do not ask for much. We put up with most things
> because we love nursing, but how much nicer it would be if
> we could be treated as human beings of average intelligence.
> The amount of bullying is amazing and a probationer's life,
> apart from long hours and hard work, is full of squashings,
> until she feels she ought to apologise for breathing. A word of
> praise or encouragement, and we will go on joyfully – but how
> seldom it comes.[16]

These are just samples of the widespread discontent
uncovered by the *Daily Mirror*. What is most striking about
the letters is that very few express discontent with
nursing as such, but rather with the poor pay, conditions
and infringements of personal liberty unnecessarily
associated with it. The opinion of most writers was that
nursing could be 'the best job in the world', if these
blemishes were removed. The influence of these articles in
stimulating nurses to action, and the *Daily Mirror*'s general
support for the campaign to unionise nurses, was publicly
recognised by George Lansbury at the historic St Pancras
Town Hall meeting of 26 November. He

> called for a special vote of thanks for the *Daily Mirror*. 'This
> paper', he said, 'has given us wonderful support. I am sure
> that everyone present will join with me in voting thanks, as we
> owe a great debt of gratitude to the *Daily Mirror* for the
> publicity we have received.'[17]

The Guild of Nurses

The Guild of Nurses was now well and truly launched, and
grew rapidly over the next year, recruiting 3,000
members. Full membership was open to registered nurses,
midwives, student nurses, and masseuses (as physiotherapists were then called). Female assistant nurses and male
nursing orderlies with two years' nursing experience could
now join as associate members. Nurses were grouped into
local branches of the guild, and an annual meeting was
held nationally in February.

The guild was launched by Mrs Drapper, the National

Organising Secretary of the NUCO, and Iris Brook as Assistant Organiser. Doris Westmacott, also a trained nurse and midwife, increasingly became the central figure in the guild, becoming its full-time organiser in 1941, staying with the union until she retired in 1967. She remembered Vincent Evans as a kind man who 'always had time for people'. In persuading people to join the guild she told me:

> It was nearly always based on facts relating to the service, keeping before their eyes the things that could happen if they didn't have an organisation to support them.

The guild had the reputation for being an organisation that nurses could go to if they were in any difficulty. The General Secretary was known as 'Uncle George' and as a sympathetic listener. The male nurses led the way in developing the union. They 'encouraged the fearful' as Doris put it, as nurses were concerned that they might not get good testimonials from the matron. She was also concerned at the effects of long hours and poor conditions, especially night duty, on nurses' health, making them prone to such diseases as tuberculosis, even though the authorities denied it.

The guild could not, of course, immediately transform the poor pay, conditions and infringements of liberty associated with nursing, but it did win improvements. Some of these came about as a result of pressure applied on authorities, particularly those with Labour majorities, to implement the TUC's Nurses' Charter. Thus in February 1938 the union's local organiser, George Esther, persuaded Carlisle Council to reduce hours from 70 to 48 and the other items on the charter were accepted in principle. He also persuaded Durham County Council to implement the charter in full. The union also persuaded other authorities such as Kent, Essex and Middlesex to implement the 48-hour week. The guild also began to win small, but real, improvements in conditions of work at many hospitals. At St James Hospital, Balham, for example, male staff were provided with lockers, while at the LCC South Eastern Hospital, 'the nursing staff now enjoy an alternative dish at their principal meal of the day'.

In other places the guild presented a more direct challenge to management's traditional prerogatives. At Gateshead, seven suspended members of the nursing staff were reinstated. Later in 1938 another suspended nurse was successfully reinstated by Mrs Drapper, which was described as 'another feather in the guild cap'. The most famous disciplinary case fought by the guild at this time, was that of the sister of Ward F2 at Forest Gate Hospital, West Ham, summarily suspended and then dismissed for 'insolence' in February 1938. She had been in dispute with the medical superintendent as to whether she should have communicated information to a woman on the state of her hospitalised baby's health, which the doctor regarded as his prerogative. What was described as 'a titanic fight' followed in which the guild sought and won support from the local Trades Council and from a 'vigilance committee' of local ratepayers. A huge protest meeting was organised at Stratford Town Hall on 14 February 1938, with messages of support read from all grades of health staff in London, and from nurses throughout the country. The town council subsequently decided unanimously to refer the case back to the Public Assistance Committee, and when the sister was eventually reinstated, the guild held a celebration dance on 11 April at the Canning Town Public Hall.

Yet the biggest struggle of all during these years was that fought by the guild with the LCC over two key demands, for the 96-hour fortnight and the abolition of spread-over shifts. Hopes had risen in September 1937 when the TUC Conference adopted the Nurses' Charter, that the Labour-controlled LCC, as the premier local authority in the country, would lead the way by adopting the Charter and implementing the two central demands. This unfortunately did not happen, and the LCC's inaction was used as a powerful argument by opponents of Fred Messer's Limitation of Hours Bill to defeat it in the Commons in December 1937.

The campaign against spread-over hours dated as far back as October 1935, when the NUCO made its first unsuccessful representations to the LCC's Medical Officer of Health as a result of the introduction of new rotas brought in because of a reduction in hours from 56 to 54. Despite being rebutted, the union did not drop the issue. In October 1936, 23 'nurses who are unfortunately AFRAID to sign their names' submitted a lengthy protest which stated that

> there is great unrest amongst the whole staff and we respectfully ask you to look into the matters and remedy them.

Not only was this appeal rejected, but the system was extended to more LCC hospitals. The issue simmered on through 1937, with a lengthy and mainly pointless correspondence which amounted to a refusal by the LCC to see a deputation from the Guild of Nurses. With the lack of formal machinery through which such grievances could be raised, and collectively solved, it seemed that the LCC was hoping that by ignoring nurses' complaints they might go away.

The guild was equally determined not to be deflected from its objectives. It called a protest meeting for 5 April 1938, combining forces also with the Guild of Ambulance and Allied Workers and the NUCO as a whole – since the 48-hour week and spread-over hours did not only affect nurses. On the day before the meeting a small group of masked male nurses paraded in uniform through central London carrying placards with such demands as 'We Demand Fair Play', 'Abolish Spread-Over System'. The following day four male nurses were joined by eight female nurses and a second demonstration was held, acccompanied by a van with a loudspeaker. They were stopped and turned away by police when they tried to march down Fleet Street. The demonstration received massive press and newsreel coverage. A new stage in the history of nursing had begun. For the first time ever, nurses had taken their grievances to the streets.

The 'meeting of protest against the reactionary policy of the London County Council', was held later that evening at 9 pm, at the familiar venue of St Pancras Town Hall.

Some 600 nurses, ambulance and ancillary workers crowded into the hall that evening to listen to speeches and pass resolutions calling for an end to the spread-over system and the introduction of the 48-hour week; the right for trained nurses to live out; the establishment of conciliation machinery for settling grievances among all hospital and institutional staffs; and for full trade union recognition to be accorded to the Guild of Nurses. The meeting enjoyed the warm support of the wider labour movement. The chairman of an unnamed Trades Council said he 'was amazed at the disclosures he heard that evening', and a delegate from the Women's Co-operative Guild said 'that the general public in London should learn the truth'.

The speeches revealed how much the campaign over hours and shift systems was a focus for a much deeper sense of unease and alienation from the employers. The spread-over system was seen as symbolic of the effects of a changed and more bureaucratic system of administration, which was the real target of many criticisms. One nurse said the spread-over system was the result of the 'bugbear of standardisation' of recent years. Another said it was 'a sign of incompetent administration', and complained that the LCC 'quite indifferently ignores our petitions and we have been forced to take drastic action to obtain some redress'. A probationer said:

> Don't talk to us about this spread-over hours of duty. I bet the matron-in-chief doesn't work it, and I jolly well know our matron doesn't work it. I don't blame them, but why push it on us?

One sister told the meeting that while the LCC had spent a great deal of money on new buildings, it had neglected the staff. She also complained that 'The life of a sister today is that of a clerical assistant,' and that 'The welfare of the patients appears to be the last thing that matters.'

Many speakers claimed that authority was also becoming more remote. As County Hall exercised more and more control over individual hospitals, the hospital system was being administered as one huge impersonal bureaucracy:

We have become mere numbers in the machine and although we are the only people who are in a position to really know and understand the working of our particular hospital, we often have to remain silent and carry out the instructions of someone who does not even know where the hospital is situated, let alone what is needed.

All these changes amounted to what the NUCO had referred to as the 'industrialisation' of the service, which an ex-MAB nurse contrasted with life before 1930:

We had no vicious system of spread-over and the staff in the main were happy and contented, for we had a spirit of co-operation between the Matron and her nursing subordinates. The individual members of the Board took a personal interest in the hospital and its staff by visitation and discussion of many issues of interest.

So behind the immediate protest there seemed to be a deeper sense of the loss of a community among staff which was presumed to exist in some previous 'golden age' of nursing, but which was now in the process of decay. The protest movement looked back nostalgically while at the same time calling for a modernisation of nursing's archaic conditions of work. But then all protest movements have their contradictions: the sense of anxiety about the present was real enough, as was the feeling of being let down by a Labour council which had been re-elected in 1937 on the promise to 'finish the job' it had begun in 1934. To be fair, the LCC was trapped in a vicious circle: the rapid expansion of hospital beds in the late 1930s had exacerbated the shortages of the earlier part of the decade. The shortfall in the number of staff nurses, 251 vacancies in June 1935, totalled 454 by June 1937.[18] The hours of staff could not be reduced until more staff were taken on, and the overworking of existing staff, combined with poor pay, unsatisfactory conditions and long hours, ensured that turnover of staff remained high. But the available remedy was there for the LCC, if it wished to use it, through the rates. Unlike some parts of the country, the local economy in the South-East was booming with the rise of industries like engineering and the expansion of office working – which was also, of course, attracting women away from hospital employment.

The LCC finally agreed to see a deputation from the guild on 13 May 1938. It was received by Dan Frankel MP, attended by members of the Hospital and Medical Services Committee, and the Matron-in-Chief, Miss Bannon. The guild's delegation was led by Mrs Drapper. The meeting was not an amicable one. The guild complained that first of all the committee had already made a recommendation to the full council to begin to implement the 96-hour fortnight, end petty restrictions and abolish spread-over hours, from 1 July 1938, *before* receiving the Guild of Nurses delegation. It had, however, received a delegation formed from other trade unions, such as NUPE, which claimed to represent nurses, before coming to its decision. It seems reasonable to presume that the LCC was trying to deny the guild the opportunity of claiming that this was a victory for its militant campaign – which, of course, it was.

The guild's deputation then proceeded to press, in detail, the resolutions passed at St Pancras Town Hall on the evening of 5 April. Its written submission detailed the kind of recognition it expected for a union with over 1,800 nurse members at LCC hospitals, such as the right to invite organisers to meetings held on hospital premises and to collect subscriptions in off-duty time without 'being regarded as agitators'. It wanted the right to wear guild badges on duty. It accused managers of keeping notes on nurses' union activities in their work records. It called on the council to allow all trained nurses to live out, since otherwise 'a sister cannot obtain that change of atmosphere which is so essential to the maintenance of health, physically and mentally'. It demanded machinery for the resolution of grievances. It wanted 'ration allowances' for staff on their days off, 'if we are away from hospital for a whole day we are paying for our food twice over'. It put forward a variety of other demands, such as the improvement of sports and social amenities. Dan Frankel gave the LCC's immediate response, which (according to the Guild's notes of the meeting), was to reject the guild's suggestion that records were kept of individual nurses' union activities. He launched into an attack on the NUCO, which had, he said, 'behaved in a disgraceful manner', and said that the submission 'was the most impertinent ever presented to a public body'. He instructed the guild to 'learn the first essentials of trade union negotiations'.

The LCC went ahead with its proposals for a 96-hour fortnight and abolition of split duties, which would involve the recruitment of an extra 1,000 additional staff at a cost of £123,000 a year.[19] It seemed that, under the twin pressures of staff shortages and militant trade unionism, the ghost of Florence Nightingale was finally beginning to be laid. By December 1938 sufficient nurses had been recruited to bring in the 96-hour fortnight in 44 of the LCC's 76 hospitals, with the remainder to follow shortly. But ghosts are not laid at one attempt. Nor did the guild make much progress on the other questions contained in its submission of 12 May 1938. The LCC would not extend the recognition asked for by the guild, nor would it make any commitment to the establishment of collective grievance machinery, alter its policy regarding residence of trained staff, allow nurses to wear guild badges or receive payment for casual meals not taken. Progress had been made, but there was still much to do if nursing was to be dragged into the modern age.

Athlone Reports

Perhaps the Athlone Committee, which had been continuing its work through all this activity, might complete the task? After all, the Ministry of Health was apparently worried about nurses 'going socialist' and joining unions 'which they are really reluctant to do'.[20] The committee did not report until 1939. Many of its recommendations closely followed the TUC's charter, including the 96-hour fortnight and the formation of a national negotiating body for setting pay and conditions. The committee also recommended universal and interchangeable pensions, and the training and certification of a second grade of nurse, the assistant nurse. There was little on offer to the probationer nurse in terms of increased pay, but the Athlone Committee did recommend government financial assistance to voluntary hospitals to meet the costs of any pay increase to trained staff. A minority of four on the committee was even prepared to suggest that this financial assistance be extended to the municipal hospitals. After a deputation from the TUC, the government's response was to encourage local authorities to make those improvements that were possible without extra expenditure, but to turn down flat any suggestion that they should interfere in the setting of wages for professionals. After all, the committee had served its purpose. Just enough MPs had been persuaded to vote against the Limitation of Hours Bill 1937, the reputation of the College had been rescued and militancy among nurses was finally beginning to die down. When the war came the focus shifted elsewhere. The work of the Athlone Committee, originally anticipated as a continuing programme of investigations, was halted.

The guild's last major protests of the 1930s took place in November 1939. With the outbreak of war the authorities took the economy measure of ceasing to resort to nursing co-operatives, i.e. agencies, as a means of meeting shortages. Some assistant nurses were offered resident posts, but many were thrown out of work. A vigorous protest meeting was held on 16 November with good attendance 'despite the teeming rain'. As a result of a war-time 'economy measure' at Paddington 30 non-resident deputy sisters (a new grade recently brought in by the LCC) were asked to become resident. Eleven of those who refused found themselves without jobs.

Those protests were not effective, however, and the 1930s closed on a note of disappointment for the guild. It had had its successes in London and the North of England, and recruited several thousand nurses, but nationally regulated pay and conditions seemed as far away as ever, and the guild was also learning, as had the PLWTU, that it was easier to recruit than retain members. As an article in the *Gazette* in September 1937 put it, nurses 'are like weather cocks. They change like the wind.' The 29,000-strong Royal College of Nursing had, partly by means of clever footwork, taken the sting out of the union's attack. It continued to be assisted by the fact that, as Ferguson and Fitzgerald put it, nursing was an hierarchical occupation in which 'the voice of organised nursing is largely the voice of those in the higher ranks.'[21]

This system worked for the College and against the unions, but for the first time an effective challenge had been made to its seemingly eternal structures, and it had begun to crumble.

For its members, the guild provided a forum for democratic representation and free expression of views, denied them in the normal course of their employment. The idea of a totally autonomous guild may have partly encouraged sectionalism and the sense of superiority among its members (although in 1938 it campaigned for reductions in hours for *all* staffs). The guild's autonomous structure did, however, give members a degree of self-government that was non-existent in the College and extremely rare elsewhere in the male-dominated trade union movement. In the process it had changed forever what the guild called the 'slaves of the lamp' image of selfless subordinated angels, whom both the public and the profession's leaders had put on pedestals. A new and more insistent demand had arisen from among nurses themselves to be, as George Lansbury had put it, 'treated as ordinary people'. It was one which would not go away, but would grow in intensity in the years yet to come.

Notes

[1] 'Not a Nurses' Bill', *Nursing Times*, 28 February 1931.
[2] *Nursing Times*, 28 November 1931.
[3] Lewenhak, *Women and Trade Unions*, Ch. 13.
[4] *MHIWU Journal*, July 1932.
[5] *Nursing Times*, 11 June 1932.
[6] Abel-Smith, *Nursing Profession*, Ch. 8.
[7] Lancet, *Commission on Nursing: Final Report* (1932).
[8] *County Officers Gazette*, 5 May 1933.
[9] See S. Ferguson and H. Fitzgerald, *Studies in the Social Services* (1954), Ch. 9.
[10] *Daily Mirror*, 3 November 1937.
[11] *Nursing Times*, 13 March 1937.
[12] Ibid., 8 November 1937.

[13] 'Nurses' Platform', *Daily Mirror*, 15 November 1937.
[14] Ibid., 29 November 1937.
[15] Ibid.
[16] Ibid., 10 November 1937.
[17] Ibid., 27 November 1937.
[18] *MHIWU Journal*, September-October 1937.
[19] *Nursing Times*, 14 May 1938.
[20] Ferguson and Fitzgerald, op. cit.
[21] Ibid.

Chapter 15
The Coming of Health Service Unionism

The Second World War placed heavy burdens upon health workers. Chronic shortages of many grades of staff persisted throughout the war, while those in cities affected by bombing sometimes worked under pressures hard for us to imagine now. The War also tested the union's organisation in other less extreme ways. While the normal business of representing members continued, the officials also had to cope with the extra work caused by the shift towards nationally determined pay and conditions, as well as responding to moves to create a National Health Service after the war – and campaigning to make sure the government implemented it. And if that was not enough, in the final years of the war close attention had to be paid to complex and difficult negotiations with the MHIWU, to achieve an amalgamation of the two organisations to form one Confederation of Health Service Employees.

With the outbreak of war, the union's structure was immediately streamlined. The NEC decided to meet only twice a year, and much of the union's business was conducted by an Emergency Committee of the three Areas in London and the South-East. Lionel Lunn remained President but never attended meetings, apparently finding the journey from Burton-on-Trent too daunting. In 1941 Doris Westmacott took over from Iris Brook as the Guild of Nurses Organiser. In the regions Bill Griffiths took over the Midlands and Wales, while Joe Richards was appointed to cover East Anglia. In 1944, W.J. Jepson took over from Councillor Webster in

Sheffield. Frank Lynch became an assistant to Ted Hardy in the North-West. Of these, Jepson and Richards and Lynch were to become future General Secretaries of COHSE, while Bill Griffiths was later a leading official in NUPE. Wartime conditions may have been stressful and demanding, but they must also have provided a good apprenticeship for the rising generation of union officials.

Membership increased steadily if not spectacularly during the war years, to reach 15,000 by 1945. At the same time the union was beginning to recruit health staffs outside the local government field. The Voluntary Hospitals Guild, under its organiser Fred Rason, had by February 1943 established 26 branches at London voluntary hospitals. It found, ironically, that the employers were more prepared to recognise and deal with the union than the LCC, as there were no other trade unions competing for recognition in that sector or any established bargaining machinery. In London there continued the long running battle between the NUCO, the LCC and unions it recognised. Elsewhere special sub-committees of NJIC Provincial Councils were set up to deal with the pay and conditions of health staffs, which made themselves accessible to the NUCO. Paradoxically, London was both the NUCO's strongest and weakest region, and thus had everything to gain from the development of national bargaining. This was in contrast with the MHIWU, which stood to lose its exclusive bargaining rights over mental nurses. Perhaps this was one reason why the NUCO became a much more forward looking union in the war than its partner in the COHSE amalgamation. One sign of this was a long overdue change of title to the Hospitals and Welfare Services Union (HWSU) in 1943.

Towards the Nurses' and Midwives' Whitley Council

The first government moves towards national bargaining for health workers were taken with the aim of relieving immediate shortages of particular grades of staff, in the first instance of nurses, and later the other grades of staff. It was not until the end of the war that permanent machinery for collective bargaining began to be established as part of a wider government commitment to establishing a National Health Service.

In August 1939 an Emergency Medical Service was created in order to prepare the health services to cope with the expected effects of the bombing of civilians in the coming war. Central government commandeered the public and voluntary hospitals, and made finance available to improve equipment and buildings. Doctors (who had to be prepared to be directed where they were needed) were recruited, and were to receive between £450 and £1,500 a year. These scales represented a big increase in pay for junior staff and the first ever uniform national pay scales in the history of the health service. The next most urgent step was to recruit the large number of trained nurses required by the scheme, which the Ministry of Health estimated to be between 34,000 and 67,000, at a time when there were only 60,000 registered nurses in the country. It was therefore decided to recruit as many trained nurses as possible and fill the gaps by recruiting untrained 'auxiliaries'. A Civilian Nursing Reserve was set up which had recruited approximately 10,000 experienced and 10,000 inexperienced nurses by the outbreak of war.[1]

The creation of a Civil Nursing Reserve was not associated with any immediate improvement in nurses' wages and conditions. The appeal to non-employed registered and assitant nurses, and those prepared to be trained as auxiliaries, was almost entirely directed towards their sense of national duty. Shortages persisted, but the health service coped because air-raid casualties were never as great as was orginally feared. The most serious problems were experienced by the general civilian services for the sick. With so many beds set aside for casualty services, sick people often found they could not get treatment. Rates of tuberculosis soared in wartime conditions, exacerbating existing staff shortages due to the work's general unpopularity and its location in remote sanatoria.[2] Such considerations eventually led the government to take action, but only under concerted pressure from the TUC Advisory Committee on the Nursing Profession, which spoke of 'the chaos and resentment which is apparent in the profession'. It had demanded pay rises and the establishment of a Salaries Committee. The immediate line of action for the Ministry lay through its authority over those hospitals participating in the Emergency Medical Service, nearly 2,400 of the total of 3,000 in the country. In April 1941 the Ministry urged the EMS hospitals to pay a minimum of £60 a year for assistant and £95 a year for trained nurses, and promised financial help to the voluntary hospitals to meet the increases. The government also committed itself to the formation of a Salaries Committee. Probationers were offered £40 a year, no greater in real terms (due to the rising cost of living) than they had been receiving before the war in municipal hospitals. Even so, as might be expected, the RCN expressed the view that the new rates for students 'were too high and did not take into account the cost of the expensive professional training'.

Both the British Hospitals Association (representing employers in the voluntary hospitals) and the RCN fought a determined rearguard action against the setting up of a Salaries Committee: the BHA because it felt that it would encourage trade unionism among nurses, the RCN because it had been trying since the late 1930s to establish a Local Authorities Nursing Services Joint Committee with NALGO. This only delayed the formation of the committee until November 1941, when the Minister set up the Salaries Committee for England and Wales under Lord Rushcliffe; a similar body under Lord Taylor was set up for Scotland. Its original brief was only to deal with the question of salaries, though under pressure from nurses' organisations the terms of reference were subsequently widened to include other conditions of work.

The Rushcliffe Committee did not, in any real sense, constitute national bargaining machinery on Whitley Council lines. Nevertheless, it was divided into employer and employee 'panels', and nurses' organisations were invited to nominate members. Despite its long standing opposition to government 'interference' in the setting of nurses' salaries, the RCN swallowed its pride and succeeded in winning more seats on the new body than any other organisation. In so doing, its leadership demonstrated yet again an ability to adapt its principles when its credibility as an organisation was at stake.

The Rushcliffe Committee Report

In 1943 there were two events of importance to the future development of nursing. First, the Nurses Act was passed, giving assistant nurses a statutory existence and admission to a 'Roll' if not a 'Register' of the General Nursing Council (GNC) after two years' training (following the final acquiescence of the RCN). They were not, however, to have access to higher posts in the nursing world. Secondly, in February the Rushcliffe Committee finally reported, nearly two years after the Minister first announced its setting up. Its recommendations largely followed those of the Athlone Committee in 1939, which in turn were based on those originally advocated in the TUC's Charter for Nurses. Trained staff were to receive substantial increases; entrance fees for student nurses were to be abolished; night duty was to be limited to six months a year for trained staff and three months for students; sick leave for staff with two or more years' service was to be 13 weeks on full and 13 weeks on half pay; nurses were to have one complete day off a week and 28 days' leave with pay each year.

Though the TUC can claim credit for many of the advances made through the Rushcliffe Report, not least the fact that it was the first ever national award to nurses, the influence of the RCN may be seen in two of the least satisfactory aspects of the Rushcliffe award. Student nurses were to be given no more than the £40 a year offered by the Ministry in 1941, and a 96-hour fortnight was to be introduced only 'as conditions permit', at a date to be determined by the Minister of Health. The Guild of Nurses produced a critical commentary on these and other aspects of the Rushcliffe Committee's recommendations. It claimed that the committee's inability to deal effectively with the question of hours was due primarily to the RCN's dominance on the Employees' Panel, the staff side of the committee. Even if a reduction in hours could not be granted because of shortages, it argued, nurses ought still to be paid for hours worked in excess of 96 in a fortnight. It attacked the recommendations on pay for being biased in favour of grades above staff nurse and ward sister. As for the derisory scales offered to students, they do

> not amount to reasonable 'pocket money' for the modern girl
> ... It is significant that the people who proclaim loudest that a
> student nurse does not seek a higher salary all come from the
> ranks of the 'higher-ups' in the profession.[3]

While the RCN justified low pay because a student nurse received a 'valuable training', the Guild of Nurses argued that it should be recognised that she 'forms an imporant part of the nursing staff'.

The Rushcliffe Committee recommendations were accepted by the government and rapidly implemented. Hospitals paying the new scales received half the cost of increased expenditure from the Ministry, and from April 1943 all those aged between 17 and 60 with some nursing experience during the previous ten years were compelled to register with the Ministry of Labour. Restrictions were placed on nurses aged between 18 and 40 in civilian employment enlisting in the armed services, and the Ministry of Labour took over nursing appointments. At the same time, an extensive publicity campaign was launched to gain recruits. Angled towards middle-class young women, its slogan was 'The War-Time Job Which Can be a Career'.

These controls were maintained until 1946, and the Ministry of Labour directed women into priority fields, such as chronic sick and tuberculosis nursing. The Rushcliffe recommendations had not been sufficiently generous or bold enough, however, and shortages persisted and continued after the war. Nevertheless the principle of national determination of pay and conditions long fought for by the trade union movement had finally been won.

Ironically, the chief beneficiary was the RCN, whose dominance on the Rushcliffe Committee foreshadowed its later domination of the Nurses' and Midwives' Whitley Council, under the National Health Service. Though unions were strong enough to force the reluctant RCN to adopt a trade union role, they were not sufficiently powerful to relegate it to the wings, especially since the RCN had grown in numerical strength during the war, from approximately 30,000 in 1939 to 41,500 in 1946. Membership of its associated Student Nurses' Association had also risen in the same period from 7,500 to 12,700.[4] The RCN had recovered from the stagnation caused by the militant trade union campaigns of the 1930s and learnt lessons from it, such as establishing a Labour Relations Committee in 1938.

Other Health Workers

Nurses were by far the largest occupational group, but the recruitment and organisation of other grades of staff was also profoundly affected by wartime conditions. We have already heard in Chapter 9 of the shortages of domestics in mental hospitals, and in fact such shortages were widespread in all types of hospitals. As the official history of the war commented:

> Few women who had a chance of finding other employment were prepared to accept domestic posts in hospitals ... Many women preferred as their war service to do what could be called a man's job rather than domestic work, which was always their particular domain.[5]

The government was much less willing to improve the pay and conditions of hospital domestics, simply issuing them with a special badge and recruiting from Southern Ireland and among Belgian refugees. Such measures were largely ineffective, and consequently standards of ward cleanliness fell, and the quality of catering also suffered as a result of shortages in kitchen staff. By the middle of 1943 there were an estimated 8,000 vacancies. The government needed a reason to justify direction of labour, and in July 1943 Ernest Bevin, the Minister of Labour and National Service, appointed a three person committee under Sir Hector Hetherington to look into the pay and conditions of female domestic workers in hospitals, institutions and the school meals service. The HWSU was quick off the mark and presented detailed evidence which called for a substantial improvement in the pay, conditions and status of domestics and non-nursing staffs in hospitals. It was virtually a manifesto for such staff in the future National Health Service. The union described its evidence as the 'Hospital Workers' Charter' and urged workers to join the HWSU in order to unify forces and 'prepare to fight' for it.

The charter focused not just on pay and conditions of domestic workers, but ranged much more widely in its recommendations than the terms of reference given the committee by Ernest Bevin, or than its members were prepared to go. For example, the union argued that portering and maintenance staff ought to have been included since shortages for these groups were just as severe. It demanded a 48-hour week, and enhanced rates for unsocial hours and for working in TB sanatoria, and compulsory superannuation for all staff. It also made imaginative suggestions to improve the status and career prospects of non-nursing staff, and it called for the systematic training of staff and the award of 'proficiency certificates' for those successfully completing them.

The report of the Hetherington Committee in November 1943 was a disappointing document. It resisted the HWSU's invitation to go beyond its specific and narrow terms of reference, and only made recommendations with regard to certain grades of female domestics, excluding those already covered by existing agreements, such as NJIC Provincial Councils. The committee introduced a new, simplified 'nomenclature' along with their suggested 'minimum' scales (which were inclusive of a cost-of-living element): non-resident cooks were to receive £3 5s a week, assistant cooks £3 0s, special maids, e.g. for doctors' residences, £2 17s 6d, general maids £2 15s and cleaners £2 12s 6d.

It endorsed the 48-hour week and suggested that hours in excess should be paid at time and a quarter, but it did not favour extra payment for Sundays or Bank holidays since 'work on these days is inevitable and is the accepted principle'.[6] It offered a paltry one week's holiday, and nine weeks' full and nine weeks' half sick-pay, a year.

The HWSU's response to the Hetherington Report was

caustic, describing it as a thinly veiled excuse for direction of labour, complaining that its 'minimum' rates – which inevitably would become 'maximum' ones – were lower than those negotiated by Provincial Councils and other local authorities. It accused the committee of setting rates low enough so as not to embarrass the voluntary hospitals, and it objected above all to a nominated committee rather than one which, like the Rushcliffe Committee, sought more fairly to represent workers' and employers' organisations.[7]

As expected, in November the Minister of Labour immediately accepted the Hetherington Report as a basis for directing domestic labour to the hospitals. However, in contrast to the policy followed by nurses, the government was not prepared to provide municipal or voluntary hospitals with any financial assistance in order to implement the award. The Minister simply directed labour to those hospitals paying the new minimum rates. He did decide to appoint a Standing Committee to look into matters of suitable training, prospects of advancement and proper welfare arrangements for female domestic workers, rather than for all non-nursing support staff as advocated by the HWSU. A golden opportunity was thus lost and, not surprisingly, chronic shortages persisted.

The best hopes for improvement lay in the achievement of national bargaining for all support staff. Although other unions, especially NUPE, were strongly in favour of national uniformity in their pay and conditions, the HWSU's action helped to speed up its arrival. In 1943 it put a resolution to the TUC's Annual Conference calling for the union's representation on the NJIC for Local Government Non-Trading Services, claiming that the main unions represented on it 'have for years frozen this organisation out'. Delegates recognised the justice of the NUCO's case when, despite the opposition of the 'big batallions', the demand for inclusion was approved on a card vote, by a two million majority. A high level meeting of General Secretaries was held at Transport House in December 1943, attended by Vincent Evans for the union, Arthur Deakin (TGWU), Bryn Roberts (NUPE) and Jack

Cooper (NUGMW), and chaired by W.P. Allen on behalf of the TUC General Council.

Bryn Roberts suggested that rather than admit the HWSU to the existing machinery, alternative and entirely separate machinery could be quickly established, given that the government was now committed to the establishment of a separate National Health Service. Evans agreed with the chairman that this fulfilled the spirit of the union's TUC resolution.[8]

With involvement from the Ministry of Labour, the National Joint Council for Staff of Hospitals and Allied Institutions was finally established by the end of October 1945, representative of both employing bodies (including the British Hospitals Association), and all unions with a significant number of members. Its scope included ambulance personnel, but excluded clerical and administrative staff. The first task set was to establish minimum rates of pay.

Ambulance Services Guild

The other major campaign on behalf of health workers was conducted by the HWSU's Ambulance Services Guild, which grew in strength during the Second World War. As might be imagined, the ambulance service was a key element in civil defence during the war. Before it a rather chaotic system had existed, with responsibility for the general ambulance service split between local authorities and voluntary associations such as the Order of St John and the British Red Cross Society, leading to frequent disputes over spheres of responsibility. In London this was further complicated by the fact that London boroughs outside the Administrative County of the LCC maintained their own ambulance services. On the recommendations of a series of reports by the Francis Committee that voluntary and public services should be unified under local authority control, this was finally put into effect by the Air Raid Precautions Act in 1937. The integration of services was not a smooth process, partly because the uniformed voluntary services resented their loss of independence, but more seriously because of the lack of standard equipment – stretchers, for example, were often not interchangeable between ambulances.

In 1939, local authorities expanded their ambulance services, chiefly by buying and converting second-hand vehicles, with financial assistance from central government. Cars were often used for patients able to sit, with larger vehicles reserved for stretcher cases. In addition to local authority services, the Ministry of Health, through the Emergency Medical Service and its regional organisations, ran a fleet of hospital trains for long distance evacuation of hospital patients from large cities, and to carry wounded service personnel, as well as ambulance coaches for local inter-hospital evacuation. In London this consisted of a fleet of 250 converted Green Line coaches.

Although ambulance work was originally a reserved occupation, controls were subsequently relaxed and many pre-war employees left for more remunerative employment, or were called up. The Ministry laid down plans for a service of 129,600 drivers and attendants early in 1939. Its original intention had been for a service entirely staffed by women, but it quickly relaxed this requirement. Recruitment by the end of 1939 had not reached near the target figures: the service consisted of 26,000 full-time and 54,000 part-time men and women.[9] There were also serious shortages in the other main division of civil defence work, the stretcher parties working from first aid posts. Earnings were poor, the work was unpopular and the service relied increasingly on part-timers and unpaid volunteers. The strain on the remaining permanent staff undoubtedly intensified, as the official history of the war acknowledges, also paying tribute to their heroism.[10]

The Ambulance Services Guild, with justification, accused the government of complacency over the state of ambulance services for civilian casualties. A deputation to the Minister of Health in March 1942 protested at the half-hearted direction of the EMS, and urged the creation of a nationalised ambulance service to be administered on a tripartite basis by Ministry of Health representatives, those of employers' associations and the TUC. It also called for the implementation of the Guild's National Ambulance Charter including national rates of pay and conditions, and state registration for ambulance workers. The union claimed that the 'cinderella' ambulance services were 'nobody's baby' administered in part by the Ministry of Health and the Home Office. It drew the Minister's attention to the fact that since 1941 a National Fire Service had been created, and claimed that this showed that the government was more interested in safeguarding property than lives. Its demands were flatly refused.

The union made better progress through the TUC, though not without some difficulty. The HWSU put a resolution to it in 1943 calling for a nationalised ambulance service, including state registration. This was referred to the General Council on the intervention of Dorothy Elliot of the NUGMW (who was also a member of the Hetherington Committee), ostensibly because it 'contained a great deal of detail' which should be the subject of consultation between the parties concerned.[11] The union nevertheless continued to press its militant campaign on behalf of ambulance staffs. It was particularly insistent that the ambulance services should be included in the post-war National Health Service and it received support from many quarters, including the *Lancet*[12] and Mr Willink, the Minister of Health in the Coalition Government[13]. Eventually the TUC's Local Government Committee was forced to accept that the ambulance service should form part of the post-war NHS, with provision of effective joint machinery for 'wages, conditions and status', despite the misgivings of other unions that this would mean recognising claims to representation by the HWSU. However, as we shall see in a subsequent chapter, the battle for a national ambulance service was far from won.

A New Beginning

The HWSU had set about the task of creating policies for the future with imagination and commitment. It could claim with some justification that, as a result of its 'specialist' character, it was far ahead of the trade union movement as a whole in developing a longer term strategy to enhance the position of all groups of staff within the

promised NHS. It also took the initiative in campaigning
for a democratic system of administration within the
proposed service, and recognised more than most that
vested interests in the labour movement stood in the way
of achieving the unity necessary to see that campaign to a
successful conclusion. Out of this realisation came its
determination to work towards the creation of one union
for all health service staffs.

We have seen how the idea of one union for the health
service dates back to the period just after the First World
War, when the Health Services Federation enjoyed a brief
life after the Ministry of Health was first created. At that
time the two largest participants, the NAWU and the
PLWTU, came close to amalgamation, but drew back at
the last moment and went their separate ways as
government plans for reconstruction in health and social
services collapsed. In the late 1930s the idea of a
federation was revived again. Following the TUC's
adoption of the Nurses' Charter in 1937, the NUCO and
the Women Public Health Officers' Association formed a
federation with the MHIWU in December of the same
year. The possible establishment of a state health service
was yet again cited as one of the major reasons. Another
was the attempt to reduce unnecessary competition for
nurses between TUC-affiliated organisations. NUPE,
however, was not party to these moves.

The first meeting of the federation was held on 7 April
1938, at St Pancras Town Hall, with George Gibson in the
chair. The meeting adopted 'an immediate charter of
essentials' which included: improved rates of pay, shorter
hours, the choice to live out, adequate superannuation and
sick pay for all employees, protective clothing for ancillary
and maintenance staff and the establishment of a Whitley
Council. Power was vested in the federation's National
Executive Committee to pursue these demands. In
practice, however, the federation did not assume the
powers theoretically vested in it. Each organisation
jealously guarded its autonomy, and although local
branches of the federation were formed, problems
occurred with existing branches of federated organisations when the federation sought here and there to do

more than organise rallies. In November 1940 the
MHIWU pulled out of the federation on the grounds that
it no longer served any purpose.

The NUCO responded by exploring the question of
amalgamation, but did not get very far. Negotiations
dragged on until, in January 1943, the NUCO declared
itself in favour of one union for the health service, arguing
that with so many organisations it was not possible to speak
with a unified voice. By March 1943 the MHIWU was
apparently in agreement with this view, for a joint
conference of the two organisations declared that 'closer
association ... leading to ultimate amalgamation is not only
desirable but essential', especially 'having regard to the
possibilities of prospective legislation'. The negotiations
continued, and as a first step along the road, the NUCO
transformed itself into the Hospitals and Welfare Services
Union.

Events had now propelled the MHIWU back into closer
liaison with the HWSU. Most important among them was
the publication, late in 1942, of the Beveridge Report on
Social Insurance and Allied Services, which the NUCO's
Executive had immediately and enthusiastically supported, not least because one of its central proposals was
for a National Health Service.

The HWSU had become a much more politically
conscious union, despite remaining unaffiliated to the
Labour Party, with a forward-looking outlook. The
HWSU's attempted balancing act between the sectionalism
of the guilds and, at the same time, a commitment of belief
in one union for all health service staffs had a very potent
appeal to radical professional workers at the time. Many
leading activists in the Medical Services Guild were also
prominent in the Socialist Medical Association (SMA)
which had been formed in 1930 for the very purpose of
obtaining a National Health Service:[14] Dr Charles Brook
was a founder member of the SMA, while Dr H.B. Morgan
was also a leading advisor to the TUC's influential Social
Insurance Committee. Lily Mitchell, a leading member of
the Voluntary Hospitals Guild, and one of the growing
number of hospital pharmacists joining the union, was the
HWSU's actual delegate to the SMA. The HWSU was also

the union favoured by Communist Party health workers, as Dr Cyril Taylor, then a member, told me.

The Ambulance Services Guild also had a strong left 'feel' to it. Like doctors and pharmacists, ambulance workers also looked forward optimistically to the future, regarding themselves similarly as 'professionals' whose mission could only be fulfilled within the context of a socialist health service. That did not mean that they had illusions that such possibilities would fall into their laps. The 'brave new world' after the war would have to be struggled for, as the Ambulance Services Guild declared in a New Year message for 1944.

For such radical professionals, the HWSU seemed to open up the possibility of uniting staff to form an organisation powerful enough to challenge the British Medical Association, and prevent any efforts it might make to sabotage or dictate the terms upon which the NHS was introduced, against the interests of working-class people.

The first step in this campaign was a successful resolution put by the NUCO to the TUC Annual Conference in 1942, prior to the publication of the Beveridge Report, which called on the government to take full central control of hospitals, ambulance and first aid services to meet wartime needs, and to extend and develop this as 'a post-war policy'. The motion called for both national pay and conditions and a 'democratically elected' system of administration.[15] In 1943 the campaign to implement the Beveridge Report began in earnest, as HWSU branches lobbied MPs to protest at any delay in adopting its proposals. To fight for the NHS, a Health Workers' Council was set up with the help of the SMA in July 1943. Its aim was 'the maintenance and improvement of the national health', and included not only health unions – the HWSU, MHIWU and NUPE, together with the SMA – but also professional associations such as the Association of Psychiatric Social Workers, the Association of Speech Therapists, the Society of Radiographers, the Society of Physiotherapists and others. On this occasion they saw their fate as linked with that of the labour movement, but sadly it was not to prove a durable alliance.

The council campaigned for the introduction of a 'comprehensive, unified health service' in which all medical skills and resources were pooled 'without any economic reservations', at the same time as calling for good conditions of employment for workers to ensure they 'are able to devote themselves to the betterment of the service through security and good economic conditions, with leisure for study and recreation'.[16]

These and other pressures eventually bore some fruit, as in 1944 the coalition government brought out a White Paper which committed it to the introduction of a NHS after the war. The proposals of Mr Willink, the Minister of Health, were a compromise: between Labour and Conservative members in the coalition Cabinet, and between the various vested interests (the medical profession, voluntary hospitals and local authorities), but they did commit the government to the principle of a free and comprehensive service for the whole nation, and this was a considerable step forward.[17] The Health Workers' Council gave 'an enthusiastic welcome to the proposals' even though they 'differ somewhat from those which the Council would like to see adopted', but the HWSU's response was less sanguine. It was disappointed that the document had only proposed a 'medical treatment service' rather than a 'comprehensive health service' and that the Minister had not consulted trade unionists in the service who were in daily contact with the people using it:

> They know what they want. They bear their complaints and grievances. They know the weakness of the present system.[18]

The HWSU called on all health workers to unite in one union and in 1944 put a historic motion to the 1944 TUC, which was ultimately adopted, supporting the principle of a free and comprehensive service, with health centres as its cornerstone, and urging the General Council to

> take such steps as are necessary to ensure full democratic control of the National Health Service, in order that the interests of all engaged in the service may be safeguarded, and bureaucratic rigidity avoided.[19]

The 1944 White Paper itself was never implemented, for with the war in Europe at an end, a general election was called for 5 July 1945. The HWSU finally came off the fence and urged its members to vote Labour, even though a number of members of the Guild of Nurses – who had become a rather subdued grouping within the union, apparently less affected by the new radicalism than other health workers – resigned in protest. The strength of the union's political commitment was evident in the fact that it sponsored five of its members as Labour candidates in the election, three of whom were elected: Fred Messer, Dr H.B. Morgan and Ted Hardy; the MHIWU did not sponsor any candidates.

Towards Amalgamation

The main reason behind the HWSU's amalgamation moves with the MHIWU were therefore political, and the latter's initial coolness was partly based on its more insular attitude. There were, however, other immediate pragmatic issues, as the HWSU was not in a very strong financial state. Its reserves were low – partly because it had put more emphasis on campaigning – and the pension fund was yet again proving a considerable drain upon its resources. The MHIWU's negotiating committee reported back to its NEC in October 1943. Strongly influenced by George Gibson, who was very much in favour of the amalgamation, it recommended acceptance, but it was still a close vote. Negotiations continued, but the MHIWU insisted in calling for a financial report on the HWSU, conducted early in 1945 by Mr Yearsley, the MHIWU's accountant. He advised against amalgamation on strictly financial grounds, but in the rapidly changing external environment such considerations only delayed amalgamation rather than stopping it altogether.

With the help of an outside chairman, W.P. Allen nominated by the TUC, a final report was prepared for both organisations and put to ballot. This outlined the proposed new organisation. The title – Confederation of Health Service Employees – had been suggested by the MHIWU at a Joint Meeting of the two unions on 22 June

1944, because it was felt that 'there was an objection, maybe a "snobbish" one, to the word "Union". ' The idea of a Confederation was seen as a suitable alternative, one which was 'all embracing', allowed for expression of the views of 'any particular or specialist service' and was broad enough not to need revision in future. It was also felt that 'COHSE' was the best way of shortening the title, because it presented the image of 'a real "cosy" and progressive organisation'.

The plans allowed for a transitional period of between three and five years in which a network of regional councils would be established throughout Britain, more or less based on the HWSU's existing areas, in addition to Scotland where the HWSU had not organised, each with officers attached to them. The councils would meet quarterly and have the power to elect NEC representatives proportionate to their members and the regional executive committees. Special arrangements were made, on the insistence of the MHIWU, to ensure that some of its ex-Executive members would definitely win places on the new NEC. The existing guild system would be preserved, with an additional Guild of Mental Nurses formed, but guilds would not be allowed an existence at branch level at the insistence of the MHIWU, which regarded the branch as an almost sacred institution and it feared that guild organisation might lead to its disintegration. Conference, the supreme governing body of the union, vested also with the power to elect the union's President and Vice-President, was to be held once every three years. A political fund was established and a 'withdrawal of labour' clause inserted. The basic structure has served the union well down the years, the main differences today being that the guilds have fallen into disuse, and that there is now an annual conference.

One of the most complex and delicate issues the negotiating team had to sort out in this, as in any amalgamation, was the assimilation of the officials and officers of the two organisations. In this instance it was complicated by the split in head offices between London and Manchester. Most, but not all, of the area officials of the HWSU were to be assimilated to Regional Secretary positions in COHSE. The exceptions were London, which became vacant, and Scotland, where Michael McBride of the MHIWU became Secretary. Regions without officers were to be covered by neighbouring regions until it became possible to appoint them. The MHIWU's Northern Regional Organiser, Jack Waite, became responsible for the northern regions and was based in the Manchester office, while Cliff Comer, the Southern National Organiser supervised southern regions from the London office. Mrs Drapper, based in London, became National Organiser for Females. The first General Secretary of COHSE was to be George Gibson, while Vincent Evans was apparently content to accept the relatively junior position of Finance and Organisation Secretary. The real hub of the union was to be in Manchester, since the MHIWU was insisting that ultimate control over finance should also be vested there, despite Evans's formal position.

In essence these plans showed the extent to which the MHIWU, as the stronger and more financially sound organisation, could dictate terms to the HWSU. Its officials were to become the leaders of the new union in the post-war period, while those of the HWSU would, without exception, be in more subordinate positions. The main influence of the HWSU was to be seen on the structure of COHSE, particularly in the creation of regions with full-time officers attached to them. These plans were embodied in a Final Report which now apparently only required the final seal of approval of the membership of the two organisations before COHSE came into being on 1 January 1945.

In fact the launch was delayed for a year. Although the HWSU's NEC enthusiastically adopted the Final Report, it was 'referred back' by a clear majority of delegates at the MHIWU Conference in October 1944. Unfortunately George Gibson – a keen supporter of the proposals – and his wife had been seriously injured in a motor accident. He was hospitalised and unable to attend the union's conference, and this may have influenced the course of events, for in his absence the NEC Report in favour of amalgamation was put in a rather uninspiring fashion by Walter Blood. In the ensuing debate, it was clear that conference was divided on the question of shifting to the HWSU's system of area full-time organisers. The weaker branches were quite attracted to the idea, and the role of regional officials in NUPE's rapid membership growth did not go unnoticed. The stronger branches on the other hand thought they were an unnecessary expense, and that they could manage quite well on their own. The chief anxiety which united many of those present was that they were being rushed into a ballot without being given the full information, especially on the state of the HWSU's finances. Rumours were flying around concerning Mr Yearsley's report, but this had not been circulated. Constitutionally, the conference could not vote against the amalgamation, but it could refer it back for fuller information, and that is indeed what happened, by 225 votes to 174.

So, to the acute disappointment of the NECs of both organisations, the planned launch of COHSE could not take place at the beginning of 1945. The episode was, however, a clear demonstration of the democracy which existed within the MHIWU and of the kind of role that a delegate conference could play in acting as a constitutional check on the national leadership. Mr Yearsley's financial report was circulated to the branches in the early months of 1945, along with an addendum, by Mark Dubury and Vincent Evans of the HWSU, which sought to soften its impact by criticising its narrowly financial assessment of union 'assets'. It spoke of the need for

the unification of ALL our resources, not only finance, but in membership enthusiasm and enterprise.

Such arguments won the day. Now in possession of all the facts, the MHIWU's delegate conference on 7 July 1945 agreed, by 306 votes to 143, to commend the proposals for ballot of the whole membership. When voting had been completed on 30 September 1945 a decisive majority of the members of both organisations had pronounced in favour of combining forces. Announcing the result to the members, George Gibson and Vincent Evans issued a joint statement which declared:

We are facing a new era. It is going to be an important one. The Minister has intimated that the changes are likely to be 'revolutionary'. What every hospital employee has wanted for years has now become a fact: a strong trade union representing the majority of organised hospital employees ... Some of the members may have personal feelings of regret at the passing, as it were, of the old Union. This we can appreciate and understand. Yet in the firm belief that through Unity comes greater strength, we now have the opportunity, providing we all have the will, of creating the strongest and most effective trade union organisation in the country. May we appeal to *all members* for that spirit of determination to go forward in strength and power, remembering all the time that our individual efforts are strengthening the power of the workers in the great collective movement for the betterment of this country and mankind.[20]

The first steps towards the realisation of these goals were merely a formality. On 8 December 1945 a historic joint meeting of the Executives of the HWSU and the MHIWU took place which approved the COHSE Rule Book, and conducted the funeral rites for the two disappearing organisations. On 1 January 1946 the Confederation of Health Service Employees came into being, with a combined membership of 40,000. The first steps had been taken. Only the future would tell whether and when the wider hopes embodied in the amalgamation, as expressed in the statement by Gibson and Evans, would be realised. The two organisations had finally come together, bringing to a close the first phase of the history of health service trade unionism.

Notes

[1] Abel-Smith, *Hospitals*, pp.426-7.
[2] Ferguson and Fitzgerald, op. cit., on which this section leans heavily.
[3] Guild of Nurses (HWSU), *The Origin and Constitution and a Survey of the Recommendations of the Nurses' Salaries Committee* (1945).
[4] Compiled from RCN Annual Reports.
[5] H.M.D. Parker *Manpower: a Study of Wartime Policy and Administration* (1957).

[6] HMSO, *Report of the Committee on Minimum Rates of Wages and Conditions of Employment in Connection with Special Arrangements for Domestic Help* (Hetherington), (1943).

[7] HWSU, *Domestic Workers in Hospitals and Insitutions: The Union's Policy in Regard to the Hetherington Committee* (1943).

[8] Minutes of Joint Meeting held at Transport House, 1 December 1943, COHSE Archive, Modern Records Centre, University of Warwick.

[9] C.L. Dunn, *The Emergency Medical Services*, (1952) Vol. 1, on which this section leans heavily.

[10] Ibid.

[11] TUC, Annual Report (1943).

[12] *Lancet*, 21 October 1944.

[13] Letter of 13 October 1944, reproduced in HWSU, No 11 Area, *Bulletins and Serving Members Letters* (1944).

[14] See D. Murray Stark, *Why a National Health Service?* (1971).

[15] TUC, Annual Report (1942).

[16] Health Workers' Council propaganda leaflet, in *Bulletins and Serving Members Letters* (1944).

[17] See P. Addison, *The Road to 1945* (1977), pp. 239-43.

[18] HWSU, *An Examination of the Proposals Contained in the White Paper issued by the Ministry of Health on the Proposed NHS* (1944).

[19] Ibid.

[20] COHSE Circular to all members, COHSE Archive, loc. cit.

Part Three

COHSE and the NHS Since 1946

Chapter 16
A Health Service Union

The National Health Service started life with an enormous fund of goodwill of its staff, its most precious resource. If this had been properly harnessed, by giving all workers decent rewards and prospects and a direct say in the running of the service, it would have grown immeasurably. Instead this opportunity was on the whole sacrificed to the government's desire not to offend the most powerful elite groups within the service – those who in fact were less committed to the principles embodied in the National Health Service. Moreover, successive governments showed greater concern with holding down the cost of the service, of which wages formed 70 per cent, than with improving its workers' welfare. They made the mistake of thinking that because the fund of goodwill was deep it was in fact bottomless. Systematically and cynically, over the space of three decades, the NHS's most precious resource was wantonly squandered. As this became more and more apparent, workers and their organisations were compelled, against their will, to confront their employers and, after much heart searching, eventually to take industrial action.[1]

But what was clear, even before its inception, was that the National Health Service and its industrial relations, would never be far from the centre of the British political stage. Whether we like it or not the NHS, its industrial relations and wider politics are interwoven to an inseperable degree. The NHS was created by 'politics' – out of the aspirations of working-class people for a better world after the Second World War – without which it could not have come into existence. And because the NHS represents the closest approximation we have to a socialist institution, it has inevitably become an ideological battleground.

The Wider Context

In 1945, after six years of living from day to day through the sufferings and deprivations of 'total war', people's minds now turned actively to consider the future. There was a general, if not specific, desire for change, that the post-war society should in some way continue to embody, in conditions of peace, the values of solidarity that had been discovered in the shelters, the factories and in the armed forces. People remembered the 1930s and Lloyd George's unfulfilled promises in 1918. War had given a practical lesson in what could be achieved through co-operation based on greater social equality. There was a feeling that the future could and should be planned, and an expectation that the government should take action on a wide number of fronts for the benefit of the people.

This was the mood of the people in 1945 and it was captured, almost to its own surprise, by the Labour Party's appeal to the electorate in its Manifesto 'Let Us Face the Future'. This claimed that the Labour Party was 'a socialist party and proud of it', and put forward a programme of extensive nationalisation measures and a commitment to implementing Beveridge's plan for social services. It was the latter, with its central feature of the National Health Service, which appears more than anything to have captured the popular imagination. The Conservative Party was formally committed to a large-scale expansion of the health and social services, but there were doubts about whether Churchill intended to fulfil his promises. The Labour governments of 1945-51 fulfilled many of these promises, although not without making compromises. By 1948 Labour's legislative programme was, with the exception of steel nationalisation, largely completed, and a certain air of inertia had set in. If 'the forward march' of Labour had by this time been 'halted', as one leading historian has recently claimed, then it was largely because it felt it had reached almost the outer limits of where it wanted to go.[2]

While a certain lack of vision and imagination may have been factors preventing the 1945-51 Labour governments from achieving more, the appalling economic condition of the country also acted as a powerful brake upon socialist aspirations. In its first year this did not prevent Labour from pursuing its programme of reforms – the memory of Ramsay MacDonald was still strong – but as time went on, as it became increasingly bogged down in the management of the domestic economic crisis, and became caught up in the ever greater international crisis of the 'Cold War', the government began to take emergency measures which hurt its traditional supporters. This whittled down its majority in the 1950 election, and led to its departure from power in 1951.

The nation's post-war economic problems were of massive proportions. During the war the country lost a quarter of its national wealth, approximately £7,000 million, through the sale of overseas assets and concentration of domestic industry upon the war effort. Without the assistance of Marshall Aid from the USA in 1948 it is likely that there would have been mass unemployment. But there was a price to be paid. The first was a drive against workers' living standards in order to restore the profitability of industry. Stafford Cripps, the left-wing Chancellor of the Exchequer, outlined the government's priorities:

> First are exports ... second is capital investment in industry; and last are needs, comforts and amenities of the family.[3]

From February 1948 the government officially issued a 'statement' adopting a policy of 'wage restraint', which was supported by majority opinion at the Trades Union Congress Special Conference of Union Executives in March 1948, including COHSE. The second effect of Marshall Aid was to tie the Labour government's foreign policy even closer to that of the USA, particularly after the Soviet blockade of West Berlin in 1948. In the restrictive atmosphere of the time, there was a crackdown against Communist and 'fellow traveller' influence in the labour movement. In April 1948 a number of so-called 'crypto-Communist' MPs were expelled from the Labour Party, and the TUC called on affiliated unions to expel Communists from any official position.

The prevailing direction of government policy was consolidated during 1949 to 1950 when Britain became a signatory of the North Atlantic Treaty Organisation (NATO), the practical consequence of which was a commitment to a massive increase in defence expenditure, which necessitated a deflationary economic policy – the devaluation of the pound by 30 per cent, a rise in income tax of 6d in the pound and the introduction of charges for medicines, dentures and spectacles. The political consequences within the Cabinet were also great. Some, like Bevan, resigned on principle, while others departed as a result of ill health or exhaustion. Finally, in October 1950, the TUC withdraw its support for wage restraint in the face of soaring profits and rising prices, and the Tories came to power in the election the following year. That the 1945-51 Labour governments achieved more for the people than any government before or since cannot be denied. But the lesson, that the labour movement courts disaster when it decides to place the welfare of the people lowest on its list of priorities, is not necessarily one that has been easily learned.

A Question of Leadership

The hopes and expectations that attended the formation of COHSE were very much part of their time, as was the faltering sense of purpose that set in by the early 1950s. First of all, however, the new union had to establish itself in difficult circumstances, and weld two rather different organisations in one.

By all accounts, the process was much smoother than had been anticipated. Reorganisation imposed heavy costs but, as ever, conference was reluctant to increase subscriptions. As membership increased, the situation eased a little. From 40,000 in 1946, it rose to above 54,000 in 1950. A more serious problem was the vacuum in leadership at the top of the union in the years immediately following 1946. Most of the figures who had dominated both amalgamating unions, and steered them through their various transformations, spanning all the important landmarks in the creation of the welfare state, soon departed from the scene. Vincent Evans died within a year of the amalgamation, his death hastened, it was suggested, by the work he had put into creating COHSE. Mrs Drapper, National Women's Officer since 1930, also announced her retirement. Herbert Shaw, who as Assistant General Secretary had for years past borne the pressure of George Gibson's increasingly frequent absences from the head office, retired in 1946. Gibson himself had been due for retirement before the amalgamation, but had been asked to stay on. In theory he had five years to serve as General Secretary. He had become a major public figure in the Second World War after he became President of the TUC in 1941, at a time when the general influence of the TUC was high because of the need to win workers' co-operation for the war effort. George Gibson was foremost among those calling for the fullest possible co-operation with the government and employers. He was a 'safe' political choice as a Governor of the Bank of England in 1946, when he was already vice-chairman of the National Savings Committee and chairman of the North-West Regional Board for Industry.

There had been some criticism within COHSE at the extent of Gibson's extra-union activities, and some eyebrows were raised concerning his right-wing political views. He had ridden most of these out comfortably, but now at his last conference in 1947 he faced two critical motions, both calling for his resignation. The first criticised him for sharing the same platform with Winston Churchill ('the arch enemy of trade unionism') in the United Europe Campaign. The second deprecated his acceptance of outside appointments 'which are of no benefit to COHSE and which take up time which should be devoted to the benefit of the members'. He survived both votes, and won over the delegates with his undoubted charm, but subsequently told the NEC that he was retiring earlier than expected, at the end of 1947.

George Gibson did not have a happy time when he retired from the COHSE leadership. In 1948 he added the chairmanship of the North-West Electricity Board, at £4,000 a year, to his list of public appointments. But he was moving into an unfamiliar world and becoming exposed to dangers of which he was only half aware. He became embroiled in a minor scandal in which he was said to have accepted gifts such as three pounds of sausages, half bottle of whiskey and a suit of clothes in return for using his influence in the Treasury on behalf of a businessman friend. By the standards of later scandals it was small beer, but in the atmosphere of austerity the Tory press was turning over every stone in the hunt for 'socialist corruption'. Gibson and John Belcher, a junior Minister in the Board of Trade, were forced to resign all public appointments in 1948. Gibson died in 1953 a 'broken man'. The *Guardian* probably came closest to the truth when it portrayed him in its obituary as a man who had got out of his depth, and 'in with the wrong sort of people, whose experience and values were remote from his own, and he made a hash of a remarkable career'.[3]

It would be a shame if history only remembers George Gibson for the hash rather than the remarkable career. His contribution at critical points to the development of COHSE, and the nursing profession as a whole, was very great. He it was who, more than anyone else, recognised in 1910 that the pensions issue could serve as a unifying force to form a National Union of Asylum Workers, and who pulled the fledgling union back from the brink of bankruptcy, after Bankart's disastrous rule as General Secretary. He played a key role in securing national bargaining for health workers after the First World War, and in the 1920s recognised the need to respond to the mental hospital scandals by developing a positive programme of reform to change asylum attendants into mental nurses, for their benefit and that of the service. In the 1930s he played the central role in the TUC's campaign to reform and unionise nursing, which challenged the Royal College of Nursing to an extent never seen before. The Nurses' Charter, which he helped to formulate, served as the model for progressive thinking on the reform of nursing for years afterwards. In the Second World War, despite all his external commitments, he played a central role in the work of the Rushcliffe Committee, which paved the way for nationally uniform standards of pay and conditions, as well as finally helping to settle the dispute between the General Nursing Council and the RMPA (about which more will be heard later in this chapter). George Gibson was at his best dealing with the problems of his members, and it is for his record of achievement over the first 37 years of his public career for which he should also be remembered, not just for the rather sad two years at the end of it.

The established leadership of both unions had therefore departed, with the notable exception of Claude Bartlett, the President. He now loomed larger than ever in the union's affairs, while elections were held to replace the General Secretary and Assistant General Secretary. Elections for a new General Secretary were held in 1948. Cliff Comer, the Southern National Organiser and the heir apparent with the most negotiating experience, won easily. Jack Waite, the runner-up, and Northern National Organiser, won the Assistant General Secretary contest in the following year. Both Comer and Waite were ex-MHIWU officials, and the elections consolidated the hold of mental nurses over COHSE's organisation.

Getting to the Root of the Problem?

The most immediate problem facing the post-war health service was staff shortages which were, in effect, a continuation and worsening of a wartime problem. As far as nursing was concerned, the National Advisory Council for the Recruitment and Distribution of Nurses and Midwives, originally set up in 1943 to advise on wartime controls, now turned its attention to peacetime shortages. It issued a Memorandum on recruitment in 1945 which declared that urgent action needed to be taken, including greater press publicity to attract both men and women to nursing, and to assimilate ex-members of the armed forces into civilian nursing. Its focus was upon dealing with the high student nurse 'wastage' during training, and called for the by now familiar improvements in hours, accommodation and a 'more modern outlook on discipline'.[4]

The incoming Labour government of 1945 moved rapidly to implement and extend the recommendations of the Advisory Council. It launched its publicity campaign with the statement, 'Staffing the Hospitals: an Urgent National Need', and the following year, 1946, announced the establishment of a Working Party on the Recruitment and Training of Nurses (the Wood Committee). 'Staffing the Hospitals' was signed by both the Minister of Labour, George Isaacs, and the Minister of Health, Aneurin Bevan, and set out the government's position with regard to nursing and domestic staffs' pay and conditions in the emerging NHS. It appealed to people to come forward to 'play their part in this great field of service', but recognised that appeals merely to a sense of national duty were not appropriate in peacetime. It rejected as 'out of date' the idea of hospital employment 'as devoted endurance of discomfort in a good cause'.

In order to improve the attractiveness of hospital work the government outlined innovative 'Codes of Working Conditions', establishing a 'reasonable minimum' standard for both nurses and domestic workers to be observed in all hospitals.

The code for nurses detailed the standards that had already been seen as desirable by numerous authorities in the past, and included: true student status for student nurses; a 96-hour fortnight and one clear day off in seven; adequate pensions; good food, accommodation and recreation; an elected Nurses' Representative Council and relaxation of discipline; the shedding of non-nursing duties; pay and other conditions in line with reports of the Rushcliffe Committee. In addition the document encouraged the recruitment of ex-service personnel, married women, part-timers and men. The hospital domestic workers' code recognised that the most urgent need was to establish joint negotiating machinery – which was in fact in the process of being set up – in order to achieve uniform pay and working conditions. Many of the details of the domestic workers' code were left to be determined by collective negotiations. The code did, however, have something to say regarding care of domestic staffs' health, including training for those likely to come into contact with infectious disease and regular screening of those exposed to health risks. It encouraged the development of better promotion prospects, proper uniforms, improved accommodation and recreation and a more relaxed approach to discipline in off-duty hours. It suggested the establishment of 'staff committees', with representatives of all grades, to discuss 'any matters affecting the work and efficiency of the domestic staff ', so long as they did not concern 'matters which fall for negotiation between organisations of employees and employing bodies'. 'Special consideration' should be given to the organisation of working methods and full use made of 'labour saving devices'. It suggested also that control and supervision of domestic staff be taken away from nurses in larger hospitals.

It appeared, then, that the new government was moving swiftly and was prepared to experiment with innovative ideas. There was, however, as much if not more emphasis in the codes on the need to educate public opinion on the extent to which hospital employment had changed as on changing the conditions themselves. It was assumed, without any evidence given, that the 'less modern and less enlightened' hospital authorities were in the minority. It was also very sketchy concerning trade union rights. The nurses' code simply urged that local management should place 'no obstacle' in the way of either unions on professional associations in seeking to represent members in the workplace. This fell short of insisting upon full recognition, and obscured the fact that unions faced many more obstacles than professional associations, which were generally favoured by management. Some Labour Councils at this time adopted a policy of more active intervention, and in 1946 both Willesden and Poplar sought to introduce a closed shop for all hospital employees, which excluded professional associations like the RCN. The moves failed after unfavourable press publicity and after pressure from the RCN brought condemnation from the government.[5] The hospital domestic workers' code referred only to trade unions, but its concept of staff committees (as outlined above) drew a dubious distinction between issues regarded as appropriate for unions, and those affecting the welfare of staff and efficiency of the service, which presumably were not.

The government's analysis and prescription contrasted markedly with COHSE's own submission on staff shortages, first put to the government by the HWSU in 1945. It first pointed out that there was a shortage of adequate buildings and equipment as well as staff, and called for better planning of facilities, including more attention given to the needs of staff. COHSE then claimed that there were two main reasons for the shortages in personnel. First, poor wages and conditions, due to the fact that the recommendations of the Rushcliff and Hetherington Reports were 'already hopelessly out of date' and no longer competitive with other forms of employment. Second, there were inadequate opportunities for consultation and promotion. The service did not seek to tap the ideas of those mass of workers who

> are daily in contact with the people for whom these services were created and know what they desire ... The majority of hospitals seem to make 'castes' of the various employees and all of them are segregated in 'water tight' compartments. This is bad for the welfare of the patients and the hospital services generally.[6]

COHSE's critique of administration followed the same lines. Authority was too remote. Chief officials 'seldom visit the hospitals and so tend to forget to look at things from the patients' point of view'. Matrons' and medical superintendents' duties were often far removed from their original training, which was 'more or less wasted', and senior staff were generally unsympathetic to the suggestions of front-line workers. It called for democratically elected health service authorities.

On trade union representation, COHSE claimed the

257 A Health Service Union

service 'is living in the past'. Where large numbers of staff lived in the matron and medical superintendent were 'all powerful', and COHSE claimed that a 'gestapo' system operated in many hospitals 'whereby the actions of a particularly spirited and independent employee are reported almost hourly'. It gave as examples the student nurse in 1945 who was fined £1 by the matron for burning the toast she was making, and the matron who rebuked a nurse for going out on her day off in a 'brightly coloured mackintosh'. It also paid close attention to the unfair treatment meted out to domestic, ambulance and engineering staffs. It called for compulsory recognition of unions, and for proper facilities to collect dues and represent members. Hospital consultative committees should be set up, but based on trade union representation.

These are just a few selected quotations from COHSE's response entitled *The Hospital Services*. It was one of the most well thought out and comprehensive statements to have appeared from within the labour movement regarding the problems of the health service, and contained positive suggestions for the future. It was calling very much for a service responsive both to the needs of the majority of its staff and the welfare of the users. Indeed it argued that there was a close connection between the two, and that the solution to the problems faced by each, necessitated curtailing the power of the senior professionals and administrators who had dominated the service for years.

Launching the NHS

The government had shown in 'Staffing the Hospitals' that it would go some way down this road, but how far? The story of the creation of the National Health Service itself has been well documented, so only the barest outline is necessary here.[7] The launching of the NHS was entrusted to Aneurin Bevan, the MP for Ebbw Vale, an ex-miner, leading member of the left and the youngest member of Attlee's Cabinet. The 1946 National Health Service Act was a mixture of socialist principle, state rationalisation and compromise with the most powerful vested interests within the service. The most radical feature of the 1946 National Health Service Act was distributional: it set out to establish 'a comprehensive health service designed to secure improvement in the physical and mental health of the people ... and the prevention, diagnosis, and treatment of illness' which was to be free at the point of use. Everyone, no matter where he or she lived, and regardless of ability to pay, should have access to the best available health care. The aim of rationalisation was to serve this end, by integrating all major services, public and private, into a single form of provision. But yet again 'vested interests' in the service prevented this aim being realised entirely. A tripartite system emerged in which the hospitals, GP services and local authority preventive and domiciliary services were administered separately until 1974. The centrepiece of the system, which came to swallow up an ever increasing part of the budget, was the hospital service. Bevan decided to separate this entirely from local government (in contrast to Willink's plan of 1944). There were good reasons for doing this if a nationally uniform system was to be created, but less justifiable was the decision to administer the system by nominated rather than elected authorities. This was a major concession to consultants who wanted state finance to fund innovations in medical technology, but feared lay 'dictation'. Bevan's plan sought to win support from consultants in order to drive a wedge between them and general practitioners. He even permitted ex-voluntary, now 'teaching' hospitals, to be administered separately from the Regional Hospital Boards, and made other concessions, such as allowing consultants to retain pay-beds. As an immediate strategy it worked, and the NHS came into being, and to that extent Bevan's heroic reputation was well earned. But there were costs. The planned emphasis on primary care, which was to be provided through locally accessible health centres, was never implemented due to medical opposition. Prevention also went by the wayside, as the traditional elites within the service tightened their grip and channelled more and more resources into the most glamorous specialties in the hospital sector.

COHSE and other organisations associated with the labour movement recognised some of these dangers. While COHSE did not openly criticise the new structure it did press for significant health worker and union representation on the Regional Hospital Boards (RHBs) and Hospital Management Committees (HMCs) to counteract medical influences. Bevan was generally against workers in the health service serving on RHBs though he appointed some union officials to them – Ted Hardy, Jack Waite and Bert Waites among them. The union wrote in complaint in 1947 to Bevan that he had appointed matrons and doctors to boards but had 'passed over a large number of subordinate grades'. His reply was non-commital. He 'took note' of the union's comments, and said that he could not in any case influence HMC appointments, as that was a matter for regions. But then in 1949 he issued Circular RHB (49) 143, which implied that all NHS staff, apart from senior medical and dental staff, were debarred from membership of HMCs, even outside their own employing authority. As a result a number of COHSE HMC members were not reappointed. The TUC passed a resolution in 1950 critical of the circular, but to no effect.

The other fear was that incorporation of the mental health services into a general medical service biased towards acute care might threaten the gains that had been made since the 1930 Mental Treatment Act. Dr Beaton, the Medical Superintendent of St James Hospital, Portsmouth, warned COHSE's No 8 Regional Council in an address early in 1949 that he was 'not optimisitc of the future of mental hospitals under the new health structure'. He discounted the 'high hopes that had been entertained in the mental hospital profession that we are at last taking our rightful place in the medical field', and warned that

> there was a tendency to want to treat mental cases in general hospitals and so still perpetuate the 'abandon hope all ye who enter here' attitude to mental hospitals.[8]

Mental nurses were also divided about the effects of merging the bargaining structure of mental and general nurses. The 'old guard' were primarily concerned with the

protection of their pay differentials. The younger 'new
guard' staff were more positive about the prospects for the
future, and more prepared to embrace professional
values. The third report of the Rushcliffe sub-committee
on mental nursing had recommended that in future
promotions above charge nurse/ward sister level should
only be open to those who had been doubly trained. The
younger generation was keen to go away to obtain SRN
and return to climb the career ladder. The old guard,
represented on the NEC by the articulate A.R. Farmer,
complained in a letter to COHSE's journal *Health Services*
that the result of this was that they would have to plug the
gaps while others went off to general hospitals.

The career prospects of the new guard, and to some
extent those of the old, had been boosted by the final
resolution of the GNC/RMPA dispute which had dragged
on since the mid-1920s. The work of the Athlone
sub-committee on mental nursing, on which both the
MHIWU and the Mental Hospitals Association were
represented, by Gibson and Feldon respectively, had been
interrupted by the outbreak of war in 1939, even though it
had been on the verge of making its report. In October
1945 it was finally delivered. It suggested that in future
there should be a single examination under the GNC,
provided that existing RMPA certificate holders were
allowed to register with the GNC, and provision was made
for greater mental nurse representation on the GNC. The
report recommended a three year change-over period,
and also called for many improvements to mental nursing,
including the granting of proper student status,
recruitment of more night staff and the granting of
greater liberty to nurses in off-duty hours. It was strongly
opposed to the introduction of an assistant nurse grade as
a permanent feature, regarding it as a form of 'dilution' of
labour. It proposed that in future the Register should be
divided threefold into State Registered Nurses, Registered
Mental Nurses and Registered Mental Nurses (Subnormality) and special branches. Discrimination against men
in general nursing, who from 1919 had only been
admitted to a *male* Register, was to be ended, and mental
nurses guaranteed the right to a two-year shortened

training for SRN. The report had a sting in its tail: if the GNC would not agree to these changes legislation would be required to create a separate statutory body for mental nurses.[8]

It could not be denied that the report was seeking to drive a hard bargain with the GNC, and behind many of its recommendations one can see the dominating and experienced figure of George Gibson. The GNC would take over mental nursing, but a high price would be exacted. George Gibson had won important concessions for mental nurses. But it was also a piece of pragmatic politics, which recognised and extended the ascendency of general hospital nursing within the nursing universe at the same time as it insisted on a fairer crack at the whip for men and mental nurses within it. The old guard had a point. There was something dedicedly bizarre about the armies of mental nurses who subsequently took their seconded training in general hospitals and returned to use not the *knowledge* they had gained but the *qualification* they had obtained as a ticket to rise in the hierarchy.

The proposals were implemented in 1949, along with many of the recommendations of the Wood Committee. As we have seen, this was set up in 1946 to propose reforms to nurse training. Its report vindicated the analysis COHSE had made in *The Hospital Services*. The best way of increasing the supply of trained nurses was to end the extremely high attrition rate of student nurses. As Abel-Smith summarises the findings:

> Wastage was attributed to hospital discipline, the attitude of senior staff, food, hours, and pressure of work, in that order. Indeed the report contributed the most outspoken and well documented condemnation of the attitudes and behaviour of senior nurses in hospitals that has yet been published. It is no wonder that the report was not well received by the Association of Hospital Matrons.[9]

The report recommended that training in future should be determined by the students' needs rather than those of the hospital; that the financing of training should be separated from hospital finance; that domestic staff should take over 'non-nursing' duties; and that students should be under the control of the training authority, rather than the matron. It also made a large number of other suggestions – notably for a large expansion in the number of ward orderlies and the phasing out of nursing assistants, and shortening training for the register to two years subject to a year's satisfactory practice under supervision – none of which the elite of the profession would countenance. But it was the proposal to separate authority over training from the matron that most angered them.

COHSE agreed with much of the report's analysis, though it said that it 'merely reiterates what had been said before, and the most important question was whether there will be requisite action at an early date'. It thought the proposed two-year training scheme was 'impractical' and would put 'serious strain' on students. Since Wood also proposed a generic training, it was worried about the marginalisation of mental nursing within the proposed two-year course. It was cautious about the expansion of ward orderlies and phasing out of assistant nurses, but eagerly supported the proposal to end the long-standing discrimination against men in nursing.[10]

The proposals of the Wood Committee were only implemented in a diluted form. Full student status was not achieved. The government regarded it as prohibitively expensive and the matrons were unwilling to surrender control over student nurses to an educational authority. Under the Nurses Act of 1949 Area Nurse Training Committees were set up in each NHS region, but as Abel-Smith observes, 'without the powers envisaged in the Wood Committee's report ... [they] served a very limited purpose'.[11] The Register was divided three ways, along the lines suggested by the Athlone sub-committee on mental nursing. The GNC itself was reorganised, with greater representation given to the state and a regional system of election for the nurse members. Yearly registration fees were replaced by a single registration for life.

An elected mental nurses sub-committee was set up and both the COHSE sponsored candidates, Claude Bartlett (the President), and Miss W.V. Walters (a Sister Tutor at St Lawrence's, Caterham), were elected. Bartlett became chairman of the committee. The GNC had already, in December 1948, drafted rules for the admission of RMPA qualified nurses to its Register. They were given until the last day of March 1952 to join it, provided that they paid two guineas and deposited two testimonials to their good character. A number of diehard RMPA loyalists refused to register, but they were permitted to continue using the title 'nurse'. To entice them in the GNC extended its registration deadline indefinitely. For the remainder, it appeared that a new era of mental nursing had begun.

Notes

[1] E. Hobsbawm *et al.*, *The Forward March of Labour Halted?* (1979).

[2] A. Sked and C. Cook, *Post-War Britain* (1979), Ch. 1.

[3] *Guardian*, 5 February 1953. For a general account of the affair see J. Gross, 'The Lynskey Tribunal' in M. Sissons and P. French (eds), *The Age of Austerity 1945-51* (1964).

[4] Ferguson and Fitzgerald, op. cit.

[5] See Bowman, op.cit., Ch. 22 for the RCN's account of these events.

[6] COHSE, *The Hospital Services: the Problem Arising out of Existing Shortage of all Grades of Staff* (1946) COHSE Archive, Modern Records Centre, University of Warwick.

[7] See, for example, M. Foot, *Aneurin Bevan 1945-60* (1973).

[8] Nursing Services Inter-Departmental Committee (Athlone), *Report of Sub-Committee on Mental Nursing and the Nursing of the Mentally Defective* (1945).

[9] Abel-Smith, *Nursing Profession*, p.182.

[10] COHSE, *Observations on the Working Party on the Training and Recruitment of Nurses* (1947), COHSE Archive, loc. cit.

[11] Abel-Smith, *Nursing Profession*, p.221.

Chapter 17
Health Workers and Pay-Bargaining 1946-51

The Road to Whitleyism

It seemed natural at the time that the NHS was set up that 'Whitleyism' should form the basis for the new pay bargaining system, with its idea of a consensus between employees and employers seeming highly appropriate for such a service. Whitleyism had in fact originated during the First World War in private industry, aiming to prevent disruption in the wartime munitions industries and to create harmonious industrial relations in the post-war world, but many of the Whitley Councils set up at this time did not survive the intensification of industrial conflict which folled. During the Second World War, however, there was a revival in notions of co-operation and involvement of unions at all levels from central government down to 'joint production committees' on the shop floor. Yet once again the idea of a common purpose which sustained joint consultation during the war proved difficult to maintain afterwards, except in the newly nationalised sectors. Perhaps these notions stood a better chance of succeeding in the NHS than elsewhere in the public sector, given broad staff commitment to service ideals.

There was, however, nothing in the National Health Service Bill of 1946 which prescribed any particular system of settling pay and conditions for NHS staff, although there was a clause which, as Section 66 of the Act, gave the Minister power to make regulations concerning 'the qualifications, remuneration and conditions of service of any officers'. This implied national uniformity in pay and conditions, and assurances were given during the Second Reading of the Bill that the government would either adapt existing machinery or set up new bodies of the 'Whitley Council type' with agreed provision for arbitration.

This is indeed what happened, though it proved a massive and complex task. This complexity had three sources. First, the difficulties of settling pay and conditions for such a differentiated workforce in a continuing process of evolution and change, and whose members were highly likely to compare each other's relative circumstances; second, the difficulty of achieving national uniformity in a service where the pay and conditions of most workers had previously been subject to wide local variations. Third, to add to these difficulties, the staff were not united among themselves but split among a multitude of competing organisations, some very small and with no previous experience of collective negotiations. The status-conscious attitudes and fragmented nature of the workforce were reflected in the workers' own organisations.

The Labour government took a pragmatic approach to these difficulties. The division of the bargaining structure into a general council to deal with issues affecting all workers and nine 'functional' councils to deal with particular grades, was affected by all three considerations. The full story of how these emerged, and how the management and workers' sides of the councils were constructed has been told elsewhere.[1] True to its promise the government took existing negotiating bodies and transformed them into Whitley Councils. The Rushcliffe Committee formed the basis for the Nurses and Midwives Whitley Council, and reproduced the dominance of the professional asssociations. The National Joint Council for Hospitals and Allied Institutions (Mowbray Committee) became the Ancillary Staffs Council, on which only trade unions were represented. As far as professional and technical staffs were concerned, a Joint Negotiating Committee for Hospital Staffs had been in operation from June 1945 and had issued scales from 1 April 1946. Yet while the employers' side included both local authorities and voluntary hospitals, the employees' side was restricted to professional associations, despite union requests to be included. The unions enjoyed more success in seeking to negotiate for medical laboratory staffs. Their professional association, the Institute of Medical Laboratory Technology, decided to surrender its negotiating role, and a separate negotiating committee was formed with COHSE and other unions. When the Whitley Council came to be formed this pre-existing system of professional/unionism separation was largely retained. Professional and Technical Council 'A' catered in the main for what were then called 'medical auxiliaries' (nowadays 'professions supplementary to medicine'), dominated by often tiny professional associations. Council 'B' covered laboratory staffs, engineers and other technicians and was dominated by unions. COHSE was represented on each. The remaining councils were entirely new creations – the Administrative and Clerical Council, which was dominated by NALGO, and the Pharmaceutical Council upon which unions had nominal representation. COHSE was represented on both of these. The irony of the union's position was that it was represented on more functional councils than any other organisation but did not exercise a decisive influence on any, a problem that would plague it for years to come. In addition there were to be separate Medical, Dental and Optical Councils, and a Building Craftment's Committee was also established.

The government had adopted a largely neutral stance towards the professional associations. They were prepared to recognise any established organisation which could show that it had members for the staff group it sought to represent. This broadly fitted in with its approach to the creation of the NHS, and its reluctance to take on the established vested interests within the service. Neither were unions in a position to mount a challenge to this approach. NALGO was still outside the TUC, the affiliated organisations were disunited among themselves and did not possess sufficient membership strength. The only major exception to the government's accommodative stance was Bevan's uncompromising refusal to recognise the newly formed National Federation of Hospital Officers, which mainly represented senior administrators, either by giving them seats on Whitley Councils or the direct negotiations they sought as a substitute.

Nor did the structure of the management sides augur well for the future. The main employing bodies, the HMCs, were originally not represented on management sides. The reason for their exclusion soon became clear: as Lord McCarthy succinctly put it in his review of the NHS Whitley system published in 1976, the employers' sides are divided between 'employers who do not pay and paymasters who do not employ'.[2] Local authorities were given strong representation as both employers *and* paymasters. As for the remainder, the over-representation of the Ministry of Health and Scottish Department indicated that there was going to be a preponderance of paymasters who would be more likely to be concerned with the containment of central government's costs rather than, say, responding to service needs such as combatting shortages of labour.

The system – and it was essentially the same on all Whitley Councils – thus became very top heavy, with management sides often largely ignorant and unresponsive to problems in the localities. The amount that they could offer was, in any case, determined by the real paymasters, the Treasury, who were not even represented at the bargaining table. Perhaps the British Medical Association (BMA), with its long tradition of suspicion and mistrust of the state, saw more clearly than most what the new structure implied. It would have nothing to do with Whitleyism, preferring direct negotiations with the state.

Whitleyism was not just supposed to be concerned with settling pay and conditions, however large they loomed in its deliberations: it was meant also to draw upon the knowledge and experience of staff as a means of improving the service for the benefit of all. Yet while local joint consultation was, for example, made legally compulsory when coalmines were nationalised, no reference was made to it in the National Health Service Act. It appeared in the NHS almost as an afterthought. Once again the Labour government appeared to be treading very gingerly so as not to upset powerful vested interests. COHSE consistently urged for joint consultation to be made compulsory, but it was not until 1948 that a Circular was finally sent out advising HMCs to set up Joint Consultative Committees with guidance on structure and constitution to come later.[3] The task of drawing up a model constitution was made the responsibility of the General Whitley Council, whose staff and management sides comprised representatives of the functional councils. They laboured until 1950 before they could produce an agreement. Under the guidelines hospital consultative committees were to include all grades of staff – including student nurses, against RCN protests – but, at its own insistence, excluding the medical profession. Committees could discuss and make recommendations on a wide number of issues (but not promotion procedures), and representation on the elected staff sides was to be restricted solely to members of Whitley Council-recognised organisations.

The same year saw the establishment of joint union-management appeals machinery at regional level, to adjudicate on disputes over the interpretation of Whitley Council agreements. There was less progress, however, on the vexed question of an agreed disciplinary procedure. Typically, there were no first or second stage warnings – sacking was usually the first stage. In fact it did not prove possible to conclude an agreement on discipline for many years. It was only the introduction of employment legislation in the 1970s which finally forced the management side's hand. In 1951 the Ministry itself issued 'interim guidance' for discipline of staff other than consultants. It said there should be a proper warning system, and an appeal system with the right to be accompanied by a 'friend' or representative of a union or professional association. But there was no machinery established to ensure that such a procedure was followed.

Ambulance Setbacks

One of COHSE's biggest disappointments in its earliest years was the failure to see ambulance staffs included within the main framework of the NHS and its collective bargaining machinery. Instead they were left to the local authorities to organise, with the cost shared equally between national and local government in England and Wales, while paid for entirely by central government in Scotland. Not inconsiderable sums were involved: the service cost nearly £8 million in 1950-51.[4]

Pressure to incorporate ambulance services within the NHS did not emanate from other unions representing ambulance personnel, as they did not want to admit COHSE to their rather exclusive negotiating club, the local government National Joint Industrial Council (NJIC) for Non-Trading Services, from which COHSE was still excluded. In 1949 COHSE pressed the Minister of Health to shift responsibility for pay determination to the Ancillary Staffs Council (ASC), but to no avail. COHSE's case was a strong one: ambulance staffs had a wider range of duties than the NJIC grading as 'motor drivers' suggested, and the ambulance services were an integral part of the health service – as official TUC policy insisted. But then strong cases do not always win arguments.

COHSE continued to press the interests of ambulance staffs, and for recognition by the NJIC. In Surrey and Middlesex it campaigned with the Fire Brigades' Union against the proposed merger of ambulance and fire services under which fire brigades staff would be expected to drive ambulances. The aim of local authorities was often to contain the accelerating cost of the service. Another management move against which the Ambulance Service Guild campaigned, at Dartford for example, was the 'increasing encroachment of the hospital car service on normal and routine work'. The Ambulance Services Guild continued to press for high professional standards, as represented by the Institute of Certified Ambulance Personnel. This was now registering fellows, associates and student members from COHSE head office, although it was formally separate from the union's organisation. Its President was Dr H.B. Morgan, a COHSE MP and NEC member, and one of the country's acknowledged experts on industrial diseases, but COHSE's lack of recognition was undoubtedly a considerable handicap in this field.

Student Nurse Campaigns

COHSE's biggest victory in these years arose out of its campaign on behalf of student nurses which was fought in 1948, just at the point at which the Rushcliffe Committee was making way for the Nurses and Midwives Council (NMC). The campaign really began the previous year with pressure on COHSE's eve of conference NEC meeting on 15 September 1947, from male and female student nurses at Claybury Hospital, Essex, for a £5 minimum wage, and an *ex gratia* 'marriage allowance' grant pending the pay settlement. Their case was put forcefully by Joe Gue, himself from Claybury and a leading left-winger on the NEC. While Rushcliffe had revised female student nurses' salaries, male students had not had an increase. The NEC agreed that an emergency resolution be put to the forthcoming delegate conference expressing the view that the existing male students' salary of £3 14s a week was totally inadequate. It called for an immediate increase or else direct negotiations would be opened up with employing authorities. The NEC was under intense pressure. Male and female nurses at Claybury, exasperated at delays in the negotiations, were threatening mass resignations from the service, and it seemed certain that other COHSE branches in the London area would follow suit. The union had to take some firm action.

The debate at conference was opened by George Gibson in one of his last major contributions. He declared that the Rushcliffe Committee in its 'death throes' now had a 'disinclination' to make settlements, despite the existence of many anomalies, like that before it. It soon became apparent that the NEC's resolution was problematic. How much was the union asking for? Others were harshly critical of the proposal to negotiate directly as 'retrograde', and contrary to the union's long standing policy of achieving nationally uniform pay and conditions. After a vigorous debate, conference adopted a simple policy of a £5 minimum wage for *all* student nurses, men and women. The union's priority for the coming year had now been set.

As part of its campaign to shock the Rushcliffe

Committee into taking action, COHSE circulated its branches in order to build up a dossier of how student nurses were managing on their meagre allowances. When sending in their budgets nurses often added comments. Helen Morgan, a pupil nurse from Greenwich wrote: 'Hairdresser not able to afford. Not able to save. Cannot afford a seaside or country holiday,' even though her parents paid her fares home and provided her with 10 shillings a month pocket money. A male pupil nurse from London said, 'Nothing to spare for holidays or occasional entertainment or even to buy seeds for garden.' A married male student nurse, an ex-serviceman, declared: 'I have been a student nurse eighteen months and pocket money is a thing of the past.' His income, including family allowance and ex-serviceman's grant, came to £4 10s a week. His listed outgoings were £4 15s 7d a week. This was a quite common feature of the budgets. The nurses were living on the very edges of subsistence and many only survived with the help of parents and other relatives.

Still the Rushcliffe Committee dallied, while nurses' debts and tempers rose. It had before it the Report of the Wood Committee on restructuring nurse training and the dominant, i.e. RCN, view was that achieving student status was more important than increases in pay. COHSE accused the RCN of deliberate delaying tactics in line with its long established policy that salaries for student nurses would attract the 'wrong type' into the profession. Then, in a parting gift as it made way for the Nurses and Midwives Council, the Rushcliffe Committee granted student nurses a paltry rise of £15 a year. This left them worse off than before as it was not sufficient to cover heavy superannuation and increased National Insurance contributions! COHSE reiterated its view that 'salaries [are] more important than status in the recruitment and training of nurses', and called for an emergency meeting of the new Nurses and Midwives Council (NMC) which had been fixed for 20 August 1948. But student nurses, especially in the London area, put the union under intense pressure to do more. More than 140 student nurses from Claybury and Goodmayes (formerly West Ham) Mental Hospitals signed forms resigning their posts, and placed these at the NEC's disposal. 1 October 1948 was fixed as the deadline by the protesting students.

The NEC was in something of a quandry. It tended to represent the older, more established staff, who were worried that the students' protests might get out of hand, or that a planned demonstration might be 'exploited for political purposes', and so decided to put itself at the head of the protests, partly with a view to controlling them. A demonstration was called for Sunday 15 August, just a few days prior to the NMC meeting. The arrangements for the demonstration and march from Trafalgar Square to Hyde Park were very strict. The police had insisted on a strictly agreed route, with no banners or posters, nor leaflets to be handed out because, according to the COHSE circular, the union had been warned that it might be prosecuted under the Public Order Act 1936.[5]

The high spirited students did not fully comply with these instructions, though nothing dire happened. The 1,000 strong march set off from Trafalgar Square bearing banners with slogans such as 'Never has so much been done by so few for such little pay'. 'Florrie's Lamp is going out. She can't afford oil on nurses' pay', 'A noble profession deserves a living wage'. Many had come straight from night duty, without sleep. When they reached Hyde Park they gathered round a coal cart borrowed for the occasion to listen to speeches from officials of COHSE and rank-and-file nurses. An estimated 20,000 members of the public gathered to listen. They heard that a group of 27 nurses travelling by bus to the demonstration had their fares paid for by a sympathetic conductor. Nurses waved their pay packets at the crowd, and Joan Syms, a third-year student nurse from Balham, jumped up on to the coal cart and told them:

> I get a wage of £4 a month after three years' training as a nurse. At my hospital we were told that the names of the nurses attending this demonstration would be taken.

To cheers, a resolution in favour of the £5 minimum was carried by the meeting.

The demonstration had gone beyond the bounds of

what the General Secretary and NEC had wanted; as Joe Soley, the then Branch Secretary of Goodmayes told me, this was due to the efforts of the Goodmayes and Clabury branches (the latter under Joe Gue), and Dick Akers, then COHSE's London Regional Secretary. But if COHSE's leadership had some private misgivings, the RCN and nursing press expressed outright condemnation of the demonstration, especially the idea of a nurse on a coal cart, as 'undignified'.[6] Undignified or not, the union pushed ahead with its threat of a 1 October deadline after which, failing a satisfactory settlement, COHSE would convene a nurses' delegate conference. Meeting followed Whitley Council meeting at the RCN's headquarters in Cavendish Square through late summer and early autumn. By the end of October new scales for students were finally agreed. A basic wage (called 'training allowance') of £200 was agreed for a first year nurse, with £100 deducted for board and lodging. Mental nurses got £230 a year, which, with free meals, proficiency allowances for passing examinations and dependents' allowances, the General Secretary claimed, 'actually exceed the £5 minimum which was the basis of our original claims'.

The first militant demonstration of nurses since the 1930s had therefore produced results, but COHSE's victory had more far reaching implications than the achievement of the immediate demand. The campaign had finally broken the age-old principle that a student nurse's allowance should just provide pocket money. COHSE had demanded a living wage for students based on the rate for the job. If the settlement fell short of achieving this, the principle itself had at last been accepted. Even the RCN now shifted its ground, and the fourth Report of its own Horder Committee in 1948 finally reversed the College's opposition to allowances which meet 'the student's financial needs'.[7] Unfortunately for COHSE it was not able to take full advantage of the situation by recruiting large numbers of general nurses into the union. The victory was not in the final analysis seen as belonging to COHSE but to the staff side of the Whitley Council as a whole, whose secretary was Frances Goodall of the RCN. In the hospitals many matrons continued to obstruct the efforts of trade unionists, and many nurses were reluctant to incur their wrath.

The Aftermath

The dispute also had a sorry internal aftermath for COHSE, because it revealed deep divisions on tactics between left and right within the union. At a rally in the Conway Hall in London on 22 September, Joe Gue had severely criticised the line being taken by COHSE's negotiators on the NMC, which appeared to him to be compromising the union's original demand for a £5 minimum. It was said subsequently that Joe Gue encouraged his branch members to intimidate members of the union's negotiating team present at the Conway Hall meeting. Whatever actually happened in the confusion of a public meeting is unclear, but COHSE's NEC decided by a majority of eleven to seven to expel him from the union 'as an example to other members not to behave in an unruly manner'. He appealed, as was his right, to a full conference of the union, on 22 September 1949, and after a seven-hour debate, won his appeal against expulsion. Not all delegates sanctioned his behaviour, but many felt that he had been treated too severely.

At the same time, the union's leadership also moved against 'Communist subversion' in COHSE, in line with TUC policy. Each member of the NEC, left and right, signed a 'solemn and truthful' statement declaring that he or she was 'loyal' to the trade union movement and not a member of the Communist Party 'or a supporter of its policy'. There is no evidence, however, of the widespread witch-hunt that was mounted in some other trade unions, such as the TGWU and the NUGMW. This was prevented by the tradition of tolerance which has always been characteristic of COHSE, as well as the strong emphasis placed on branch autonomy. The only action which appears to have been taken was against Dr Cyril Taylor, who was rebuked by the NEC for referring to his membership of COHSE when standing for the Communist Party in municipal elections in Liverpool in opposition to the official Labour candidate.

Despite this unfortunate aftermath COHSE could claim that its campaign on behalf of student nurses had been a victory. Its efforts on behalf of other staff met with more mixed results. An agreement for trained staff was negotiated by May 1949 when staff nurses were granted a minimum salary of £315 a year, with a board and lodging deduction of £120, ranging up to a maximum of £415. Ward sisters' scales were also agreed, but negotiations then got bogged down for mental nurses, midwives, tuberculosis nursing and local authority staffs. Some of the complex negotiations were resolved in late 1949, but those for nursing assistants and local authority staffs continued to drag on. For the first, but not the last time, they appeared to be snarled up in the employers' desire to pursue the government's 'wage restraint' policy. The management side refused point-blank to settle for local authorities' nursing staffs, and the dispute was not resolved until the staff side went outside the system to win an arbitration award from the Industrial Court in April 1950. Negotiations for nursing assistants and other senior grades dragged on into 1951, and nursery staffs did not have any scales until 1952, four years after the setting up of the NMC!

Some of the problems were 'teething troubles' due to the assimilation of a large number of highly differentiated workers from Rushcliffe to Whitley Council scales, a mammoth undertaking. However, as negotiations for unqualified and more specialist grades of nurses dragged on, the delays seemed to be deliberate government tactics. At the 1950 conference tensions between negotiators and the membership at large emerged again.

COHSE registered a more decisive victory on its long standing campaign to have tuberculosis scheduled as an industrial disease. It had been known for some time that nurses suffered more from this deadly disease than the general population, but little had been done. When Doris Westmacott became the Guild of Nurses Organiser in the early 1940s she began assembling a dossier on nurses who had contracted tuberculosis through their work. At that time the most they could hope for was an *ex-gratia* payment, depending on the generosity of their employing authority. Hopes rose with the passing of the National Insurance Act of 1946 which allowed for payment of industrial injury benefit where illness could be shown to be due to an 'accident' or 'series of accidents' arising out of and in the course of employment. It now depended on whether it could be established in legal terms that tuberculosis was an 'accident' or a disease whose onset was gradual. The breakthrough came when, after a four-year battle, the Appeal Court in 1949 upheld the decision of a County Court in a case brought against Doncaster Corporation by Nurse Pyrah that tuberculosis was an 'accident' and she was therefore entitled to compensation. Unfortunately Nurse Pyrah died of TB, but the principle had been established and other successful cases followed. The next stage of the fight took place in the wider political arena. A TUC deputation (which included COHSE) was 'sympathetically received' by Edith Summerskill at the Ministry of National Insurance, and in November 1950 she accepted that tuberculosis should become a scheduled disease.

Ancillary Staffs' Negotiations

For nurses the first years of the NHS had brought immediate gains, but later a growing sense of frustration. For ancillary staffs there was much less to cheer about. In their case any problems in determining their pay were not due to occupational complexity, for the Ancillary Staffs Council (ASC) had inherited a relatively simple pay structure from the Mowbray Committee. At first matters progressed smoothly, and despite the existence of wage restraint new scales were agreed from November 1948, giving men in Group 1 a basic rate of approximately £5 a week and women between £3 14s and £4 2s. Above this, Groups 2-7 received additional pay on top of their basic rates, according to grading and supervisory responsibilities.

Thereafter they received no increases for two years because of the wage freeze. The management side also turned down claims for a 44-hour week in the autumn of 1949. The Labour government's budget in 1950, with its increase in income tax to finance the massive growth of defence expenditure, hit the lowest paid particularly hard. Unlike manual workers in the private sector, those in the NHS could not negotiate incentive pay schemes, which the government exempted from its freeze. A further blow came in October 1950 when the Industrial Court made an unfavourable decision on the ASC staff side arbitration claim for a 44-hour week for 120,000 full-time and 32,000 part-time hospital ancillary workers. The court accepted the employers' arguments that it would cost too much to implement and lead to similar claims for nurses.

Not surprisingly ancillary staff began to get restless, feeling that they were a forgotten army about which the union cared little, compared to nurses. The union's leadership did respond to this growing discontent. Cliff Comer was active within the TUC in 1950 criticising the one-sided nature of the government controls on wages while profits and prices were allowed to soar. Pressure was also mounting throughout the labour movement and in autumn 1950 the TUC withdrew support for the wage freeze. The staff side now pressed ahead with its claim for ASC workers, who received two arbitration awards during 1951, with their pay levels becoming linked in the process more closely with those of local government manual workers, where they would remain until they were rudely dislodged in 1973 – but that is another story.

The Dimming of the Dream

The withdrawal of TUC support from the Labour government's economic policy in 1950 foreshadowed its electoral defeat the following year by the Conservatives. Its record of achievement increasingly became the basis of its claim to power, and it consequently failed to map out an imaginative programme for the future. NHS staff, however, had benefited both as citizens and workers from that government's greatest achievement, the creation of the NHS. By 1950 the *News Chronicle* had already described the NHS as 'a bold achievement noted with awe by the whole world'. The Ministry of Health admitted that it had underestimated the 'vast amount of inarticulate misery and pain' which had existed prior to its inception. The transfer of staff and buildings had gone smoothly, and the service was now universally accepted despite continuing problems. People understood, as Hugh Ferguson put it in a *Tribune* article in 1949, that 'decades of insufficient development, of a class outlook in medical care, cannot be made good except over a period of years', despite concerted efforts by the Tory press to discredit the health service.[8]

Health workers understood both the achievements and the remaining problems more than most. They therefore gave an enthusiastic welcome to Aneurin Bevan, as Minister of Health, when he addressed delegates at the end of COHSE's Hastings conference in 1950. He said he accepted the need for economies, justifying (against his own private beliefs) the recently threatened 1 shilling prescription charge. However, he declared that this was an exception and that he regarded a free medical service as a 'sacrosanct' principle, no matter what 'sacrifices' might be necessary in the national interest. He congratulated those present for having done a 'pretty good job, very much more than we are given credit for', declaring that:

> We are starting off an entirely new thing. We were seeing what people medically need, and in so far as we can provide it, we provide freely. The result was Himalayan demands for spectacles, the dentists invaded ... the pharmaceutical service swollen to most extraordinary proportions.

Yet, despite Tory alarms, NHS workers were 'working off the backlog' and demand had now stabilised. To loud and prolonged applause he ended his speech by saying

> I do not ask you to set aside any of your own personal and professional preoccupations; nevertheless I ask you to remember that the full citizen is not only a person who looks after his own interests, but manages to make his own interest and the public interest one.[9]

As we have seen, the 1950 conference's 'preoccupations' were increasingly the desperate material ones of the members. Claude Bartlett, now COHSE's representative (in place of Gibson) on the General Council of the TUC, had told delegates in his presidential address that there were growing dissatisfactions with the Whitley Council system. Already he was arguing that:

> The time has come for a review of this machinery. It is cumbersome and completely unbalanced so far as the basis of representation is concerned, and much can be done to improve its efficiency and regain the confidence of those whose conditions of employment and remuneration are regulated by its decisions. I know of no other set of workers in this country where the procrastination and delay in reaching agreement and implementing awards would have been accepted with the patience and tolerance displayed by the nursing, domestic and other staffs of our hospitals and institutions.

He especially singled out ancillary workers for comment: 'Quite frankly, I am amazed how many of them find it possible to make ends meet.'

The following year, the government broke Bevan's 'sacrosanct' principle and introduced charges for NHS dentures and spectacles. He resigned, along with two junior Ministers, John Freeman and Harold Wilson. This was a factor in the defeat later that year of a Labour government which had set out boldly, but had lately lost its way. Now health workers' concern over their squeezed living standards was compounded by uncertainty over the future of a Health Service which was now in the hands of the Tories.

Notes

[1] H.A. Clegg and T.E. Chester, *Wage Policy and the Health Service* (1957), Ch. 1.
[2] W. McCarthy, *Making Whitley Work* (1976).
[3] HM (48)1, cited by A.W. Miles and D. Smith, *Joint Consultation: Defeat or Opportunity?* (1969).
[4] *Health Services Journal*, (COHSE's official journal referred to henceforth as *HSJ*), May 1950.
[5] Circular to Branch Secretaries, Joe Soley file, COHSE Archive, loc. cit.

[6] Abel-Smith, *Nursing Profession*.

[7] Ibid.

[8] H. Ferguson, 'Health Service: the First Year', reprinted in *HSJ*, August 1949.

[9] 'Conference Proceedings', *HSJ*, November 1950.

Chapter 18
The Lean Years, 1952-59

From the desolate vantage point of the 1980s it is almost possible to be taken in by the mythical image of the 1950s as 'golden' years. The economy was booming, standards of living were rising and the poverty and unemployment of the 1930s seemed to have been banished forever. With the years of austerity over, people had begun to enjoy themselves again. Like all mythologies, the image has elements of truth to it, and when Harold Macmillan, the Tory Prime Minister, told the electorate in 1959 that they had 'never had it so good' it was, for many of them, a statement of truth. But there was another reality to the 1950s, lurking in the shadow of its affluent image: the reality of growing poverty among those who did not share in the boom – the elderly, single parents, large families and the low paid.[1] Of the last many were to be found working for the government, with NHS ancillary workers among the lowest paid occupational group of all.

The main reason was that the Conservative government continued and intensified the policies of cost containment pioneered by the Labour government at the end of the 1940s. One result was a vicious circle of abysmal pay and deteriorating working conditions which exacerbated existing staff shortages by leading to massive rates of turnover among nursing and ancillary staffs. The other was a lack of investment in the deteriorating stock of buildings, many of them dating back to the nineteenth century, which also adversely affected health workers' working conditions. Yet although the Tories took a rather niggardly view of the NHS, they were finally compelled to preserve it and even, against their inclinations, to start to increase the funds allocated to it each year.

Doubts about their original intentions had first been manifest in the Tory *Campaign Guide* of 1950 which expressed 'alarm' at the cost of the NHS in its first year of operation.[2] Few people were surprised, therefore when in 1952 it implemented the 1 shilling prescription charge put on the statue book by Labour, brought in charges for elastic hosiery, wigs, surgical footwear and abdominal trusses and imposed a massive £1 charge for a course of dental treatment. The government moved next to curb the rising cost of the hospital service, which was swallowing up an increasing amount of the NHS budget. In late 1951 it had already sent out a circular outlining the procedure to be followed when, 'from time to time', HMCs find it 'necessary' that 'the services of a certain number of staff have to be dispensed with'.[3] Then in 1953 Iain Macleod, the Minister of Health, circularised health authorities calling on them to make economies of 5 per cent in certain categories of staff, amounting to 7,500 in all, in order to effect savings of £2.5 million. COHSE and other health unions protested vigorously and the circular was not on the whole acted upon. More alarming still was the government's decision, also announced in 1953, to institute an official committee of enquiry into the cost of running the NHS, which produced the Guillebaud Report in 1957. The trade union movement's evidence to the committee was centrally co-ordinated by the TUC, which argued in 1954 that the £400 million spending limit, imposed by Labour in 1950 and maintained since by the Conservatives, had 'retarded the development of essential services'. It drew attention to the gross overcrowding, long waiting lists and poor after-care facilities in the mental health sector. It criticised the failure to build the health centres which were supposed to be an integral part of the service, and the lack of space in hospitals to treat growing numbers of elderly people who might be fit to return to the community after a short course of treatment. It criticised the low priority given to prevention. It opposed prescription and other charges and said that any abuses in the NHS were due to profiteering by suppliers.[4] The

Guillebaud Report itself, much to everyone's surprise, largely cleared the NHS of the accusation that costs were accelerating out of control. In fact it congratulated the NHS on achieving so much within such tight budgets, and suggested that more resources should be devoted to it.[5]

The report's impact was twofold. For a generation it protected the service from right-wing forces which had sought unsuccessfully to undermine its most fundamental principles. Now the Conservative government had in 1957 accepted that the NHS was a desirable estate of the realm, to be financed in the main from taxation, just as it accepted the main framework of the welfare state and the mixed economy. Yet, as the *New Statesman* commented, the report also allowed the service to become 'a promising but neglected child' of the welfare state.[6] Since it refrained from outlining any coherent plans for the future development of the National Health Service, the practice continued of financing, and largely squeezing the health service, on a year-to-year basis.

The percentage of the national wealth spent on the NHS declined prior to the publication of the Guillebaud Report, and only increased marginally thereafter.[7] As far as health workers were concerned, then, the report was a mixed blessing. It helped to arrest the decline of the NHS that had taken place under the Tories, but did not guarantee much else.

The associated squeeze on health workers' living standards in a period of apparently 'free' collective bargaining followed a now established pattern. Pay negotiations would become the subject of interminable delays, due largely to management sides' inability to conclude agreements without their broad financial contours being the subject of Treasury approval which was rarely forthcoming. Finally, with staff frustration growing to danger levels, both sides would agree to go to outside arbitration, which might or might not resolve the problems upon which the two sides of the Whitley Councils could not agree. This pattern not only helped governments to operate an informal policy of pay restraint, but also (through the convenient arbitrationn mechanism) to get themselves off the hook where necessary.[8] The pattern varied between Whitley Councils but was discernible in all of them.

Mental Nurses' Pay and Conditions

The biggest stumbling block of all occurred with negotiations on mental nurses' pay. COHSE wanted to protect the differential between the pay of mental and general nurses which they had enjoyed prior to the NHS. The opportunity came when nurses at the Ministry of Health Special Hospitals of Broadmoor, Rampton and Moss Side were granted an extra or 'lead' payment of £50 a year. COHSE immediately put in a claim asking for the same for all mental nurses.

These are the bare facts, which seem dry now, but they were of very real material concern to staff at the time. Behind them lay an appalling story of staff shortages and growing discontent among the staff. Between 1952 and 1953 there was actually a decrease in the number of student nurses from 45,000 to 44,000, although the situation improved in subsequent years as a result of efforts made to recruit nurses from Eire, the Commonwealth and colonial countries. Student nurse training declined in popularity during the 1950s among domestic female school leavers, and the supply of male recruits also began to dry up. As ever, nursing did not seem able to retain the recruits it did attract. One in three general student nurses failed to complete his or her training, many leaving before the end of the first year. A large number of studies in the 1950s and 60s sought to explain this phenomenon. While many focused on the supposed deficiencies of the recruits themselves, some did suggest the obvious truth that rigid and outdated authority relations, and the pressures of work in comparison to the rewards offered by outside work, played the most significant part.[9]

The increasing recruitment of overseas nurses created some tensions in the union. The National Executive Committee was forced to define its position in 1954 when members at Cafn Coed branch, Swansea, opposed the recruitment of six young women from Barbados as student nurses on the grounds that if wages and conditions were improved, 'we would be able to get enough student nurses in our own country without recruiting them from elsewhere'.[10] After much agonising the National Executive Committee in December 1954 passed a resolution opposing a colour bar in any shape or form, but expressed concern that recruitment of overseas nurses might erode standards of pay and conditions still further. Nevertheless when the issue blew up again in 1955 when members from Storthes Hall in Yorkshire met with their Regional Secretary, then David Williams, to oppose the recruitment of 29 student nurses from Nigeria and Jamaica, they were told by the National Executive Committee that they were out on a limb. Along with other unions, COHSE was under pressure from the TUC to act to remove 'causes of friction and preventing exploitation'. Wherever possible COHSE wanted to let sleeping dogs lie, as did most other unions. Not until the 1960s was a concerted effort made to recruit overseas health workers to the union.

The shortages of nursing staff were greatest in the mental hospitals, and were in fact symptomatic of a profound state of crisis in the whole system of mental health care. The hopes of a new era after the settlement of the GNC/RMPA dispute had simply not materialised. As the Conservative government's economies bit deeper, the mental hospitals suffered worst of all as their staffs sought to cope with both a deteriorating stock of buildings and growing overcrowding. More patients were being discharged, especially with the introduction of new drugs, yet still the numbers of patients continued to rise, due largely to the fact that mental hospitals were being asked to become one of the main coping agencies for Britain's growing elderly population.[11]

The Labour Party started to become active on the issue. Kenneth Robinson, a Labour MP who was to become a future Minister of Health, published an article in *Tribune* in 1954 which declared that mental hospitals were 'in danger', saying that in some areas overcrowding was so bad that voluntary admissions had been restricted or even stopped, and that the Victorian buildings were unsuitable for modern treatment methods. He also drew attention to the staffing crisis which had led to the recruitment of more untrained assistant nurses to plug the gaps.

Unless something was done he predicted 'a breakdown of our mental health service within a few years' and warned that 'to repair the neglect of a hundred years will cost a great deal of money'.[12] The recruitment of more untrained staff was the direct result of what COHSE called the 'dilution' Circular RHB (53) – the government's alternative to solving the recruitment crisis by improving pay, conditions and prospects. The union described the Circular as 'putting the clock back thirty years' by reversing the trend, fought for by the union since the 1920s, of making mental nursing an increasingly trained profession, but its protests were to no avail.

The recruitment situation worsened, while negotiations on mental nurses' salaries dragged on and on . When the whole issue went to arbitration the Industrial Court's decision acted as further inducement to dilution of labour. While management's offer of a £15 increase to student nurses was confirmed and the pay of trained staff increased by £25 a year, many assistant nurses received increases of £30 a year. COHSE's claim had been for an all-round increase of £50 a year to bring the mental nurses' lead up to the £90 a year now paid to nurses at the 'special' hospitals of Broadmoor, Rampton and Moss Side. Eventually, after more frustrating negotiations, COHSE felt driven to take industrial action. Unfortunately, this uncovered the fact that the union, as well as the mental health service, was facing something of a crisis.

The revolt of mental nurses

COHSE had begun in 1946 with bold aspirations of becoming an industrial union for the health service. By the mid-1950s the campaign to recruit general hospital staff was not getting very far. The union was increasingly squeezed on nurses by the RCN, on ancillary workers by NUPE and the TGWU, on administrative staff by NALGO and on laboratory and professional staffs by the Association of Scientific Workers (later ASTMS). Instead of responding to COHSE's campaign for industrial unionism, health workers were increasingly organising on the basis of grade. In these circumstances COHSE was increasingly seen as the union for mental nurses, and particularly as the union for those in charge nurse positions and above who dominated its NEC. The union's preoccupation in the 1950s with the critical problems facing the mental health service only served to reinforce this tendency. As the situation worsened, with COHSE apparently powerless to change it, membership of the union even fell a little in the mid-1950s.

A large part of COHSE's problem lay in the absence of an effective and united leadership at the centre. Cliff Comer had resigned as General Secretary in April 1953 for what he told the NEC were 'purely personal' reasons. But he was also tired both by the conflicts over strategy between left and right within the union and by COHSE's failure to realise the aspirations which led to its creation in 1946.[13] His resignation could not have come at a worse time for COHSE, just when the Ministry had issued the 'dilution' Circular (53) 54. Jack Waite took over as Acting General Secretary and won the subsequent election. Then in his late fifties, he had been a Yorkshire miner before the First World War and a mental nurse at Wakefield in the 1920s. Like Comer, he had risen to prominence in the MHIWU during the 1930s, and his approach had been formed in response to the circumstances of the time. He was the last of the interwar generation of mental nurses to lead the union.

Jack Waite certainly took over at a time of mounting anger among mental nurses. At the 1953 delegate conference a resolution harking back to the past was carried, calling for separate negotiations for mental nurses, either through the Whitley Council or directly. Pressure also increased on the NEC to sanction an overtime ban in pursuit of the £50 claim, which it resisted in favour of its own emergency resolution empowering it 'to take such steps as they may deem to be necessary and advisable' if the claim was not met.

The Industrial Court ruling of 1954 resulted in a rather desultory award, and when more or less the same thing happened in 1955 the NEC came under pressure from

Region 3 (North-west) to implement an overtime ban. On two occasions arbitration had failed the union by largely upholding management's offer. The NEC responded at its March 1955 meeting by deciding to lodge a new claim for a £50 increase for student nurses failing which 'we have no alternative but to consider the banning of overtime'. Negotiations crawled on through 1955, and in November student nurses were finally offered yet another £15 a year increase. Membership discontent was now seething and unofficial action spontaneously erupted in Lancashire and then spread elsewhere. According to the NEC Minutes of March 1956 'the first indication that the General Secretary had of it was through the press'. He had circularised branches in January and then in February asking them to suspend their action, as Mr Turton, the Minister of Health, had agreed to see a COHSE deputation on its demand for a separate Whitley Council. According to COHSE's own estimates the 'Ban Overtime' movement, though strongest in Lancashire, had spread by February 1956 to 33 hospitals in many parts of the country, with 10,000 of its members taking part.

The spread of industrial action had taken place after a 60-strong demonstration of COHSE members at the opening of a government sponsored 'mental health exhibition' on 30 January 1956. Their placards included ironic comments on it, such as 'Mental Nurses wanted: to Work Themselves to Death'. The aim of such exhibitions, which took place throughout the country in the mid-1950s, was to influence favourably public attitudes to mental illness and its treatment in mental hospitals, and to create a positive image of mental nursing in order to recruit more nurses. The philosophy behind them was that the public's idea of conditions inside mental hospitals was lagging behind the changes and improvements that had been made. The publicity material used for them showed no overcrowded wards or apathetic, neglected patients and over-worked staff.

COHSE was adamant that such exhibitions were no substitute for material improvements in pay and capital investment in buildings. It virtually accused the government of using exhibitions as a cover-up of scandalous conditions in mental hospitals. It praised the *Daily Express* for a series of articles in September 1955 exposing conditions inside mental hospitals, saying that they were 'a realistic antidote to the slushy sentiment which the newspapers usually reserve for nurses', and that 'mental hospital staffs prefer the unvarnished truth'. They had, for example, described how 83 women slept in a corridor nine feet wide, and how 140 men were herded into a ward designed for 75, with one nurse and an orderly to look after them. They talked of hospitals which were 'more or less rotten', with peeling plaster and damp streaked walls, and drew attention to the desperate staffing situation. Merrick Winn, the author of the articles, described how in such circumstances the minimal resources were concentrated on acute cases, with a large 'chronic' population receiving no psychiatric treatment at all, locked up in overcrowded wards primarily because of staffing difficulties.[14]

The demonstrations against the exhibitions continued through 1956 and 1957. In the meantime, however, the NEC had been under intense pressure to institute an official overtime ban in support of a twelve-point claim which included a 44-hour week, six weeks' holiday, enhanced overtime rates, a substantial salary increase and a separate Whitley Council for mental nurses. In the desperate staffing situation of many hospitals the ban would have had a dramatic impact, but would not have required nurses to break their contracts. The NEC, however, did not act decisively. In March 1956, it ruled out the possibility of strike action because it 'would offend the public'. Instead it threatened an 'official ban on overtime from May 1 next', unless there was 'satisfactory progress in negotiation', and meanwhile called on all branches to suspend their action.

What happened subsequently is a rather messy story. The NEC met again on 26 April 1956, the day on which the NMC agreed revised salaries of £20 a year for a student nurse, £30 for a staff nurse, £35 for a charge nurse and £40-65 for those above them in the hierarchy. But no settlement was reached on the claim for enhanced overtime rates of pay. The Minister had also refused to intervene to create a separate Whitley Council for mental nurses, following the convention that such matters were for the staff side of the NMC alone to determine. The majority of the NEC wanted to hold fire. It was worried that there would be a less than 100 per cent response to a ban, and that the GNC would discipline those taking part for engaging in 'unprofessional conduct'. On the advice of the General Secretary the NEC decided finally to defer the ban until the union's conference later that summer, but one-third of its members – those from the London area and the North – voted for its immediate implementation.

The NEC faced a motion of no confidence at the June conference in Llandudno, supported among others, by Bob Vickerstaff, representing Gosforth branch, who said that the NEC had backed off from the ban when there was 'a hundred per cent support for it'. The left-wing Joe Soley defended the NEC and its policy – to which he was actually opposed – and the no-confidence motion was 'overwhelmingly' defeated.

Conference then voted for an immediate overtime ban, against Jack Waite's advice. Even so, the NEC still held off from implementing it, then only selectively, until a year later in September 1957. In the meantime the NMC staff side had reluctantly accepted a 5 per cent increase, which only compensated them for the rise in the cost-of-living, rather than their claim for 'a revaluation of the services of the nurse to the community'. Discontent was now seething within the union, especially in the North and Scotland. There had been a brief sit-down strike at Rainhill in Lancashire. There was even talk of some regional councils breaking away from COHSE. In the face of these pressures the General Secretary was forced to concede to demands for a special delegate conference 'to iron out misunderstandings'. Yet calls to extend the ban throughout the union were rejected by the conference, when it was held in St Pancras Town Hall on 15 January 1958, only because, as Albert Spanswick from Lincoln put it, the time when it could have been effective was now past. COHSE did not win its central demands, except for the 44-hour week, which as usual was to be implemented 'as conditions permit'. The call for a separate Whitley Council fell by the wayside, as did enhanced overtime rates, at least for the time being. Jack Waite retired due to ill health in September 1958 and he was succeeded, in a closely fought election, by John Jepson, the Southern National Officer and an ex-HWSU official. Mental nursing's monopoly on the leadership of COHSE had finally been broken.

The State of Mental Nursing

The discontent beneath the revolt of mental nurses ran far deeper than simple dissatisfaction over rates of overtime pay, or even pay and staffing problems. Against the background of overall neglect changes were taking place in the apparently ordered world of the mental hospital, fracturing the timeless and self-contained community with its firmly defined hierarchical relationships. The uncertainty created by these changes added to the problems experienced by nurses, and formed an important background factor to their militancy.

The traditional structure of the mental hospital was by this time crumbling under the pressure of a new philosophy emphasising treatment, liberalisation as a result of being part of the NHS and the so-called 'drugs revolution' of the 1950s. Wards were unlocked, military-style uniforms with brass buttons and peaked caps abandoned, ancillary workers recruited to replace patient and nurse labour, rates of both admission and discharge rose, and the hospital farms – pride of the former asylums – were run down and eventually sold off. But these were merely the surface appearances of deeper changes in the authority relationships involved in a shift from a custodial to a more treatment-based regime. As Dr Denis Martin argued in his perceptive book about Claybury Hospital in the 1950s, the traditional basis of relationships in mental hospitals was 'authority and submission', particularly among the nursing hierarchy. He described male nurses as especially reluctant to risk criticism from above because their whole lives were built around the hospital: 'Any apparent threat to his promotion prospects therefore strikes economically at the roots of his security, his home life.'[15] This was perhaps one reason why COHSE was so internally divided about imposing an overtime ban.

By the time COHSE was agonising over taking collective action, this traditional system, with its inbuilt bias against innovation, was in decay. Among the principal causes was the fact that the principle of 'clinical freedom' for individual consultants, so much a part of Bevan's deal with the medical profession in 1948, cut across the traditional managerial authority of the medical superintendent. In addition, the superintendents lost out to the Hospital Management Committees. The superintendents' days were numbered and from 1960 it no longer became a requirement to appoint one. Nurses were, of course, likely to be profoundly affected by these complex changes in the authority structure and the expectations now placed upon them. The whole way of life, particularly of the older generation of nurses, was undergoing a transformation. Many staff were worried about how to adapt to the new situation. Audrey John undertook a study of nurses in four Scottish mental hospitals in 1958 and talked to one

> male nurse, almost due for retirement, who told of 18 consecutive years labour in the gardens, during which time he become a registered mental nurse without ever working for a single day in the wards of the hospital ... His main problems had started when promoted by senority, he was expected to assume responsibility for a number of treatments with which he was totally unfamiliar.[16]

Another study of mental nurses, undertaken by Maddox in the Liverpool area in the early 1950s, found that nursing staff responded rather differently to these changes according to whether they tended to belong to the younger or older generation of nurses. The staffing crisis was used by the older generation as an 'excuse for inaction', while the younger generation quickly became disillusioned when they realised it was not possible to put their ideals into practice. In addition, some therapeutic aspects of the nurses' role had been transferred to a new set of specialist groups – occupational therapists, art therapists, etc. Thus it seems that the role of the mental nurse was in fact becoming more restricted in the 1950s, despite the general aura of 'progress'. In addition, as Maddox also observed, their training did not equip them with the new psycho-therapeutic skills they now required, being based too heavily upon general nursing due to a common first year syllabus across all nursing disciplines.[17] His critique was later confirmed officially by the Clark Committee in 1968.[18] Many of the idealistic spirits soon left the service, one publishing a highly critical personal account of his experiences as a student nurse at Shenley Hospital near St Albans.[19] Many of the idealists who joined after the war did stay, however, convinced that the unsatisfactory state of mental nursing could be changed through the union; among them were two future general secretaries of COHSE, Albert Spanswick and David Williams.

These changes, and the contradictions associated with them, were bound to generate conflicts. As well as forming the background to the national dispute, localised tensions and discontents surfaced publicly in a number of instances. At Lancaster Moor and Napsbury Hospitals staff went as far as to threaten strike action. Although industrial action did not actually take place in either case, it provided more evidence that the overtime pay issue was symptomatic of deeper discontents. At Lancaster promotion procedures formed a very large part of staff grievances, particularly the appointment of Miss Hill, the Deputy Matron. Staff also claimed that Dr Silverstone, the Medical Superintendent, was introducing changes without making use of the joint consultative machinery, and refusing to hear representations from COHSE. In 1948 staff passed a motion of 'no confidence' in Dr Silverstone, and gave 21 days' notice of intention to strike and only suspended it when an official inquiry was set up.[20] This reported in 1953 and blamed the workers rather than management, but in its margins the report did admit that management had not used the JCC machinery fully, and that Dr Silverstone had an 'obvious preference for the disciplinary route to the co-operative route' in his dealings with staff.[21] A 'near strike' over promotion procedures at Napsbury in Hertfordshire was symbolic of the older generation's fears that they would be bypassed by younger 'high-flyers'.

The scarcity of properly established joint consultation machinery was undoubtedly often a hindrance to winning staff co-operation to the great changes taking place in mental hospitals. COHSE tried to remedy matters through its first Educational Conference, held in October 1958 and organised by its new Educational Department, which associated the union with the movement for change in the mental health services at the same time as calling for greater consultation over its implementation. The impending changes in the law relating to mental health and the associated shift to community care undoubtedly acted as a stimulus to COHSE.

The 1959 Mental Health Act

The Mental Health Act itself was passed in 1959 with support from all political parties. It was the result of the Report of a Royal Commission set up in 1954 at the height of the crisis in the mental hospitals. Its members included COHSE's President Claude Bartlett, who had long called for the dismantling of the restrictive lunacy laws, and the report's recommendations along these lines were finally put into effect. The Board of Control was abolished and the legislation for 'mental illness' and 'subnormality' – as they were now called – merged, and a new controversial category of 'psychopathy' added. It was anticipated (correctly) that in future most patients would be treated informally. A minority would continue to be compulsorily admitted in a variety of ways. Patients' interests were said to be safeguarded by the creation of an independent Mental Health Review Tribunal.

The Act was a major step forward giving formal legality to the changes that were already taking place within the service, but there was a catch. The emphasis was now on 'community care' but, despite the recommendations of the Royal Commission, the Tory government had made no specific financial provision to help local authorities to develop their community mental health services. COHSE was extremely doubtful that local government would build these up and staff the necessary community services unless provided with the cash by central government. Two MPs closely linked with COHSE – Bessie Braddock and H.A. Blenkinsop – had pressed Derek Walker-Smith, the Minister of Health, on these points without success. Although the impetus for change was genuine, there was therefore more than a suspicion that the government was climbing on the bandwagon of 'community care' because it presented a cheap solution to the mental hospital crisis of the 1950s. By the 1960s these intentions had become blatantly apparent.

There were other implications, too. As well as the shift to the community, the Act was bound to hasten the further integration of the mental health service into general medicine, with an increasing transfer of acute work to general hospital units. Though some nurses would follow their patients in both directions, the job prospects for most staff remaining in the traditional mental hospitals was not particularly rosy. Left to care for a largely chronically ill and increasingly elderly population of patients, the de-skilling process begun in the 1950s would in fact accelerate, leading to a further decline in morale and, by an almost inevitable series of steps, to the mental hospital scandals of the late 1960s.

Whitleyism: The Plot Thickens

COHSE was very preoccupied with mental nursing matters during the 1950s, but the union was also active on a number of other fronts. Here too the Conservative government manipulated the bargaining machinery in order to obtain what it wanted, and when this failed to produce the required results it resorted to other means. As one of the leading historians of the welfare state has put it:

> The Whitley Council machinery would deserve several chapters in any text book written on the art of government manipulation.[22]

The one group who formed something of an exception to this rule were ambulance workers. Although the ambulance services were formally part of the National health service, they were by the 1950s administered by local government and came under the NJIC for Non-Trading-Services. This had a double-edged effect. In terms of status they were now largely regarded as local government manual workers, but with material conditions which were superior to those that they would have obtained had they been subject to the underhand pay policies that operated in the NHS. This was one reason why NUPE had supported their transfer to local government, while COHSE had objected largely because it thought that recognition of the ambulance workers' place in the health team was of more strategic importance. In consequence COHSE tended more often to represent those ambulance workers with aspirations for professional status, while NUPE and the TGWU attracted those who felt less uncomfortable at being associated with manual workers. Because of the circumstances of their jobs (like psychiatric nurses they formed something akin to an 'occupational community'), ambulance workers tended to regard themselves as a race apart, whatever union they belonged to. COHSE's bargaining position in relation to ambulance workers eased a little from 1954 when the NJIC made informal arrangements to hear representations from COHSE when ambulance matters were being discussed. COHSE's lack of full recognition on the NJIC nevertheless remained a severe disadvantage in the competitive struggle to organise ambulance workers.

The growing competition between NUPE and COHSE for ambulance workers was part of a general heightening of tension between the two organisations. The NHS labour force expanded rapidly in the 1950s, which intensified recruitment competition between unions. NUPE had long enjoyed a reputation for aggressive recruiting tactics, and the growing problems this was posing for COHSE were highlighted in the case of Mr R.H. Andrews, an ambulance driver in Truro who had resigned from COHSE to join NUPE in 1951, along with six of his colleagues. A complaint by COHSE led to a ruling from the TUC Disputes Committee that NUPE should expel them from membership. Mr Andrews took NUPE to the High Court to test the legality of the expulsion and won his case. As a result NUPE declined to implement this TUC ruling and others made in response to COHSE complaints. The TUC felt that NUPE was being obstructive, and in December 1955 even threatened to expel NUPE from its ranks. In January 1956 NUPE's NEC agreed reluctantly to implement the TUC's recommendations 'to the best of its ability'.[23] This was a compromise rather than a climb-down by NUPE, as the original TUC disputes ruling against it was never implemented. In the longer term the Andrews case probably encouraged the spread of poaching and the adoption of an 'if you can't beat them – join them' attitude by other NHS unions.

COHSE's lack of membership of the NJIC inevitably pushed it further into promoting itself as the union which took on the wider issues affecting the service, heightening its already pronounced 'professional' ethos. Through a close association with the Institute of Certified Ambulance Personnel it continued to press for proper training and professional recognition of ambulance workers. It won representation on the Ministry of Health's Committee under Dr Lillico, whose report on training led to Circular 30/51 which recommended that every entrant to the service should possess a first aid certificate and that local authorities should provide refresher courses. The Institute argued through its General Secretary, Mrs N.E. Berger, that this did not go far enough; even so, this recommendation was not observed by many authorities.

COHSE also campaigned against the continuing efforts by some authorities to amalgamate the ambulance and fire services. The biggest struggle was waged at Blackpool where the majority of staff were in COHSE. In 1954 the Fire Brigades Committee of Blackpool Corporation proposed the merger of the two services in order to achieve economies. The COHSE ambulance workers set about a concerted campaign of protest, issuing an appeal for support to the local labour movement. They won in this instance, even though some 20 ambulance authorities had already been merged with the fire service.[24]

COHSE believed that the most important problems facing the ambulance service were due to poor co-ordination of requests for transport, which could only be remedied by its proper integration into the NHS. It therefore resumed its mission to convert the TUC to this cause, but its motion to Congress in 1954 was remitted to the General Council and became subject to the complex and interminable negotiations involved in that process primarily because the interests of other more powerful unions were affected.

These developments were not occurring in a vacuum. Both management and workers were responding to fundamental changes in the ambulance services during the 1950s. Put briefly, there was an increased volume of work, much of it absorbed by the more intensified exploitation of the existing workforce by cost-consious local authorities with encouragement from circulars from central goverment. In 1950-51 there were some 4,200 ambulances in England and Wales. By 1959-60 this number had only increased to approximately 5,000 despite the fact that the number of patients carried increased 82 per cent, from 9 to 16.5 million. Much of this had been achieved by the use of centralised radio control which had revolutionised the service and done away with the need to keep a fleet of vehicles and personnel on permanent standy-by in case of emergencies. Most of the increase was in 'routine' cases, particularly the ferrying of patients back and forth from their hospital out-patient appointments. Due to bed shortages hospital stays were shorter and more patients were being treated from home. By 1960 only 6 per cent of ambulance patients were classified as emergencies.[25] True, the skills demanded of personnel involved in this kind of work were rising dramatically, but they were a relatively small elite section within the workforce.

COHSE's appeal was pitched very much to the latter group rather than the growing army of semi-skilled ambulance drivers, increasing numbers of whom were women, employed largely on out-patient work. As with mental nurses, this situation helped to highlight the stagnation affecting COHSE during the 1950s compared with other unions eager to recruit health service staffs.

Among hospital ancillary workers the biggest battle was over the attempt to reduce the basic working week from 48 to 44 hours. NHS ancillary workers' hours were longer than those workers in comparable jobs, and there was an exodus of staff to industry and local government attracted by the superior pay and conditions. The hours of ancillary workers contrasted unfavourably with most other groups of employees in the NHS. A survey conducted by George Paine in 1955 into the 'lost legions of hospital staffs' showed that while management was resisting the claim for a 44-hour week for ancillary staffs, laboratory staff and pharmacists enjoyed a 39-hour week, administrative staff 38, radiographers 35 and speech therapists 33.[26] Only nurses were also working a 48-hour week – and management would not concede to ancillary workers because it would have led to a similar claim from nurses. Exactly which section of management was opposed, however, needs to be made clear. The employing authorities – the HMCs and Boards of Governors of teaching hospitals – were very much in favour of a 44-hour week, because it would ease their increasingly desperate staffing situation. The management side of the Whitley Council, however, was dominated by Ministry of Health officials, who were in turn responsible to the Treasury.

The Whitley 'charade' or 'roundabout' (as it was variously called by COHSE members) presented itself yet again. The management side refused the claim, which went unsuccessfully to arbitration three times between 1951 and 1956. The claim was not conceeded until 1959, and then only after the intervention of the TUC's Economic Committee and massive rank-and-file pressure on all the unions involved. For example, regional protest rallies within COHSE urged the NEC to take 'drastic action to secure the 44 hour week'. Even then the agreement of 1957 was for implementation in two stages, and not until July 1958, seven years after the claim was first submitted, did ancillary workers actually obtain the 44-hour week.

Nurses gained from the efforts of ancillary workers. The 44-hour week was also conceded to them in 1958, the year that it became operational for ancillary workers. But there was, as usual, a catch. It was to be implemented at individual hospitals, as so often in the past, 'as conditions permit'. A further blow occurred when the government made it clear that it was not making any money available to enable hospitals to employ the extra staff needed to implement shorter hours and still maintain the same service.

It was clear that action would at least have to be taken on these anomalies and a major review of salaries was in fact overdue. After years in which their pay had been subject to interminable delays, and fallen behind other comparable groups, what COHSE described as 'the biggest ever overhaul by the Nurses and Midwives Council' finally materialised in March 1959. Increases ranged from 5 to 22 per cent and the mental and mental deficiency nurses' lead had, 'after tough bargaining', been increased to £50 a year. Nurses had now got something like a reasonable pay deal, one that at least restored the ground lost during the 1950s. But it had been a long time coming and the refusal to grant extra financial resources to implement the 44-hour week contrasted with arrangements that had been made in relation to ancillary staffs.

This shoddy treatment of nurses led inevitably to comparisons of the relative effectiveness of the two staff sides, the one Council composed solely of trade unions, the other dominated by professional associations. Yet COHSE was experiencing considerable difficulty in attracting general nurses in the 1950s. This was partly because it was preoccupied with mental nursing matters, but the RCN's stranglehold of training schools enabled it to fend off COHSE's attempts at incursion in this field; also, anti-union attitudes were still widespread among general nurses. The 1953 COHSE conference had declared 'total war upon the Royal College of Nursing'. It was not, however, a war which at that stage COHSE had much chance of winning. Only when matrons and assistant matrons, able to use their influence to inform staff about the advantages of union membership, could be persuaded to join COHSE, did the union make break-throughs. One long-standing matron member was Mary Burns of Barnsley who took a very active part in COHSE from its formation in 1946 and was a prominent member of its NEC during the 1950s.

There was in fact a spate of disciplinary cases involving matrons in the late 1950s, and COHSE was directly involved in some of them. In 1958 COHSE successfully defended Matron Theresa Reid of Winwick Hospital near Liverpool, for 'insubordination'. Then in 1960 Mary Burns herself was sacked because she wrote to the group secretary complaining that the hospitals in the group were functioning 'a hundred per cent inefficiently' and demanded an inquiry. After an appeal her reinstatement was 'requested' by Sheffield Regional Hospital Board. Local management initially refused until ordered to comply with the request by the Minister of Health.

These cases highlighted yet again the inadequacies of the disciplinary appeals system and the continuing failure of the General Whitley Council to conclude an agreement on such a vital issue. The Ministry memorandum 'permitted' a dismissed employee to appeal to the region as an outside disinterested body, but it did not establish this as a right and only the Minister could insist that the HMC implement its findings. The cases also showed that matrons themselves were now not immune from the arbitrary justice they had, as a group, often handed out to others in the past: in the final analysis they too were only employees. The growing sense of vulnerability experienced by nurses with the removal of authority away from the hospital – Mary Burns had been sacked by a Group HMC – was to be one factor that led eventually to the growing unionisation of general nurses. In both cases, the General Secretary, W.J. Jepson, authorised the defence of the two individuals concerned and won. More nurses now began to wonder whether, if they were to find themselves in such circumstances, they might be better off with a trade union rather than the RCN.

Nurses were, of course, not the only workers whose strong sense of 'professional dignity' provided very little real protection against a cold employment climate in which management was increasingly treating professional workers as simply another group of employees. In 1956 this was amply illustrated by the case of a sacked radiographer who approached COHSE for help after having been refused assistance by the Society of Radiographers. She was successfully defended before the Group Committee by Jepson. The growing remoteness of authority and the drive for greater 'efficiency' seem to have been significant factors in a number of these cases. Both represented a decline in more personal forms of supervision, due to the growth in scale of the NHS and the pressure to squeeze as much out of the existing (human) resources that could be obtained.

Health workers' relationships with the central state were more transparently obvious. The story of manipulative obstructions, delays and parsimony is a thread connecting the negotiations for all the groups we have so far considered in this chapter. The Whitley 'charade' continued, especially since the Guillebaud Report of 1956 had, in COHSE's words, 'whitewashed' the Whitley Council system. Although it had called for some streamlining to deal with delays and for a substantial increase in HMC representation on management sides, it defended to the hilt the right of the Treasury to determine in advance the financial framework of management's offers. In general the committee seems to have thought that although the system needed a bit more flexibility it was working quite well.

Health service staff knew otherwise, to their cost, and in November 1957 experienced another shock. Not content with normal practices of underhand manipulation of the system, the government intervened directly and refused to implement a 3 per cent award to administrative and clerical staff. The government was using health workers to set an example to others in the current pay round. The Minister of Health's intervention directly violated assurances firstly given by Aneurin Bevan in 1948 and maintained by other ministers since then, but broken again by the Thatcher government. At NALGO's invitation all unions on the Administrative and Clerical (A & C) Council joined forces to impose an overtime ban with the proviso that it should not harm patients. Although staff were united the limited nature of the ban meant it made little impression on a government which saw this as a 'test case' for its new policy of wage restraint. After nine weeks the ban was lifted and a new claim submitted based on the Noel-Hall Report on restructuring the A & C grades. After the usual process of negotiation, delays and finally references to arbitration, a compromise settlement in 1959 – as with nurses – went some way towards restoring their economic position.[27] Nothing could disguise the fact that the Minister's overt intervention had fundamentally changed bargaining relationships. A crossroads had been reached.

As far as the two relatively generous deals in 1959 for nurses and A & C workers were concerned, both were influenced by the fact that 1959 was an election year and the government had received much unfavourable publicity and disapproval in opinion poll ratings for its treatment of health workers. It was an election in which Harold Macmillan astutely turned round the government's recent setbacks on domestic and international fronts, transforming them into a handsomely increased majority for the Tory government and earning himself – for a while at least – the nickname 'Supermac'.

The image successfully projected by Macmillan and the Conservatives during that election has remained the basis for our picture of the 1950s ever since. It was supposed to have been a time of affluence when the Tories were willing guardians of Labour's welfare state, a time also when NHS workers had not yet resorted to 'bloody minded' militant tactics but were contented and well cared for. This chapter has confronted this seductive image with the reality and found it wanting. The source of the militant trade unionism of the 1970s can therefore be traced directly to the shoddy treatment of health workers first established as the norm during the 1950s.

Notes

[1] B. Abel-Smith and P. Townsend, *The Poor and the Poorest* (1965).
[2] Quoted by A. Lindsey, *Socialised Medicine in England and Wales* (1961) p.100.
[3] RHB (51)101, quoted in *HSJ*, November-December 1951.
[4] See *HSJ*, September-October 1954.
[5] *Report of the Committee of Enquiry in the Cost of the National Health Service* (Guillebaud), (1957).

[6] Quoted by Lindsey, op. cit., p.121.

[7] HMSO, *Royal Commission on the National Health Service* (Merrison), (1979), Table E.

[8] See Clegg and Chester, *Wage Policy*.

[9] See the review of this research by J. Macguire, *Threshold to Nursing* (1969).

[10] *HSJ*, March-April 1955.

[11] K. Jones, *Mental Health Services*, p.358.

[12] Reprinted in *HSJ*, March-April 1954.

[13] *NEC Minutes*, 28 April 1953.

[14] *Daily Express*, 19, 20 and 21 September 1955.

[15] D.V. Martin, *Adventure in Psychiatry* (1962), p.9.

[16] A. John, *A Study of the Psychiatric Nurse* (1961), p.40.

[17] H. Maddox, 'The Work and Status of Mental Nurses', *Sociological Review* 2 (1954), pp.195-208.

[18] Ministry of Health, *Psychiatric Nursing: Today and Tomorrow* (Clark), (1968), Ch. 3.

[19] P. Warr, *Brother Lunatic* (1957).

[20] *HSJ*, December 1948.

[21] *HSJ*, September-October 1953.

[22] Abel-Smith, *Nursing Profession*, p.201.

[23] TUC, Annual Report (1956).

[24] *HSJ*, November-December 1954.

[25] W.C. Virgo, 'The Ambulance Service', in J. Farndale (ed.), *Trends in the National Health Service* (1964).

[26] Quoted by *HSJ*, January-February 1955.

[27] The full story of the overtime ban is told in Spoor, *White Collar Union*, Ch. 23.

Chapter 19
A Union in Transition, 1959–65

The Turning Point

Turning points can rarely be located precisely, but 1959 seems to mark some kind of watershed for COHSE. This was the year when its acknowledged identity as the union for male mental nurses began to change and the embryo of its new character began to form. Many of these changes were set in train by the chastening experience of the overtime ban 'fiasco', and they were shaped further by trends in the development of the NHS, the trade union movement as a whole and in British society at large. Just as the mental hospitals in the late 1950s ceased to be so isolated and inward-looking as in the past, so a breath of fresh air was blown through the union most associated with those who worked in them.

In 1958 Jack Waitc was succeeded by 'Jack' Jepson, a man not much younger in years but who came to power promising 'a more dynamic leadership'. He was acutely aware that COHSE had become a too narrowly based union, most representative of the interests of the older generation of male psychiatric charge nurses. To renew itself the union had to develop more appeal to the younger generation of health service staff who had been recruited to the NHS since 1948. If COHSE wanted to recruit them, it had to show what it could do for them *now*, not trade on past achievements. If it could do so, there was a vast army of unorganised general nurses who were ripe for capture.

The change in style of leadership associated with Jepson was crucial in liberating the energies which transformed

COHSE from a stagnating to a growing union. Head office, which had previously been preoccupied with the minutiae of Whitley Council negotiations and left recruitment up to the branches and regions, now saw building the membership as a major responsibility.

Symbolic of these developments was the long overdue shifting of head office itself from Manchester to Banstead in Surrey, a direct result of Jepson assuming the mantle of power within COHSE. Now the union's centre was closer to the centres of power in the NHS, rather than its own traditional areas of strength. It was now poised to become a more broadly based union, geographically and occupationally.

There was a touch of irony in the fact that these changes were occurring on the eve of COHSE's celebration of its fiftieth anniversary in 1960, but in a way it was appropriate. The problem for COHSE and the labour movement as a whole was to recognise the value of tradition yet at the same time be able to respond effectively to present events. It was a quandry faced by both wings of the labour movement in 1959: male manual workers of the traditional sort who provided the trade unions and the Labour Party with their bedrock of support were a declining part of the labour force. The future of the labour movement lay in the hands of unions like COHSE who were seeking to capture the growing army of previously unaffiliated white collar, professional and welfare state workers, many of them women, to convince them that they were workers and needed the collective protection of the movement.

The year 1960 also marked the summit of the career of Claude Bartlett, himself the embodiment of the service-oriented trade unionism which had emerged from mental hospitals during the interwar period. President of the union for more than 30 years, in 1960 he became the first ever lay TUC chair, presiding over one of its most acrimonious ever conferences. Significantly, he called in his address for renewed efforts to recruit 'those black-coated white collared workers who at present stand a little aloof from us'. Bartlett finally retired at COHSE conference in 1962 after 35 years as the union's President.

He was succeeded by A.R. Farmer, the existing Vice-President, a charge nurse at West Park Mental Hospital, Dorking, who had long been associated with the view that the union should broaden its recruitment base.

Within just two years of COHSE's fiftieth anniversary celebrations the union would be forced to conduct a strike ballot of the members in the face of a government intent on depressing health workers' living standards. The years following 1959 mark another transition, from the disguised 'Whitley charade' of the 1950s to a much more overt form of control – government income policies, already anticipated in the Ministerial veto of the A & C award of 1958. The continuing attempt to contain the rising costs of the NHS by squeezing the incomes of those working for it also took place within a wider context of mounting economic difficulties. The Macmillan government initially dealt with the inflationary effects of its pre-election budget through hire purchase controls. However in July 1961, as Britain's balance of payments crisis worsened, the new Chancellor of the Exchequer, Selwyn Lloyd, went a stage further. As well as cutting public spending by £300 million, raising interest rates and indirect taxation, he called for a six month 'pay pause', which would be enforced rigorously in the public sector but which would be left to employers to apply in the private sector. This involved blocking 35 wage claims, including those of nurses and other health workers, civil servants and teachers, even to the extent of vetoing Wages Council awards and delaying Industrial Court decisions. The way that these decisions had been announced was particularly inept politically, for no attempt was made to secure union support for the government's measures before they had been taken, and they blatantly and unfairly discriminated against public service workers.[1] It was a rude awakening for workers to the new era of public sector industrial relations.

The other significant impact of the Macmillan era on the NHS was the steps that were taken to restructure the management of the service and establish goals based on notions of 'efficiency', after the publication of the Hospital Plan of 1962. Both incomes policies and growing managerialism led to shifts in staff attitudes that assisted the growth of unions such as COHSE. Incomes policy destroyed the paternalistic relationship between health workers and the central state, while the growth in scale of hospitals and associated shift to more remote and impersonal styles of management broke down traditional relationships based on direct contact. This was not an entirely new development, as we have seen from previous chapters, but it undoubtedly accelerated in the 1960s prior to the 1974 reorganisation of the NHS, creating uncertainties favourable to the spread of trade unionism.

The Battle against the Government

The effect of the pay pause was to turn the staff discontent, already prevalent in the mental hospitals, into a much more general phenomenon. COHSE rejected the pay freeze, restated its belief in free collective bargaining and condemned the interference with the arbitration machinery. The NEC co-ordinated its protest activities with other public sector unions such as the National Union of Teachers (which played the leading role in calling unions together) and NALGO. Many of these were not at the time affiliated to the TUC, but this and similar experiences subsequently brought many of them in.

All unions were agreed that their claims should go ahead as normal. By December 1961 a number of issues had been impeded on the A & C Council which might normally have gone to the Industrial Court. Management on the Professional and Technical (B) – Council actually concluded an agreement with the staff side, only to declare that it could only be implemented at some future date. Luckily ancillary workers had concluded deals on several important issues, such as overtime rates for weekend working, before the pause was announced. The most serious trouble was brewing on the Nurses and Midwives Council. The relative economic position of nurses had slipped badly again since the last major award of 1959. There had been considerable controversy on the council at the majority decision to accept 5 per cent from December 1960. Five COHSE regions pressured the NEC in March 1961 to do more. One of them suggested that it should also press for a Royal Commission into the Nursing Profession, on the precedent established for the police service, and this was adopted by the NEC as policy. Meanwhile in August 1963, pause or not, a major claim for the reconstruction of nurses' salaries was put on the table, amounting on average to 35 per cent.

Despite a promise by the Minister of Health, Enoch Powell, that certain grades merited an increase despite the country's economic difficulties, nothing materialised for nurses despite the strong arguments in their favour. The pay of ward sisters of between £656 and £840 a year was less than that earned by many typists, while at the base of the pyramid were student nurses paid as little as £299 a year. In the autumn of 1961 COHSE submitted its proposal for a Royal Commission into the Nursing Services to the TUC. In moving COHSE's resolution Jack Jepson pointed out that within the past year the number of nursing vacancies had increased from 20,000 to 26,000 and that they wanted the commission to look at all aspects of nursing, not just pay and conditions. Jack Cooper (General Secretary of the NUGMW) opposed on behalf of the General Council. Because it included pay issues, TUC policy was that it would bypass existing negotiating machinery.[2] The motion was lost, but COHSE doggedly brought back the resolution to the 1962 Congress after it had been adopted by the Labour Party, this time tactfully omitting mention of pay and conditions in the motion. In his speech Jepson criticised the TUC for not taking a stronger lead. Enoch Powell had claimed that the number of nurses was increasing. This was true, but it was the familiar problem of demand seriously outstripping supply. In any case, much of the increase was due largely to the recruitment of part-timers. When this was taken into account the real increase in staffing was much less than the Minister was making out. COHSE had done its homework thoroughly, producing statistics to back up its case which all pointed to a massive shortage of staff due to a combination of low pay and government stringency measures on recruitment.

COHSE's motion to the TUC was passed, but only narrowly, after the General Council had asked for it to be remitted. They had argued that it was 'not ... the function of the General Council to initiate propaganda campaigns on behalf of the workpeople of a particular industry'.[3] This was a sad retreat from the position it had taken in the 1930s when it had led the campaign for the reform of nursing pay and conditions through its 1937 charter. The Nursing Advisory Committee was still in existence and could have conducted the necessary campaign, but it was a pale shadow of its former dynamic self, when George Gibson had been its leading light. The narrow majority for the COHSE motion meant that the issue was not pursued with any vigour by the TUC General Council, and the labour movement lost a golden opportunity to throw its weight behind a campaign to improve the lot of nurses.

While all this had been going on, nurses had been pitched into a fierce struggle with the Tory government, and in particular with Enoch Powell, its Minister of Health. Powell was even then a right-winger. He had previously been responsible for the notorious 1957 Rent Act[4] and came to the Ministry of Health determined to make his mark. He won a position in the Cabinet in 1962 when health had previously been regarded as a minor department. He undoubtedly had a greater personal influence than any Minister of Health since Bevan, though only within the tight financial margins imposed on him from outside, which he did not dispute.[5] As T.E. Utley, one of Powell's admirers, put it in 1968, he was faced as minister with the regrettable fact that the National Health Service existed. The assumption on which it was based – that it would be free at the point of reception and that it should be universal – were at the time politically unchallengeable. Decades of sustained persuasion might be necessary before these assumptions could be modified.[6]

Powell's importance as minister lay in the fact that he pioneered managerialist methods of solving the NHS's problems which have been increasingly adopted since, and in the process have progressively eroded its socialist principles.

We can therefore easily see why he so stubbornly resisted the nurses' pay claim of 1962, until compelled to do so by the most determined protests ever mounted by nurses, and the effect these were having on the government's declining popularity. When the pay pause ended in April 1962 the government sought to establish a 'guiding light' of increases of no more than 2.5 per cent for 1962. Once again low paid public sector workers were chosen to serve as the example to others, and in February nurses were offered the paltry sum allowed for under government policy. The reaction of staff side organisations was swift and determined. There were in fact two protest campaigns, one run by the RCN and that initiated by COHSE. Most staff side organisations, including NALGO and NUPE, were content to let the College take the lead. COHSE, however, decided to push ahead on its own. When the negotiations on anomalies had broken down in 1961 COHSE had been the only organisation which did not agree that a new claim for 35 per cent should be submitted. Instead it had urged the staff side, without success, to press for a Royal Commission. When the claim was submitted the staff side refused to incorporate COHSE's proposal for hours comparable to those of other professions and additional pay for split shifts. Of course, when we say the 'staff side' we mean the RCN which dominated its affairs, and through Felicity Goodall, held the chair. In launching its own campaign against the 2.5 per cent offer COHSE declared that it

> was not prepared to sink its own ideas and bow meekly and respectfully to others who in COHSE's opinion should not be regarded as negotiating bodies.

This represented a distinct shift from its approach in the 1950s when COHSE had been primarily concerned to protect its autonomy in what it regarded as its own sphere – hence its demand then for a separate Whitley Council for mental nurses. COHSE knew it had to establish its own separate identity within the Whitley Council if more general nurses were to see any point in joining it. Rather than continuing to modify staff side claims in the privacy of Whitley Council meetings, so that the RCN got credit for COHSE's efforts, it now began openly to criticise them. Jepson, for example, argued in an important *Journal* article of March 1962 that the present sorry plight of nurses was the fault of both successive governments *and* the College. He had announced the beginning of a new era of competitive struggle between COHSE and the RCN.

The first protests were initiated by the RCN. On 13 March, more than 1,000 nurses crowded into a meeting in London to which 'all trained nurses' had been invited to discuss the response to management's 2.5 per cent offer. The chair was taken by Dame Irene Ward, the Tory MP for Tynemouth, who according to the *Nursing Times* report 'set the whole tone of the meeting', and introduced 'a distinguished panel of representatives' from nurses' professional associations.[7] Under pressure from the floor, the meeting voted to get up a deputation to see the Minister of Health.

The deputation met Enoch Powell on 29 March, but did not budge him. The Prime Minister also refused to intervene, despite the pressure of a twelve-and-a-half hour debate on the pay of nurses and 'medical auxiliaries' in the House of Commons on 27 March 1962. The culmination of the College-run staff side campaign (in which COHSE participated) was a rally in the Royal Albert Hall on 29 May attended by 7,000 nurses and addressed by MPs of all three parties.[8]

Early on in the campaign all organisations representing nurses had made it clear that industrial action was 'out of the question' – all, that is, except COHSE. While COHSE went along with the actions already proposed, the writing of letters to newspapers and MPs, the telegrams to the Prime Minister and so forth, it also insisted on organising its own national and regional rallies and demonstrations. It went further still in threatening to conduct a strike ballot if the more accepted forms of protest activity 'failed to break the deadlock'.

COHSE's meetings and demonstrations were a resounding success. The opening meeting at the Caxton Hall, London on 4 April, exceeded all expectations. 4,000 nurses turned up and had to be accommodated in overflow rooms. They were in a militant mood, as Joe Soley told me, and insisted on moving on afterwards to lobby MPs at the House of Commons, despite the reservations of the General Secretary. According to the May issue of the union's *Journal*:

> police intervened when about 150 crowded into the central lobby at the House of Commons and warned against disorderly behaviour when argumentative groups formed around MPs.

In the following weeks thousand marched and protested in more than a dozen cities as far apart as Newcastle, Manchester, Leicester, Bristol, Southampton, Glasgow, Lincoln, Aberdeen, Norwich and Stockton-on-Tees. Enoch Powell faced demonstrations wherever he went. At Lincoln, for example, six or seven nurses sat down in front of his car and 'he was nearly mobbed' when he came to visit the county hospital to see what all the indignation was about. The demonstrators showed their usual genius for street theatre and devising arresting slogans. At Bristol nurses marched to the central hall carrying a black-draped coffin, with the inscription 'Dead of Whitleyism', which lay on the table throughout the meeting. At Liverpool a young nurse in a padlock and chain headed the 2,000 strong demonstration. Slogans included the familiar variations on themes of lamps and Florence Nightingale, as well as:

> 2½ per cent – NOT TO BE TAKEN
> Our Wages Have Paused But We Haven't
> Defend and Extend the Health Service
> We Appeal to the People
> Should Midwives Restrict Productivity to 2½ per cent?

At the 1962 South Wales miners' gala a banner read 'Empty Purses Mean Less Nurses – Less Nurses Mean More Hearses', while the Lincoln branch used 'Pause or No Pause – Angels Must Eat' as its slogan.

The climax of COHSE's contribution to the staff side campaign was the London March on 28 April from Marble Arch to Trafalgar Square, which was described by COHSE as 'Britain's biggest ever demonstration' by health workers.

At the rally in Trafalgar Square Jepson and Mary Burns received an ovation.

An historic feature of the demonstrations, which must have worried the government, was the outbreak of unofficial sympathy strikes in support of the nurses by many engineering workers, initiated by workers at Ford's Dagenham plant. COHSE was the only health service organisation which seriously considered taking industrial action. Although it was something of a publicity stunt, it showed that nurses were finally thinking the unthinkable. Staff shortages were the spur. As Dick Akers, recently elected Assistant General Secretary of COHSE, told a rally in Aberdeen on 14 May:

> Nurses who quit the profession because they want no more to do with its pay and conditions represent a 'silent strike' that has been going on for years.

The results of COHSE's strike ballot on 14 August 1962 showed the depth of militant feeling: 7,296 voted in favour, 5,375 voted against and 16,068 voted 'in principle' in favour of a strike 'but on conscience grounds could not do it'. In any case, the campaigning had obtained its desired effect by this time. After an abortive attempt by the Minister to reopen negotiations, the staff side proceeded to arbitration after 12 June. The award of the Industrial Court in September followed the demands of the staff side, almost to the letter. A 7.5 per cent interim increase was granted, backdated to 1 April. Staff and management sides were ordered to open negotiations on the rest of the claim and complete them by March 1963, failing which it would again intervene. The nurses had taken on a government and won a famous victory.

COHSE claimed that the victory as its own. The union had certainly led the most dynamic campaign of all the staff side organisations, and took the whole nursing community nearer to the brink of national industrial action than it had ever been. The government was worried on two counts: firstly the strength of public opinion, as an opinion poll had shown that 90 per cent of the population was solidly behind the nurses, and secondly, revolt from within, as increasing numbers of Conservative backbenchers put pressure on their government, especially during the second Opposition-staged debate in the Commons on 14 May. It was at this point that Powell first raised the possibility that more than 2.5 per cent might be available, the first signs of a crack in his stern resolve that would eventually lead to victory. COHSE had played the greater role in mobilising public support in general behind the nurses. The RCN had concentrated more on exploiting internal divisions within the Conservative Party. Both had been influential in securing a victorious outcome. A fragile coalition had been established during the campaign that could not survive for long after it, not least because COHSE had recruited thousands of general nurses.

A Changing Union – A Changing Membership

COHSE emerged from the 1962 nurses' pay dispute stronger and more confident than ever before. It was a vindication of Jepson's leadership and the decision to go for a more broadly based union. He received a rapturous reception wherever he went and became the first leading official of the Confederation since Gibson to become a nationally known figure. His other main achievement was less public: he had succeeded in re-establishing the authority of the General Secretary over a divided Executive Council, divisions which had played some part in dispatching his two predecessors. By 1963, within five years of Jepson taking over, membership of COHSE had risen to 67,000.

There were also dramatic changes in the composition of this membership. The protests and demonstrations of 1962 had been dominated by women general nurses, and this was also reflected in membership figures. In 1956 women formed only 41 per cent of the membership. By the mid-1960s they were in the majority. Interestingly, it was in the North of England and Scotland, and the new areas of Northern Ireland, that saw the biggest influx.

The Northern Ireland Region was given an independent existence in 1962, as a result of the initiative of Fred Green, COHSE's Regional Secretary in the North-West of

England. Previously COHSE members in the province had been attached to Liverpool and were often secretive about their membership for fear of victimisation. The earliest Northern Ireland branches were in psychiatric and mental handicap hospitals, but membership subsequently spread to general hospitals and then into the social services sector. Bill Jackson was given charge of the new region, and has remained in post to the present day. Originally an activist in the engineering union in his previous employment at Shorts and Harlands in Belfast, he later became a driver at Purdysburn psychiatric hospital in Belfast. Appointed because of his previous negotiating experience in the private sector, he certainly needed it in his new position because at that time there were no standard pay and conditions in Northern Ireland's health service. Management did not observe British Whitley Council rates of pay and conditions, so there were wide variations across the province with marked differences in pay between rural and urban areas. During the 1960s, then, the new region faced an uphill struggle. It was not until the 1974 reorganisation of the NHS brought parity of pay and conditions with the remainder of Britain that these difficulties eased.

At first COHSE was less successful in attracting women in the South of England. Perhaps one reason for this was the more solid strength of the RCN in London and the Home Counties. Women were beginning to play a greater part in union affairs, mainly at branch level, although not in proportion to their growing numbers. The union had one female Regional Official, Kath Daly in charge of No. 6 (West Metropolitan). In May 1965 Rose Lambie was appointed as Assistant Woman Officer. She had formerly run the shops at Hartwood psychiatric hospital in Scotland where she had been active in the COHSE branch. When Doris Westmacot retired in 1967 she succeeded her as Woman Officer. Women were encouraged to come forward to participate in union affairs, but it was not at this stage felt necessary to take special steps to facilitate the process.

Another striking feature of some of the pay pause protests had been the participation of black nurses, especially in Birmingham. The union was beginning to overcome the hesitancy which had characterised its approach to race issues during the 1950s. The numbers of overseas nurses in the NHS increased dramatically. Enoch Powell, while publicly denying that there was a staffing crisis, was encouraging their recruitment as a cheap and convenient way out of it. The number of auxiliary nurses was increasing at a much faster rate than numbers of registered staff.

Overseas Nurses

The role expected of the black nurse was to fill the most unpopular spaces in the labour force – the low paid, low opportunity and low status areas that were shunned by others. A survey of the Oxford area in 1961 found that only 3 per cent of student nurses in teaching hospitals were non-European, compared with 21 per cent in non-teaching hospitals. Nationally only 1 or 2 per cent of student nurses in teaching hospitals were from overseas, leading to accusations in Parliament in 1965 that this might partly be the result of overt discrimination.[9] The hospitals where overseas staff were concentrated tended to be the less glamorous, dealing with more 'run of the mill' illnesses, caring for the elderly and the chronically physically ill and mentally impaired. In the teaching hospitals themselves, they were concentrated in auxiliary grades.

The most acute problems were probably experienced by those overseas nurses who were lured to this country to undergo pupil nurse training for 'the Roll' with the promise that they would receive a valuable training. They often found that the training was inferior and that they were exploited as cheap labour. An article which appeared in *Nursing Times* in 1965 was one of the very few which examined their plight. Though many became disillusioned with their training this was not reflected in 'wastage', as it was with English trainees, because once here they were stuck with the job. After training they found themselves with a qualification which gave them no opportunities of advancement within the NHS, and which was unlikely to be recognised in their home country. Not surprisingly, it was reported that the first thought of many of them was to obtain a place as a student nurse to retrain for the Register.[10]

White nurses often did not understand that the black nurses' growing resentment and anger had justifiable cause. Black nurses themselves rarely voiced their grievances publicly as they were in a vulnerable position,[11] but we can begin to understand their feelings from complaints of white nurses to the nursing press that, for example, they had 'chips on their shoulders' and did not, as a letter to *Nursing Times* put it in 1965, accept discipline as a result of them 'having little desire to integrate',[12] and that their 'aspiration levels [were] set unrealistically high'.[13] In other words, white nurses thought that the problems largely lay with the attitudes of overseas nurses themselves, not British racism.

A combination of conscience and reality forced COHSE to review its policy on overseas nurses. The reality was that overseas nurses were here to stay and that if COHSE was to maintain its new dynamism it would need to recruit them. COHSE's own new awareness was also linked to the more general anti-racist awareness of the early 1960s, spurred by the revulsion at South Africa's apartheid system (which forced it to leave the Commonwealth in 1961), and labour movement opposition to the legal restrictions on Commonwealth immigration in 1962. In 1959 COHSE's conference had voted through a motion calling for language tests and a 10 per cent limit of foreign staff at any one hospital, but in 1961 Jepson publicly praised the positive role played by overseas nurses in alleviating the NHS staffing crisis and countered accusations from some quarters that they were responsible for declining standards of care, saying 'We welcome them into membership'. In the same year COHSE was issuing recruiting leaflets in four languages. Then the 1962 COHSE conference overwhelmingly rejected a motion calling for the discontinuation of recruitment of 'foreign nationals' as nurses.

COHSE Versus the College

If a changing membership composition was one consequence of COHSE's success and growth as a union, the
other was a renewal of conflict with the RCN. There were
three main areas of contention: representation on the
Whitley Council, policies adopted on the Nurses and
Midwives Council (NMC) itself and COHSE's criticisms of
the RCN plans for the future of nurse education.

The claim for greater representation on the NMC arose
out of a conference resolution of 1962, but it was not until
May 1965 that agreement was reached to reallocate seats,
largely by reducing the number of seats held by the RCN
and the Royal College of Midwives. Since the number of
seats held by NALGO and the NUGMW were also reduced,
the professional associations continued to hold the balance
of power – by one seat. Nevertheless this was a considerable
morale boost for COHSE, which claimed that its nursing
membership was closely approaching that of the RCN.

The years following the 1962 arbitration award also saw
a concerted challenge to the RCN by COHSE on
substantive issues of policy. The first sign was a
disagreement over the Industrial Court's further arbitration award to nurses in the April 1963 pay round. Hailed
by the RCN as a good award because it 'recognised
qualification and responsibility and improved career
prospects', COHSE described it as

> a raw deal for student nurses, nursing auxiliaries and nursing
> assistants who are actually worse off through higher
> board-and-lodging charges.

At the same time COHSE was pushing its policy of
enhanced rates of pay for time worked in excess of 44
hours per week and for Sundays, rest days, nights and split
duties. Management would not budge beyond the offer of
a £1 special payment for grades below ward sister level for
Sunday working and night duty, but which excluded
student nurses. The offer was opposed by the RCN which
had always been against any form of overtime payment or
shift allowance, whatever euphemism was given to it, on

the grounds that it was 'unprofessional'. The College sought without success to have the money incorporated into basic pay scales, and eventually accepted the deal with reluctance. Payments of between £1 5s and £1 10s were introduced in June 1964. The College then engaged in one of its periodic heart-searchings. Its Branches Standing Committee in 1963 rejected the extension of enhanced rates to other grades, yet in 1965, when it felt compelled to conduct a referendum on the matter, there was a 74 per cent majority in favour of them, as long as students (who they still did not regard as workers) were excluded from the scope of such payments. By the time the staff side could table a claim for enhanced duty payments in 1967, however, the whole issue had become caught up in the sticky web of the 1964-70 Labour government's incomes policy due to the College's dilly-dallying. It is likely that the pressure of competition from COHSE played at least a part in the College's change of heart.

As well as demand for enhanced payments, which had arisen out of a decision at COHSE's 1962 Torquay Conference, the union was also pressing forward with its policy of a 39-hour week. The staff side adopted the claim although nursing staff had to be content with a modest reduction of hours to 42, to be implemented (in theory) by the end of 1965.

COHSE exploited the RCN's prevarication about overtime payments to the full. The agreement brought 'a storm of protest from members who pointed out that ward sisters and charge nurses are excluded' and Jepson also said that it was 'unforgiveable to exclude students'.

The NEC meeting in June was also angry that students' economic position had declined in recent pay deals. It decided that 'COHSE must do something about it' and launched a series of campaign meetings up and down the country. The most successful was that held in the familiar protest venue of St Pancras Town Hall in London on 7 July 1964. It was chaired by veteran campaigner Joe Soley, by now Chief Male Nurse at Goodmayes Hospital. He claimed that COHSE's 37,000 nurse members were not getting a 'square deal' and that there was still 'too much Victorianism' in the treatment of student nurses. The colourful Mary Burns also encouraged student nurses to protest. She described the missing overtime payments ironically as 'Beatle money' after the group's current film *A Hard Day's Night*:

> Those four boys haven't a bigger fan than I am, but I want you to think of the money they're getting and the money the students are getting ... How many of you in this hall haven't done one hard day's night? You do four or five every week.

The meeting was also addressed by Kenneth Robinson, Labour's Shadow Minister of Health, who promised 'to review the whole National Health Service Whitley system' if Labour were to beat the Tories in the forthcoming election. Labour did win the 1964 election but the promise was not fulfilled. The RCN's embarrassment was compounded in October 1965 when the medical profession accepted the principle of overtime payments.

The RCN's alternative approach to the problems of student nurses was embodied in its proposals to reform nursing education, as expressed in its Platt Report of 1964. This revived the periodic demand for full student status with student nurses receiving a much more academic education over the first two years of training in independent training schools. Instead of wages they would receive lower maintenance grants on the understanding that they would no longer be treated as pairs of hands. Their place in the hospital labour force would largely be taken by enrolled nurses, while auxiliary nurses would largely be absorbed into a 'ward assistant' grade, which looked more or less like a ward orderly.[14]

To COHSE this appeared to be pie in the sky, and no excuse for failing to deal with the problems students experienced because they were part of the hospital labour force. In any case opinion in the union was generally against the whole philosophy of the report. It would reinforce and widen the already apparent class distinctions between registered and enrolled nurses, and exclude nursing assistants from the nursing team by relegating them to an ancillary status. The Platt Report was, therefore, permeated by an elitist philosophy. Jepson noted that the committed had been influenced by the 'nurse consultant' and education system that had emerged in the USA which, he believed, did not necessarily lead to a better standard of care. He defended the apprenticeship system on the grounds that 'nursing education must be related to what happens in the wards'.[15]

COHSE was not the only critic of the proposals and, given their expense, the Labour government was also reluctant to act. It was, however, prepared to act on the recommendations of the official Salmon Committee on restructuring nurse management which had been packed with College representatives together with a sprinkling of management 'experts', because it thought that these might be 'cost effective'.[16] The Salmon Report proposed to sweep away the whole traditional matron system and replace it with an impersonal nursing officer system which would extend upwards beyond the hospital to group level. Administrators would be relieved of control over the 'non-nursing' labour force, e.g. cleaners, linen rooms, home sisters, but would continue to have minimal 'sapiential', i.e. only advisory, power over them.

At this stage COHSE had very little to say about the Salmon Report. Its NEC was critical of details, thought that it displayed a general hospital bias and was concerned that the most senior posts should be open to men. In contrast to its analysis of the Platt Report, however, it had little to say, positively or negatively, about the managerialist ethos of the report.

Of course the Salmon Report was only part of a wider set of changes which had begun with the Hospital Plan of 1962 and culminated in the 1974 reorganisation. Against a general background of expansion, the government was seeking to get more efficiency – larger hospitals, bigger administrative units, faster throughput of patients. Also central to the strategy was the increasing concentration on acute facilities and high technology medicine and the closure of older hospitals, especially the run-down of the mental hospitals prophesied in Powell's famous 'water tower' speech of 1961. The guiding idea was that the NHS should be treated as a business like any other, and the first target for trying out these ideas were the ancillary

workers, because they were not sufficiently powerful to
resist it. Some voices were raised against these tendencies,
particularly by COHSE's Vice-President Tony Marshall. In
a far-sighted article he attacked the growing 'industrialisation' of the NHS and the growth of an 'assembly line'
mentality, which ignored the fact that 'human relationships
are a very important part of this most human of services'.
He urged a return to 'basic principles', which unfortunately
has largely gone unheeded.[17]

The Ancillary 'Cinderellas'

The problems faced by the hospital ancillary 'Cinderellas'
– as one branch secretary described them in 1961 – had
always been severe. Appalling pay and conditions were
compounded by the lack of recognition of their worth by
almost every other grade above them in the hierarchy. In
the status-conscious environment of the hospital there was
a pronounced and long established tendency, from the top
downwards, for each group to search desperately for some
'other' to which it could feel superior. Most ancillary
workers had always been in the unfortunate position of
being at the end of this process, with no one that they
could feel superior to.

No attempt was made to alleviate ancillary workers'
inferior economic and social conditions in the 1960s, and
their work was to be subjected to a ruthless efficiency drive
that began during Powell's era and accelerated throughout
the 1960s and beyond. The first omens for the future were
already appearing in 1960. Enoch Powell's Advisory
Committee for Management Efficiency had begun its
work with a flourish that emphasised the need for
consultation over change in order to 'foster a climate of
opinion throughout the service in which better methods
are not only accepted but welcome'. It was chaired by a Sir
Ewart-Smith, formerly of ICI, and its vice-chair was
COHSE's President Claude Bartlett. It promoted the idea
that the new emphasis on 'improved working methods'
would benefit health staff rather than lead to an
intensification and a deterioration in their conditions. Also
in 1960, the National Association of Hospital Management

Committees (NAHMC) issued a paper which called for outside work-study consultants to be brought in to study ways of improving ancillary services, as well as calling for the expansion of the Ministry of Health's own Organisation and Methods of Division. Yet despite the cosy assurances given when Manchester Regional Hospital Board appointed a number of work-study officers, a study at one hospital produced the startling conclusion that

> fifty per cent of the domestic staff could be dispensed with by natural wastage, providing that mechanical cleaning and washing-up machines were obtained.[18]

There was a pronounced division of opinion within the union over the value of work study. The leadership appears to have been generally in favour so long as no redundancies were enforced and protocols of consultation were observed, and this was the view taken by the other unions on the Ancillary Staffs Council in 1960. But there were critical voices from the branches, some rejecting the idea altogether as 'industrial' methods were out of keeping in the health service, with others insisting that workers should receive some form of financial compensation for co-operating with work-study engineers.

There was no difference of opinion, however, over the second innovation of Powell's era, the introduction of outside contractors. Again, Powell's economic orthodoxy – a kind of monetarism in chrysalis form – regarded monopoly, of which the NHS was an example, as inherently inefficient. Contracting out of services provided one way out of this assumed dilemma. By 1962, ten out of the fifteen Regional Hospital Boards in England and Wales had recently contracted out some of their catering, cleaning and garden services, according to a NAHMC Report. This saw some advantages, but pointed out that 'a fee has to be paid' in terms of loss of control or pride, and that commercial enterprises would not take the well-being of the patient as their first objective.[19] HMCs may have had mixed feelings: unions and NHS ancillary staff were united in opposition. Joe Richards, COHSE's Assistant General Secretary, said in 1961 that their introduction was leading to 'a highly explosive situation' over which ASC staff 'are becoming very restive'. In some hospitals contracts were signed without consultation, leading in at least one instance to a short strike by cleaners who were persuaded to return by the matron. In 1963 the TUC adopted a motion opposing private contractors, put by NUPE's General Secretary Sidney Hill with the support of Dick Akers of COHSE.[20]

Management misgivings and worker opposition stemmed the growth of contracting services at this stage, and this might have encouraged the increasing use of work study as the more acceptable alternative, but the introduction of these techniques was also hindered by the lack of any financial incentive for the workers. There matters lay for the time being. Like other health workers, ASC staff were more immediately concerned with their pay levels. Some thought that COHSE was too preoccupied with the problems of nurses and was neglecting their interests. One branch secretary argued in the September 1964 *Journal* that nurses regarded themselves as

> the elite of COHSE. Seemingly the union does very little to alter this state of affairs. Ancillary staff are always last in the queue for increases.

He was particularly incensed at the three-year deal recently negotiated with the ASC for November 1963. Such deals were a fad during the 1960s, imported from the USA in the hope of controlling inflation by creating more predictable wage costs, and similar deals were negotiated for other grades. Male ancillary workers would receive £1 1s in three equal instalments of 7s by November 1965; women were to get 15s 9d in three instalments of 5s 3d a year. The branch secretary criticised the deal severely, suggesting that it 'does no credit to the negotiators', and at the end of it 'ancillaries will be even further behind the average wage'.

These and similar suggestions that ancillary workers were being neglected were strenuously denied by Frank Lynch, who was then the national officer leading COHSE's negotiating team on the ASC. Although COHSE had extended its recruiting ambitions from the mental nursing field to the whole of nursing, the truth was that it had been lagging behind in seeking to recruit other grades, particularly ancillary staffs.

COHSE's most concerted campaign in this period was over the issue of equal pay for men and women. Equal pay had been established for most other groups of health workers, although nurses' low pay and that of other female health workers was clearly linked to the general undervaluing of women's skills in a male dominated society. But for ancillary workers sex discrimination was overt. At the beginning of 1961 there was a glaring difference between men's and women's national minimum rates, even when they were doing the same work: men received £8 17s 8d and women just £6 13s 3d

In cash terms the gap had been widening in recent years. The situation had not changed by 1963 when Dick Akers put a motion to the TUC Conference that autumn calling for an end to such blatant discrimination. In 1961 Enoch Powell had refused COHSE's request to allow the issue of equal pay for supervisory grades to go to arbitration. As Akers pointed out in his speech, equal pay for other grades in practice meant a man doing a woman's job and getting as little as she did. He then went on to give examples of overt discrimination:

> If you telephone Brighton General Hospital and inquire about a patient, and if a man answers that telephone, I can assure you that his basic rate of pay is £11 9s. If you telephone the Royal Sussex Hospital and a woman answers the phone and probably says, 'Can I help you?' her rate of pay if £9 1s – roughly 50 shillings difference ... We now come to the more crazy part of the National Health Service business: we come to what we call the supervisory grades, the women in charge of very large and major departments – kitchens, laundries and so forth – and here we get the fantastic position that women in charge of these large departments which employ men as well as women are in many cases getting less than the men they control.[21]

In the hierarchial structure in which ancillary workers

were at the bottom women were one level lower still, even when they held responsible positions. The pressure yielded some small results. The three-year pay deal agreed in November 1963 raised the women's rate to 82 per cent of the men's. Despite the arrival in power of a Labour government in October 1964 no further improvement was made until the passing of the Equal Pay Act of 1970. None of this dealt with the fundamental problem that women were segregated into occupations such as cleaning that received lower pay because they were defined as 'women's' work; this, of course, is a problem which has still not found a solution.

COHSE was also maintaining its efforts on behalf of ambulance staffs through David Williams, the responsible national officer. The 1962 Conference reiterated its support for a nationalised ambulance service, and Dick Akers put a motion to this effect on COHSE's behalf to the 1964 TUC conference. It faced vigorous opposition from the unions on the Local Authorities National Joint Industrial Council – NUPE, the NUGMW and the TGWU – who were still primarily seeking to maintain their exclusive bargaining rights. The General Council wanted the resolution to be remitted. In theory this was because a working party (the Platt Committee) had been set up to examine training and equipment for the ambulance service, and this was said to be a reason for holding fire.

In fact it appeared to be protecting the interests of the 'big batallions'. COHSE's arguments were strong. The working party had been set up as a result of the need to rationalise accident and emergency services into larger units to cope with modern demands and developments in medicine and surgery. There was no better way of achieving this than through a nationalised service, as already existed in Scotland, which could standardise equipment and training. These arguments won the day, and despite the powerful opposition COHSE's motion was passed by a sizeable majority.[22]

Encouraged by this success COHSE pressed ahead with a mass lobby of the House of Commons on 20 May 1965. It was the first ever national protest rally by ambulance workers, who now numbered some 13,000 in England and

Wales. The union's hope was that the recently elected Labour government, in the shape of its Minister of Health Kenneth Robinson, might be sympathetic to COHSE's case. Prompted by a Parliamentary question arising out of the lobby, Robinson promised to review the issue. In 1967 he recommended in his written evidence to the Royal Commission on Local Government in England that the ambulance services should be transferred to the Regional Hospital Boards. Although this did not bear immediate fruit, it did set in motion the series of steps which led to the final merger of the ambulance service into the NHS in 1974 as part of the general reorganisation of that year. As in the 1950s, the issue of nationalisation was symptomatic of deeper discontents over manual workers' status and pay. In May 1965 unofficial industrial action in the form of an overtime ban spread among ambulance staffs. Although short-lived, it was a sign of things to come.

With hindsight we can now see that discontents of all kinds and varieties among health workers were mounting during the 1960s. Two social scientists conducted a survey of professional and technical staff for Welsh Regional Hospital Board, interviewing a cross-section of physiotherapists, occupational therapists, psychiatric social workers, almoners, pharmacists, bio-chemists, orthoptists, chiropodists, radiographers, medical laboratory staffs and others. Although there were variations between professional groups, a clear pattern emerged. Underlying the widespread dissatisfaction with pay levels was a concern by workers that they often did not possess the facilities to do their job properly. This, combined with what they felt were the attitudes of doctors and nurses towards them, meant that 'the potential value of their work as they envisage it is not recognised'.[23] They had 'disappointed expectations' – a conclusion which could have been applied to nearly every group of health workers. It was a warning of trouble to come that should have been heeded, especially with a Labour government in power from 1964 to 1970. Yet little positive action was taken to avoid the crisis which finally hit the service in the mid-1970s. We must now turn to examine how this came about and the role COHSE played in the dramatic sequence of events.

Notes

[1] Sked and Cook, *Post-War Britain* (1979), pp.180-4.

[2] TUC, *Annual Report* (1961).

[3] TUC, *Annual Report* (1962).

[4] For its effects, see N. Ginsburg *Class, Capital and Social Policy* (1979).

[5] He claims never to have been 'at variance ... with either of the Chancellors of the Exchequer with whom I served', in E. Powell, *A New Look at Medicine and Politics* (1966), p.2.

[6] T.E. Utley, *Enoch Powell: the Man and his Thinking* (1968), p.52.

[7] *Nursing Times*, 23 March 1962.

[8] *Nursing Times*, 1 June 1962.

[9] Quoted by B. Hepple, *Race, Jobs and the Law in Britain* (1970), p.274.

[10] J.L. Martin, 'West Indian Nurses and their Problems in Training', *Nursing Times*, 6 August 1965.

[11] M. Thomas and J.M. Williams, *Overseas Nurses in Britain* (1972).

[12] Letters, *Nursing Times*, 26 March 1965; see also 23 April 1965.

[13] Martin, op.cit.

[14] RCN, *A Reform of Nursing Education* (Platt) (1964).

[15] *HSJ*, September 1965.

[16] Ministry of Health, *Report of the Committee on Senior Nurse Staff Structure* (Salmon), (1966).

[17] T. Marshall, 'Powell's Progress', *HSJ*, November-December 1963.

[18] *HSJ*, January-February 1960.

[19] National Association of Hospital Management Committees, *Hospital Services: Contract or Direct Labour?* (1962).

[20] TUC, *Annual Report* (1963).

[21] Ibid.

[22] TUC, *Annual Report* (1964).

[23] A. Crichton and M. Crawford, *Disappointed Expectations?* (1963), p.51.

Chapter 20
The Road to Halsbury, 1965–74

On Tuesday 17 September 1974 Britain's nurses received their biggest ever pay award from a specially appointed committee of inquiry chaired by Lord Halsbury. It gave them the kind of deal that it had never proved possible to negotiate through the Whitley Council system. The road was thereafter paved with very few signs of government good intentions. Nor was it a permanent settlement. Within a few years its value was quickly eroded by inflation and nurses found themselves back to square one. Nevertheless the report and the militancy which preceded it marked a turning point in COHSE's development, propelling it on a path of growth as rapid as any union since the end of the Second World War. This was not simply a happy accident, for we have seen how COHSE had transformed itself under Jepson into a union that would be ready to seize such opportunities when they were presented.

The Battle for Leadership

The late 1960s saw a renewal of a competitive leadership battle within the union as Jack Jepson's period of office came to a close. This did not affect the presidency, a position in COHSE which has always been somewhat above the fray. A.R. Farmer had been President since 1962, but had seen himself as a transitional figure holding the ring until a more likely looking 'younger man' emerged. When he retired in 1965 his place was taken by the 53-year-old Bob Vickerstaff, a charge nurse at St

330

Nicholas Hospital, Gosforth, near Newcastle-on-Tyne. Bob was one of eight children in a mining family in Spennymoor, County Durham. Initially he had followed his father down the pits at the age of 14, but later emulated his sister to become a student mental nurse in the 1930s. He won a place on the NEC in 1958, partly as a result of his stern criticism of the leadership's bungling of the overtime ban. He remained in office as President into the 1970s, exercising considerable sway over the NEC in the tradition established by Claude Bartlett.

Among the full-time officers there was a long-running jostle for ascendency within the union. Jepson retired in 1965 on reaching the compulsory retiring age of 65 years of age, fulfilling his election promise to serve the full term. There were four contenders for his successor; in terms of seniority they were Dick Akers, Frank Lynch, David Williams and Albert Spanswick. Dick Akers the Assistant General Secretary, was aged 62 and a veteran campaigner who had played a leading role in the nurses' protests of 1948 and 1962. He also had considerable experience of Whitley Council negotiations. His previous career had been highly colourful; from a boy clerk in the telegraph office of Barking station, he became a steward on transatlantic liners and then valet for a rich family on Long Island, New York. Only when he could not get a work permit to return to the USA in 1930 did he take a 'temporary' job as a mental nurse at Goodmayes Hospital. It was there that he was schooled in trade unionism by Joe Soley, then the local MHIWU branch secretary.

Frank Lynch was his most likely rival. Aged 57, his background was in Labour Party politics in Salford where he had served as a councillor from 1935. When Ted Hardy was elected Labour MP for Salford South in 1945 Frank was encouraged to take his place as Area Secretary of the HWSU, and Regional Secretary of COHSE in 1948.

Both Albert Spanswick and David Williams were much younger men, aged 47 and 39 respectively, swept in by Jepson's new broom to strengthen the full-time officer contingent at head office. Albert Spanswick had entered nursing through his wartime experience in the Royal Army Medical Corps. He was schooled in trade unionism by Herbert Hough, leader of the 1922 Radcliffe strike. He came to notice as a campaigning branch secretary during the overtime ban and was selected to succeed Kit Esther as secretary to the North-East region in 1959. Thereafter he rose rapidly to become national officer with special responsibility for A & C staffs in 1962. David Williams's rise to prominence was equally rapid. Like Albert Spanswick he trained as a mental nurse on being demobbed after the Second World War. He chaired the COHSE branch at Denbigh Hospital in North Wales and became a Labour councillor. In 1955 he was appointed Regional Secretary, and national officer with special responsibility for ambulance staffs in 1962.

The results of the election were close. Akers scraped through to take office in January 1967, and Lynch took over in 1969 when Akers retired. Since Lynch was by then 60, a fiercely competitive contest arose between Spanswick and Williams to occupy the position of heir apparent, that of Assistant General Secretary. Spanswick won, but only after a second ballot due to objections that the Scottish region's methods of voting contravened the rules. One of the factors which probably swung the election his way was the prominent role he had played in defending COHSE members against allegations of cruelty to patients in the inquiries which followed the publication of Barbara Robb's book *Sans Everything* in 1967.

Dick Akers' achievements during his short period of office were not outstanding. With typical good humour he gladly accepted the nickname some gave him as 'the caretaker pope', and performed the role reasonably well. By the time Frank Lynch took over COHSE was beginning to lose the initiative. Health workers' discontent with the Labour government's incomes policy were mounting, yet membership was stagnating around the 70,000 mark and a more streamlined RCN was beginning to gain a tactical advantage.

Lynch had not served an apprenticeship as branch secretary. Having entered on to the scene as an official he regarded himself primarily as a general adminstrator. As a man of the 1960s he saw the problems of the union largely in terms of the need to reorganise it along more efficient lines. Central to his strategy was the transformation of the General Secretary from the chief negotiator to the chief administrator of the union. Responsibility for nursing matters was delegated to Albert Spanswick, who also took over from Frank Lynch on the PT (B) Council, while David Williams assumed overall charge for COHSE's efforts on behalf of ancillary workers. All his other proposals for change derived from this fundamental break with the union's previous tradition so that he could concentrate on what he regarded as the 'first essential' – to 'ensure that head office is organised to provide the service which our membership demands'. Lynch strengthened the officer force in 1969 by appointing Terry Mallinson as an additional national officer whose union and health service career had been remarkably similar to those of Spanswick and Williams.

Frank Lynch had the foresight to see that the pace of change was accelerating in the NHS with the development of new forms of bargaining linked to incomes policy and the impending reorganisation of the service itself. He wanted to create a structure which could anticipate and respond to these developments. Hence the decision was finally taken to establish a research department early in his period of office. He also wanted to devolve more power upon the branches because the battle for membership would be won or lost there, and he felt that Whitleyism had made branches too reliant on the head office.

There is no doubt that his general instincts about the directions in which COHSE should go were correct, at least in organisational terms, and his period was the most innovative in the history of the union. He was not a charismatic figure and tended to see the union primarily as a machine. This, combined with his lack of extensive experience of the NHS, and of campaigning, were his chief handicaps. In general terms, however, Lynch's approach was a demonstrable success. When he took over in 1969 COHSE was approximately 75,000 strong. When Albert Spanswick was elected in the summer of 1973 he assumed control of an organisation with 120,000 members.

As always in such circumstances, it is difficult to know how much to attribute to the influence of one man. The late 1960s and early 1970s were a period highly favourable to the spread of trade unionism among NHS staff. Management at the centre was seeking to encourage greater trade union recognition at the local level. The first signs of this came in 1966 with the introduction of the Deduction of Contributions at Source (DOCAS) scheme, which overnight transformed the role of those staff organisations like COHSE able to take advantage of it. Henceforth branch activity would no longer be dominated by chasing up members in arrears, thus giving the opportunity of taking on a more enhanced role in representing members in the workplace. It also began to give COHSE the edge in the intensifying recruitment battle with the RCN, which continued with yearly subscriptions. Then in 1968 the General Whitley Council concluded an agreement that local managements should grant staff organisations 'all reasonable facilities for keeping in touch with their members in hospitals'.

The Minister was careful to emphasise that what this meant in practice would be 'dictated by local circumstances', and the term 'reasonable' was deliberately vague and open to interpretation. It also encouraged local managements to set up the Joint Consultative Committees (which they had failed to do after 1950), suggesting the discussion of facilities was an appropriate issue for getting them off the ground. Of course local managements still tried to place obstacles in the union's way, but the agreement acted as a real lever which local activists and regional officials could use.

Why did central government intervene more directly in this way? There was of course a Labour government in power between 1964 and 1970, and one might expect that it would accord greater rights to NHS trade unions. NHS management had reasons of its own and was finding it increasingly difficult to consult individually with employees over the changes in working methods which it wished to bring in. In other words their desire to foster union organisation was linked to the managerial transformation in the service, which was well underway by that time. As for the workers, my own research in the 1970s into local union organisation at a number of general and mental hospitals, some of them with COHSE branches, revealed that managerial changes since the 1960s had generated considerable anxiety. Authority over decisions was shifting from the hospital to more remote bodies which they felt they could not personally influence, but a union branch secretary or full-time regional official might.[2]

Frank Lynch certainly grasped the importance to unions of the growing sense of uncertainty, insecurity and vulnerability that began to grip health workers from the late 1960s.

'Sans Everything' and After

Uppermost in Lynch's mind was the uncertainty created by the publication of Barbara Robb's book *Sans Everything* in 1967, which accused staff looking after old people in psychiatric hospitals and other long-stay institutions of neglecting and even ill-treating patients. In its wake inquiries at a number of hospitals had been highly critical of the nursing staff, as a result of which, Lynch argued, 'morale in the nursing service is at its lowest'. During this period, COHSE came to the fore as the union which defended nursing staff in such circumstances and, as Lynch put it, placed the blame for neglect 'at the right door', asking:

> Why should nursing staff be compelled to work in the conditions that exist? Who is responsible for allocation of funds to these hospitals? Why has the allocation of funds to psychiatric hospitals been so low in comparison with the allocation to other types of hospitals.[3]

This points to a much deeper neglect, which had profound social, economic and political roots. The danger was that making scapegoats of a few nurses would help solve society's conscience while failing to deal with the underlying causes. Barbara Robb's rather sensationalist book contributed in some measure to such a scapegoating, though to be fair *Sans Everything* did not simply restrict itself to allegations of neglect and ill-treatment of patients. Its proposals for reform included a much more comprehensive psychogeriatric service, improved community care and the creation of a special hospital 'ombudsman' to investigate complaints. The press, however, dwelt upon the complaints of ill-treatment.

If the background to the scandals of the 1920s had been the deliberate neglect of asylums during the First World War, those of the late 1960s can be traced back to Enoch Powell's cost-cutting policy of closing mental hospitals. No extra provision of resources were to be provided to finance community care, and the savings were to be used to upgrade acute medical services envisaged by the Hospital Plan of 1962, which exaggerated further the existing bias in the NHS. High technology acute hospitals were seen as 'good': they produced 'cures' and hence were worthy of investment.

Mental hospitals were 'unnecessary' or even 'bad' since they did not produce cures, and even displayed anti-therapeutic tendencies. They cared for those who had either made their contribution to society (the elderly), or those who couldn't or wouldn't (the chronically mentally ill and the severely mentally handicapped). Lavish state expenditure on their well being was thus not justifiable in 'cost-effective' terms in the new, managerialist NHS.

The effect of all this on staff working in mental hospitals was devastating. Starved of resources, they found themselves attacked on all sides. Victims of government policy, yet publicly blamed for the defects of the system they had to operate, they were isolated geographically and socially and inevitably tended to close ranks and react defensively. No one ever asked them their views on the future of the mental hospitals, nor were they consulted over innovations in treatment, but were expected to follow orders, whether from 'radical' or 'conservative' psychiatrists. Powell simply announced his intentions without consultation. Confused about which way to turn, they sometimes sought to defend the status quo, and looked increasingly to their union for support.

By November 1967 Dick Akers as General Secretary was promising that COHSE would defend members accused of ill-treatment. He stated clearly what became the definitive COHSE position on the scandals. While all incidents should be investigated, and dealt with, many of the problems derived from staff shortages. So 'if some of these enquiries result in an increased nursing establishment at many understaffed hospitals then they will have done some good'.[4]

It had emerged that in some instances COHSE members were the subject of allegations made in *Sans Everything*. Kenneth Robinson, the Minister of Health, acted very cautiously, instituting internal rather than independent enquiries at the hospitals named in the book. COHSE was most actively involved in St Lawrence's, Bodmin, where there had been a 17-day inquiry, at the end of which COHSE successfully obtained the reinstatement of a suspended ward sister, while another member 'took the opportunity' to resign his post. The result of the various inquiries were published as a White Paper in July 1968 which found that most allegations were either unfounded or exaggerated. COHSE members breathed a sigh of relief.

The inquiries did not, however, go away. Both the media and the authors of *Sans Everything* regarded the White Paper as a 'whitewashing' exercise.[5] An arbitrary pattern was established whereby an aggrieved member of staff would go to the press or else a journalist would work undercover as a nursing assistant. Publicity would then lead inevitably to the setting up of an official inquiry. The scope of public concern widened to take in the mental handicap hospitals, which had been virtually ignored since the 1930s when most of them had been set up. Also significant was the departure of Kenneth Robinson, with the mantle of power now transferred to Richard Crossman, Secretary of State of the new 'umbrella' Department of Health and Social Security (DHSS). Crossman took the crucial decision, against the advice of his civil servants, to publish in full the report on Ely mental handicap hospital near Cardiff, which substantiated *News of the World* accusations of theft and cruelty.[6]

The report on Ely was published in the spring of 1969. COHSE members involved in the inquiry were represented by David Williams. He did not criticise the report as such, which he described as 'searching', but was concerned that the focus on 'bad conditions' would detract from all the good work that went on at the hospital. But his overall comment on the report was courageously one of approval:

> However painful the report is to members of staff at Ely Hospital, in the end it will lead to many improvements for patients and staff.[7]

In the event this proved over-optimistic. Crossman managed to get some resources diverted to upgrade mental handicap hospitals, but the combined resistance of civil servants, Regional Hospital Boards and the medical profession largely frustrated his plans.[8]

The Ely report had also highlighted the problems of junior staff who had the courage to complain of bad conditions. A student nurse who made accusations against a charge nurse – which were later substantiated – found himself dismissed by the HMC, even though the charge nurse had previously been warned about his behaviour. According to most criteria, management had failed in its task, so Crossman wanted to create an independent inspectorate. The powers of the new Hospital Advisory Service (HAS), however, fell far short of his original intentions. He was also prevented by medical opposition from creating an independent hospital ombudsman to whom complaints could be submitted. It took more inquiry reports, Fairleigh in 1971 and Whittingham in 1972, for Keith Joseph as Minister to announce finally that an ombudsman would be established, albeit with limited powers.

The roots of abuse were complex and did not have a single source. The persistence of the traditional deferential power structures in which staff were discouraged from making suggestions let alone complaints, played a big part. The high degree of dependency of residents and their isolation from the wider society did not help, especially in a siuation in which work was highly routinised and performed with minimal support, training or appreciation from seniors, let alone society at large. Years spent performing such work were likely to produce the apathy out of which abuse could develop. Custodial attitudes at least minimised the demands made on staff time, even though they reinforced low levels of job satisfaction. The policy of discharging ambulant patients and transferring the acutely disturbed to general hospital units only served to increase the proportion of chronically ill, dependent patients in the hospitals. As the Whittingham Inquiry Report observed, the policy

> of running down and closing existing out of date hospitals could lead to a two tier system of psychiatry – well staffed 'acute' units and 'long-stay dumps' which are professionally unattractive and hence understaffed, yet indispensable.[9]

Ancillary Workers Come of Age

Before the 1970s nurses led the way among health workers in campaigning for improved pay and conditions, with psychiatric nurses playing the dominant role. From the late 1960s there was a rapid development in the collective organisation of ancillary workers which was simply in line with the expansion in the size of the workforce. In 1949 there were 157,112 such workers in England and Wales; by 1968 their numbers had grown to 226,804.

But this was only part of the story, for alongside growth went changes in social relationships, as staff were massed together in the much larger district general hospitals that were being built in the 1960s. The policy of the day was centralisation, which was magically expected to achieve efficiency. This was combined with a policy of relieving nurses of 'non-nursing' tasks and of managerial responsibility over them.

Two things were happening: first, the work was often becoming more remote from the point of patient-contact, and second, those doing it were becoming subject to a more impersonal and 'functional' style of management. Such changes, as two far-seeing commentators predicted in 1970, were likely to give rise to forms of work organisation which were prone to disputes, and to lower staff inhibitions about taking industrial action.[10] Centralisation, as Roger Dyson observed in his analysis of the

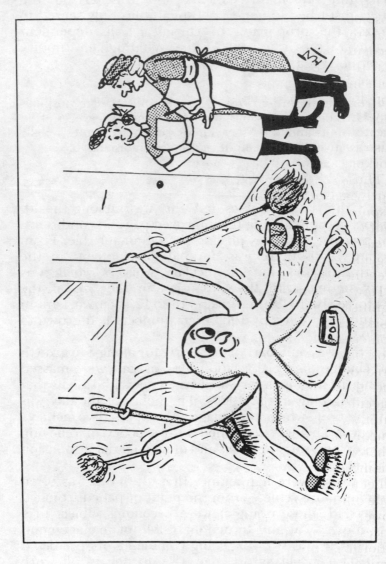

Cartoon satirising management's view of the ideal ancillary worker, *Health Services Journal*, November 1968

effects of the 1972-73 ancillary workers' dispute in the Leeds region, also gave workers immense potential power to strike at the jugular veins of the district general hospitals.[11] Once it was exercised workers would realise that they possessed an informal collective power not recognised within the formal structures. The realisation that they were 'important' was a fundamental shock for both management and ancillary workers. As Dyson also noted, management was compelled to negotiate with stewards about emergency cover over areas which they previously regarded as their prerogative. Once this power was discovered it fundamentally changed the pattern of workplace industrial relations.

Thus the foundations for the 1972-73 pay dispute were partly laid by management policies in the 1960s, and the dispute itself raised job control matters rather than being confined to purely economic issues. The spread of incentive bonus schemes was also a factor encouraging local organisation – sometimes to fight for, sometimes against their introduction, and also raised issues of control.[12]

However the question of low pay was the most significant cause of the dispute. The revolt of ancillary workers was part of a much wider rebellion of men and women low-paid workers in 'dirty', low status jobs which took place from the late 1960s. It was highlighted by the strike of local authority manual workers in 1969 and 1970, and the strike of women sewing machinists at Ford's Dagenham and Halewood plants in 1968. Although the latter was less of an outright victory than was hailed at the time, it nevertheless served as 'a source of inspiration for other women workers', and it is reasonable to assume that this included many women hospital ancillary workers.[13]

Let us now retrace the steps that led to strike action. The scale of the economic crisis facing Labour when it came to power in 1964 initially enabled it to negotiate a voluntary prices and incomes policy with the TUC and Confederation of British Industry (CBI), to be supervised by a National Board for Prices and Incomes (NBPI). Although seen at first as a temporary expedient, incomes policy remained in one form or another until it collapsed in 1970, the year that Labour departed from power. The crucial stage was reached in 1967 when, unable to secure co-operation with the trade union movement, the government had imposed a six months' compulsory freeze to be followed by a similar period of severe restraint. COHSE was among those unions which warned that the continuing rise in prices and the more restrictive effects of policies on public sector workers were testing their loyalty to the limits.[14] In 1966 there were even limited strikes by ancillary workers in London which put their unions under considerable pressure. At Claybury Hospital a *Health Services Journal* article reported one member as saying: 'Freeze? We ancillaries have been out in the cold so long we're losing our sense of feeling.' It went on conducting a series of revealing interviews with members, some of whom were on wages set below unemployment benefit levels. Miss Bakhurst was a cook earning £10 10s 8d including payment for four hours' standard overtime. She worked split duties most days:

> 'The job is heavy on clothes, particularly stockings,' she says. Entertaining is important to a single woman, but Miss Bakhurst says: 'You can't entertain friends on my money. I would like to have my sister down from Hertfordshire more often and visit my father more often.'

Miss Bakhurst did exactly the same job as John Frazer, yet he got £2 14s 8d a week more than her. All the same, he

> does not live in the lap of luxury. He is a young married man and, of course, he does not relish living all his life with in-laws however well they get on. So, in order to find the money towards the day when he, his wife and their baby can have their own home, he works five out of six Sundays and often several hours overtime at night. And after all that he has slightly over £14 to show for it. 'You've got to work full out or you couldn't exist,' he says.

Such was the reality of low pay in the health service, with thousands of decent and vitally important workers barely managing to scrape a living in the midst of the supposedly affluent 1960s.

Harold Wilson had promised that when the freeze was

over the low paid would receive preferential treatment in the thaw that was to follow, and COHSE took him at his word. As a first step, the NBPI had undertook an in-depth investigation of the pay and conditions of hospital ancillary workers. The report discovered that women ancillary workers vastly out-numbered men, making up three-quarters of the total. Although half were part-time, many worked more than thirty hours a week. As one might expect, shift working was widespread but – at this time at least – very little overtime was worked. The NBPI researchers uncovered one of the largest concentrations of low paid employment in the country. Rates of pay were scandalously poor. Of 129 industries listed by the Ministry of Labour, only six paid men lower weekly wages. What is more, hospital ancillary workers were fast losing ground in comparison to other workers. They had not received an increase since November 1965.[16]

They thus had a seemingly unanswerable case for special treatment. Yet they did not obtain justice. The board argued that the reason for the low earnings was the predominantly unskilled nature of the workforce, as if that somehow justified inaction, despite the weight of its own evidence. The real reason for the board's caution was given later in the report. It was concerned that if a higher than average increase was granted to NHS and local authority manual workers 'an unreasonable burden would be placed on the ratepayer and taxpayer'. As board member Joan Mitchell candidly admitted several years later, the NBPI was 'concerned at the repercussion that such an increase might have generally for other low paid workers'.[17]

There is also evidence that behind-the-scenes govern-ment pressure was put on the 'independent' NBPI. Local authority workers were due an increase on 6 March 1967 since their previously negotiated settlement had been postponed for the maximum six months allowed by Government policy. Strictly speaking NHS ancillary workers were allowed an increase on the same grounds, and the board initially granted it to them. After government pressure, the board delayed implementation of its 11s 8d a week award for health workers until 1 May, judging that NHS unions were weak and did not expect special treatment![18] Neither the board nor the Labour government was moved by considerations of social justice. The cause of low pay, in their view, was not due to the employer's miserliness but the workers' own 'low productivity'. The only hope they could offer for improvement in the short or long term was by means of productivity improvements. The board concentrated its criticism on management and recommended the wider introduction of interim bonus schemes until proper work-study based schemes could be established.

Health service unions, including COHSE, were on the whole taken along with the report's reasoning. Frank Lynch urged members through the pages of the union journal to make use of opportunities to establish bonus schemes and to co-operate fully with management in introducing them. The extent to which the road to productivity led to the end of low pay depended in part on how quickly schemes could be introduced. The record is not an impressive one. By the beginning of 1971 only 2 per cent of NHS ancillary workers were covered by fully work-studied schemes, with another 4 per cent likely to be covered in the near future; an additional 1 per cent were covered by interim schemes. It proved extremely difficult to get schemes off the ground, largely because local managements were unenthusiastic about them.[19]

Meanwhile the problems of low pay remained. The effects of the government's post-devaluation economic policy after 1967, with its heavy increases in indirect taxation, hit lower paid workers particularly hard. In November 1969, however, a breakthrough did occur. The regrading of ASC workers advocated by the NBPI finally emerged into the light of day. Seven groups from A to G were established up to charge hand level, and staff were distributed to them according to their job evaluation ranking. In addition, eleven supervisory grades were enumerated. Supervisors as a group gained in the exercise, as did certain other groups, like porters, whom it was generally agreed had been traditionally undervalued. All staff received a minimum increase of 15 shillings (men) or 13 shillings (women).[20]

But even as the deal was being concluded, the euphoria which attended it was rapidly evaporating. As David Williams told the union's Biennial Conference in June 1970:

Changes in the economic climate since and increases granted to other workers inside and outside the health service makes the agreement look considerably sicker than it did in November last year.

In 1969 the government's incomes policy collapsed and the pent up frustration of public sector workers finally vented itself in a massive pay explosion. Electricians in the NHS had conducted a successful wage campaign, even employing limited industrial action. Nurses had followed them and, as we shall hear later, successfully 'raised the roof'. But most influential of all was the action of local authority manual workers, spurred on by striking dustmen, who had demanded an extra £2 10s a week in the famous 'dirty jobs' dispute of 1969. In November 1970 male manual workers in local government received £2 10s (and women £2 2s 6d) as a result of Jack Scamp's Court of Inquiry Report. For the first time COHSE's NEC threatened industrial action if NHS ancillary workers did not get the same. In at least one COHSE branch, St James, Leeds, ancillary workers worked to rule. This time ancillary workers got what they were asking for.

By this time, however, there had been a change in government, with the Conservatives under Edward Heath voted in because of the disillusionment of Labour voters. At first there was no official incomes policy, but informally public sector workers were selected to serve as an example to others. The most recent investigation of the (almost defunct) NBPI into the pay and conditions of ancillary workers, showed that even after their large rise in November 1970, 25 per cent of male ancillary workers were in the lowest tenth of the earnings league. Women ancillary workers, who still earned considerably less than their male counterparts, fared on the whole better than did women manual workers generally. By a perverse logic, the board argued that this meant that women ancillary workers 'are not low paid'! The report also provided a fuller picture of ancillary workers on the eve of their explosion of militancy. Most apparently enjoyed their jobs. The men, many of whom were aged over 50, had typically been in their jobs for a long time although there was a higher turnover among the younger newcomers. They felt their work 'was of positive value to society'. Many of the women, who were also older than those found in other industries, felt the same way about their jobs, and especially valued the friendliness of their workmates. Nearly 70 per cent of men and a majority of women were members of unions, but a significant proportion of the men – 25 per cent – were reported to be highly critical of the unions to which they belonged.[21]

From April 1972 efforts were made to speed up the introduction of bonus schemes by a deal negotiated through the ASC which allowed for self-financing lead-in payments of £1 a week pending the introduction of full work-study based schemes. Workers now had the right to request such schemes, although in doing so they would concede a number of rights to management including the reorganisation and reallocation of the work concerned.[22] This did little, however, to remove the more immediate pressure for an improvement in the basic rates, which surfaced at COHSE's Morecambe conference, which was in many ways one of the most significant in the history of the union. Following a 1971 ASC agreement recognising stewards, COHSE finally decided, despite the reluctance of some conservative-minded branch secretaries, to sanction the election of union stewards and demanded that they should have time off with pay to carry out their duties. There was a call for day nurseries to be introduced for staff on a national basis. A motion critical of 'the absence of any effective consultation between our negotiators and the membership in matters of vital importance, such as pay claims' was remitted to the NEC for further discussion. Conference rejected yet another motion in favour of amalgamation with another union after considerable behind-the-scenes 'discussions' with NUPE and the NUGMW.

But perhaps the most momentous decision of all was to

support the NEC's decision to register as a union under the Tory government's anti-trade union Industrial Relations Act 1970. COHSE did not support the Act itself, and indeed condemned it in the most forthright terms possible. The issue was whether COHSE should support the TUC campaign of non-compliance with the legislation out of loyalty to the movement or allow more 'pragmatic' considerations to win the day. COHSE activists were worried about competition for membership from the RCN who as non-affiliates would be bound to register and take advantage of the privileges offered registered unions. The motion to deregister was put by Bernard Morgan from Tooting Bec Hospital, who called the Act 'a sugar-coated pill full of poison'. So-called pragmatists won the day and as a result COHSE was expelled from the TUC at its Brighton conference later that year. TUC discipline as a whole held firm and the Act was made unworkable. By the end of 1973, soon after Albert Spanswick was elected General Secretary, the NEC reversed its earlier decision and by 1974 COHSE was back in the fold.

The other most memorable event of COHSE's 1972 conference was the commitment to take drastic action, if necessary, in support of the low paid. As Bob Vickerstaffe told the delegates:

> We have long heard the cry that doctors cannot function without the support of nurses, but is it not equally true that *none* of the professional services can function without the supporting services of technicians, clerks, porters, cleaners, cooks or labourers?

The ASC claim was duly submitted later that year, the demands including £4 a week on the basic plus 'threshold' payments linked to changes in the cost of living, a 35-hour week, and four weeks' annual holiday. The aim of the £4 increase was to restore the value of the 1970 award which had been eroded by inflation. In addition the unions were demanding a £1 'lead-in' payment for *everyone* as compensation for the fact that few productivity schemes had been introduced.

It was probably the most ambitious claim ever launched

by the staff side of the ASC, but it suffered a rather undignified fate when Edward Heath imposed a wage freeze (Phase One of his incomes policy) from December 1972, several weeks before the existing agreement ran out. It is likely that industrial action would have been taken in pursuit of the claim, freeze or not, but local authority manual workers, with whom ancillary workers' pay had always been linked, managed to squeeze a £2.40 a week agreement out of management just before the incomes policy came into effect. All health unions came under intense pressure from below. The recent expansion in the number of stewards (and their enhanced status) was creating a much broader band of activists who could potentially mobilise for industrial action. Committees of such stewards, sometimes cutting across unions, were formed in localities such as London and Manchester. There had already been unofficial action over the original claim in Bristol and a body calling itself the London Alliance of Stewards for Health Workers (LASH) called a one-day stoppage on 27 November 1972.

It soon became clear that all unions would now have to take some form of national action if the seething discontent was not to get out of hand. The COHSE leadership in particular felt, perhaps reluctantly, that it should match the militancy of other NHS unions who as a result of COHSE's expulsion from the TUC now regarded its members as 'fair game'. In addition, David Williams had recently been elected to chair the staff side of the ASC. The staff side decided to organise a one-day strike and demonstrations throughout the country on 13 December 1972, the day the settlement had been due. The strength of militant feeling shown – some 150,000 ancillary workers went on strike – encouraged the NEC in February 1973 to test the extent to which members were prepared to take industrial action. COHSE joined with NUPE, the TGWU and the NUGMW in setting up a National Co-ordinating Committee, with regional offshoots, charged with the responsibility for waging the now inevitable campaign of industrial action. The plan was that workers would be brought out at selected hospitals in 'rolling' strikes of short duration, and emergency cover would be provided.

By the beginning of March 1973 it was apparent that a large majority of ancillary worker members were in favour of taking industrial action. In the ballot every single region of COHSE, and a resounding 80 per cent of those voting, was in favour. The battle lines were therefore drawn in hospitals up and down the country, and the face of hospital industrial relations was permanently changed. The depth of militant feeling took the union's leadership by surprise. Frank Lynch reported to the NEC on 14 March that 'the dispute is widespread and far greater than could have been imagined earlier'. Militant action was being taken, especially in the Midlands and the North, and the union's instructions were not always followed to the letter. The tendency was for much longer 'once-and-for-all' strikes to take place, and in some instances emergency cover was not provided. The union was having some difficulty in meeting its strike pay commitments, particularly in the Midlands due to an unauthorised three-week long strike at the East Birmingham hospital. The predominant opinion in the NEC was that

> having made our point, the action should be discontinued and the offer [under Phase Two of incomes policy] accepted with the addition that the ASC wage claim should be referred to the Pay Board [the new body set up by the Tories].

But COHSE could not withdraw unilaterally from the joint staff side campaign and decided 'to continue at present and try to exert a proper control within our own organisation'.

Eventually the strike was called off on 5 April by the inter-union National Co-ordinating Committee, and the employers' offer under Phase Two of incomes policy (£2 for men and £1.80 for women) was accepted in an atmosphere of some recrimination. Unless the unions had been prepared to step up their action they could not have forced more from the government. Many branches were also beginning to waver by the end of March. The appropriate time for militant action, if it ever existed, had by this time passed.

Many of the newspapers had, of course, condemned the

dispute, but not always from a serious understanding of the position of ancillary workers. As the Sheffield Labour MP Joe Ashton put it, ancillary workers before the dispute were

> expected to get on with the job in the true British stiff-upper-lip tradition with a cheery tug of the forelock, and to take their greatest pleasure out of an ounce of twist or a day in the country. Like the Hindu untouchables, they are expected to act as sweepers and silently shout unclean while the rest of us praise the surgeons and the dedicated nurses and assume that somebody waves a magic wand to get rid of the surplus guts and garters. There is no glamour in it. No 'Emergency Ward Ten' and 'Dr Kildare'. No perks like the surgeons get by doing cosmetic nose jobs at £200 a time. No recruiting adverts on TV, just an automatic assumption that the pollution shifters will be there forever. Well, they won't.[23]

The strike itself was not a resounding victory, but its true significance was that it announced to everybody that the days of being taken for granted had gone forever: by the nurses who in some places abused and even threw water over demonstrating ancillary workers; by the doctors who suddenly found that essential services to their private patients had been suspended; by the managements which were having to negotiate not just emergency cover but the jealously guarded prerogatives that they never thought would be questioned by such underlings; by the successive governments which gaily presumed that the camel's back was broad enough for any load. A dispute had ended, but a new era of health service industrial relations was just beginning.

Nurses' Pay: The Long March

Nurses did not stand idly by while all this was going on. Their pay had suffered from the effects of government incomes policies and their patience tried to the limits. The spirit of revolt which swept through public servants, the low-paid, among women and those doing 'dirty' jobs was also felt in nursing. Student nurses were to some extent influenced by the rise of student militancy. Many of the oppositional currents of the 1960s and early 1970s therefore found echoes in the ranks of nurses.

After the reasonably generous 1965 pay deal nurses found it increasingly difficult to get much out of the Labour government. They experienced, along with other public sector workers, the tight clamps of incomes policy at a time when workers in the private sector devised ever more resourceful means – such as bogus productivity deals – of getting round state attempts to limit the growth of earnings.

When the two-year wage settlement ran out in 1967, in the middle of the government's period of 'severe restraint', the staff side's pay claim was referred to the NBPI for investigation and report. The claim, which showed the influence of the professional associations, was biased strongly in favour of the higher grades. While increases of between 40 and 50 per cent were claimed for matrons and approximately one-third for trained staff, others – enrolled staff, auxiliaries and students – would have got much less, 16.5 per cent at most. This was justified on the basis of comparisons with other workers and to provide an attractive career structure with decent remuneration at the middle grades of nursing management. The NBPI Report showed how after devaluation in 1967 the aim was to tighten the incomes policy noose even further in order, as it put it, not to 'fritter away the advantages of devaluation by cost increases incurred directly or indirectly'.[24] Whereas labour shortages had previously been one reason for an 'exceptional' increase, the only relevant reason for an increase now accepted by the board was whether new salary structures would promote greater 'economic efficiency'. This was interpreted to mean pay levels which encouraged nurses to stay in post or return to nursing, and to provide sufficient incentive for individual nurses to take on extra responsibility.

The board's report in March 1968 found that there were shortages, particularly of staff nurses and of all grades of staff in psychiatric and geriatric hospitals. To deal with the latter they introduced an increased 'lead' of £100 a year throughout the grading structure, which COHSE had been demanding for years. Its more general proposals were for 9 per cent over two-and-a-half years, with 4 per cent backdated to October 1967 and running on in instalments until the end of March 1970. The next instalment would not be paid until January 1968, some ten months later. Like all percentage increases it generally favoured the highest paid, widening differentials all the way down. What was to become one of the most controversial recommendations concerned student nurses' board and lodging charges. The report advocated that in future student nurses should only be charged rent and laundry, and be charged for meals only as taken and no longer receive free meals on duty, as was the practice in many hospitals. All staff would now receive enhanced pay for Sunday and night work at the princely rate of time-and-one-tenth.

Nurses' pay was not the only issue tackled by the NBPI. It tried also to reform nursing institutions in order to achieve 'no cost' solutions to the problems which it had identified. These might alleviate staff discontents at the same time as promoting greater 'efficiency'. It argued that on the whole the problem was not so much recruiting as retaining staff, which it felt could be tackled by other means than a pay increase. With a perverse logic it suggested that because recruitment was on the whole being maintained nurses were not being underpaid! This illustrated how its definition of low pay looked at the issue from the management's rather than the workers' point of view. The report also urged the more rapid introduction of the system of nursing management advocated by the Salmon Report in 1966, especially the appointment of chief nursing officers at hospital group level, in the hope that this would lead to more efficient allocation of staff resources between different types of hospitals. It also called for the creation of a national staff committee to train nurse managers, and pioneer more efficient working practices, on the lines of that already formed for hospital administrators. It suggested that split shifts should be ended, greater efforts be made to recruit part-time married women as staff nurses, that nurse banks should be set up as an alternative to agencies and that more hospitals in remote areas should pay travelling expenses or provide

transport for staff. It also strongly advocated the lifting of
petty restrictions in nurses' homes, at least for second- and
third-year student nurses, who should be given a choice
over living in or out, as the restrictions caused 'resentment'
and 'contribute to low morale and wastage'. All in all, the
non-pay proposals of the report amounted to the biggest
package of reform measures for nursing since the creation
of the NHS in 1948.

COHSE generally reacted favourably to the report. The
increased leads of £100 (previously £50 a year) for all
grades up to ward sister and charge nurses, and the
extension of overtime pay to these grades in mental
hospitals, helped to 'buy off' those nurses traditionally
represented by COHSE. Perhaps the union was impressed
by the apparently scientific investigation which underpin-
ned the board's recommendations, but a closer examination of the report shows that many of its proposals are
simply asserted to be necessary, with very little hard
evidence provided to back them up. This was particularly
the case with its suggested speed-up of the Salmon
reforms, which were implemented in some haste and
confusion. On the whole, though, the reforms – especially
for students – appeared to be progressive, although there
was some concern at the board's straightforward refusal to
reduce hours below 42 a week or extend overtime pay to
nurses in general hospitals. When examined closely the
pay part of the package only amounted to an average of
3.5 per cent a year, and a condition of the award was that
there should not be another review of nurses' pay and
conditions before the end of March 1970. The two years
following the publication of the report in March 1968 saw
an unprecedented wage explosion which wiped out the
value of the award, such as it was. Unrest spread among
nurses, especially student nurses in general hospitals, initially and rather briefly harnessed by the United Nurses
Association (UNA), a publicity seeking break-away from
the RCN led by the flamboyant Sister Patricia Veal, members of which unashamedly called themselves 'bed-pan
bums' and thought that 'genteel' methods of protest had
not got very far. Her biggest success was in August 1968,
organising a 2,000-strong demonstration from Hyde Park

to Millbank, handing in a petition to 10 Downing Street on the way.[25] At last somebody seemed to be doing something. Ms Veal was mainly a thorn in the flesh of the RCN. Among the 'happenings' that she staged was a demonstration outside the College headquarters on 15 May 1969, where she turned up with a broom, sweeping dirt from the pavement under an old piece of carpet, saying: 'The College has been sweeping so much dirt under the carpet recently, I thought this was appropriate.'[26]

When the RCN closed the door on her and her broom she went off to the offices of the General Nursing Council to present the Registrar and Education Officer with a pair of rose-tinted spectacles.[27] On 22 April she had demonstrated outside the DHSS and even managed to drag Richard Crossman, the Minister himself, out to address the chanting nurses. The Minister, as his diaries reveal, was clearly concerned about his media image. He had gone out because he was worried

> about a problem which might turn into serious trouble ... Sister Veal was refusing to let me have the microphone and I seemed friendly, though harassed and unhappy about it all, as we stood shouting in the cold April wind.[28]

The 'trouble' was the new 'pay-as-you-eat' scheme introduced in 1969 as a result of the recommendations of then NBPI report. Despite receiving rebates there were protests from student nurses throughout the country that at the end of the day they were out of pocket. They were already reeling from increased and backdated board-and-lodging charges when they had received their first 4 per cent pay deal instalment. The *Daily Mail* was instrumental in fanning the flames of discontent with an article by Olga Franklin on the 'Scandal of Britain's Hungry Nurses' which said that the scheme should perhaps be renamed a 'pay-as-you-starve scheme'.[29] The *News of the World* also joined in with its own 'Our nurses must not go hungry' campaign of letter writing to Richard Crossman.[30]

COHSE was in something of a quandry regarding the new scheme which it had helped to negotiate through the Whitley Council, and Dick Akers defended it as progressive through the letters column of the *Nursing Times*.[31]

The immediate problem was resolved after a fashion with an extra 10 shillings a week allowance for student nurses under 21 years of age. Protests died down and were harnessed into the RCN's 'Raise the Roof' campaign which, to the College's relief, eclipsed the efforts of Sister Veal and her dwindling band of followers. The roof was to be raised in two senses. First, the sedate 'flowery hat' image of the College was to be exorcised by a determined publicity campaign of meetings and demonstrations to convince 'the public', and through it the government, of the justice of the nurses' pay claim. Second, the pay claim submitted by the RCN assumed that 'raising the roof' by concentrating on massive pay increases for senior nurses would, in the wake of the implementation of the Salmon Report, restore nursing's attractiveness to career-minded middle-class girls.

At the top of the scale the RCN was demanding an extra £1,500 a year for a chief nursing officer, while it was only claiming an extra £325 maximum increase for staff nurses. The 'Raise the Roof' campaign was therefore an odd combination of pressure from below in the service of a salary demand biased considerably in favour of those at the top. It had originated out of senior nurses' discontent that the NBPI had given them a lower percentage increase than many clinical nurses. Nursing tutors were also angry at the effects of the report in depressing their pay. The report thus united the two wings of the nursing hierarchy and the 'Raise the Roof' campaign was launched in the summer of 1968 – at least a year before the unions started preparing for the end of the agreement in March 1970. This gave the College the competitive edge, especially since tutors would be bound to encourage their students to participate in the College's campaign. Students were urged to join the protests to secure the extra £1,500 for their matrons ('Hammer hard upon that door, for fifteen hundred more') in order, as it was put to them, to get the ceiling raised and thus to provide more headroom for everyone.[32]

The campaign's militancy was strictly controlled from

above,[33] although it was not always easily contained: at a demonstration in Edinburgh, for example, there had been scuffles with police as some nurses attempted a 'sit-down' strike outside Woolworths.[34] The College had undeniably seized the initiative, though some critical voices were raised against the tenor of the RCN's campaign; a COHSE branch chairman, for example, wrote a letter to the *Guardian* complaining that:

> Many nurses deplore the 'Raise the Roof' campaign, and believe the claim submitted by the RCN to be unrealistic and not in the interests of nurses generally ... The campaign appears, to some of us, to be an attempt to use public sympathy to gain large increases for senior grades at the expense of the lower grades.[35]

Unrealistic or not, the campaign succeeded in winning the RCN considerable publicity as the organisation which appeared to be campaigning on behalf of student nurses. Although all staff side organisations were demanding a large increase, it was the College which grabbed most of the headlines.

As in 1962, COHSE organised its own demonstrations, but they were rather late in the day and tended to be overshadowed by those of the RCN. On 13 January 1970 COHSE organised a 200-strong demonstration outside the Whitley Council meeting at the DHSS offices at the Elephant and Castle. It included nurses from hospitals in the London area and COHSE industrial nurses on Fleet Street. They marched round the building headed by two Irish pipers, Liam O'Sullivan and John Murphy, both charge nurses at Leavesden Hospital, while the Joint Negotiating Committee of the NMC met inside. This was followed by other pay campaign meetings and marches up and down the country in Norwich, St Albans, Colchester, Harlow, Carlisle, Lincoln, Maidstone, Northern Ireland, Manchester and elsewhere. The efforts of all organisations led to a successful resolution to the pay campaign. Management initially offered a pay deal averaging 22 per cent in January, but phased in two stages of 15 per cent in April 1970 and a further 9 per cent to be paid in April

1971. As a result of further staff side pressure, including a lobby of the House of Commons attended by thousands of nurses, the management conceded a single 20 per cent pay rise a fortnight later. COHSE's efforts appeared late in the day, but when the deal was concluded it announced to the press that the 20 per cent increase was only

> ... a beginning. We were determined the offer should be without strings and this we have achieved. Now we can and shall press for urgently needed reforms in overtime, split duties, and the often horrifying conditions of work in hospitals.[36]

It was clear that the figure of Albert Spanswick, the newly elected Assistant General Secretary who had only just taken over COHSE's responsibility for nurses' pay, lay behind COHSE's late spurt towards the finishing line. The demonstration on 13 January had departed from the union's previous cautious practice because it had been staged even though the union was only negotiating and not technically in dispute. There was wide support in COHSE for this new militancy, and at the union's conference later that year Albert Spanswick received a 'rousing ovation'. Although few realised it outside the union, it had been announced to the world that COHSE would not be upstaged by the RCN next time around.

The preparation for battle began in earnest in 1972 with the formulation for the so-called 'revaluation' claim. This took account of the impending NHS reorganisation, the likely future of nurse education following the publication of the Briggs Report in 1970, growing shortages of staff and the extent to which nurses' salaries had slipped back in relation to comparable occupations at a time of increased inflation. The claim lodged on 12 January 1972 ranged from 26 to 40 per cent according to grade and was (for once) biased towards the lower rather than the upper end of the scale. The claim, which Albert Spanswick played a major part in formulating, therefore commanded considerable support among rank-and-file nurses.[37] An interim award of 8 per cent was granted in 1972 on the

assumption that negotiations would proceed on revaluation. These negotiations were halted in November 1972
by a statutory pay freeze imposed as a result of a 'U-turn'
by Edward Heath's Conservative government. The claim,
periodically updated, was trapped by the three 'phases' of
Tory government's incomes policy until Heath's defeat in
the February 1974 General Election.

Ironically, negotiators on the Nurses and Midwives
Council had settled under Phase Three. It was not until
the appearance of the incoming Labour government
which concluded a favourable deal with striking miners
that signs of dissatisfaction among nurses began to appear.
As Barbara Castle, Minister of State for Social Services,
wrote in her diary at the height of the subsequent dispute:

> I really do seem to have walked into a pack of trouble. Unions
> always seem to let their pent-up frustrations explode as soon
> as there is a Labour government.[38]

The material basis for the militancy lay in the fact that
between April 1970 and the end of 1973 nurses' pay had
risen by approximately 24 per cent while prices had risen
by 35 per cent and average earnings by 50 per cent.[39] The
dispute was detonated by delays caused by the Conservative government's Pay Board which had not yet been
abolished by the new Labour administration. By the end of
April nurses had still to receive the interim pay increases
promised for 1 April, let alone any promise for a wider
review of their pay and conditions. Meanwhile the
government sanctioned the implementation of higher
canteen prices due to come into effect in April.

The first salvo in the campaign was fired within the
RCN – and to some extent at it. At the mid-April meeting
of the RCN's Representative Body in Blackpool the chair
of its student section, Brian Lamond, proposed an
emergency resolution that Mrs Castle be sent a telegram
asking her to come to Blackpool to 'hear about the gross
injustice to which we have been subjected'. When this
resolution was threatened by a proposal to move to next
business Brian Lamond threatened that the students
section might 'consider withdrawing support from the

RCN'.[40] Finally a compromise demand was made for a 44-strong delegation which the government agreed to see on 13 May.

Trade unionists did not stand idly by, however, and NALGO and COHSE organised a demonstration at just a few days' notice for the meeting of the Nurses and Midwives Council on 30 April at which the staff side was to demand an independent review of nurses' pay. The demonstration attracted 1,500 nurses, mainly from London hospitals, who were turned back by a cordon of police as they tried to force their way into the DHSS; they then set off to march to Parliament to lobby MPs but were stopped by police at Putney Bridge as Parliament was sitting.[41] This demonstration more than any other event sparked off the nationwide campaign. It was addressed by Albert Spanswick, COHSE's newly elected General Secretary. His speech, for the first time in the campaign, raised the possibility of industrial action if the government did not move swiftly.[42] A few days later, at Storthes Hall psychiatric hospital near Huddersfield, the first token walk-out took place, and similar actions soon took place elsewhere. The RCN momentarily recaptured the initiative on 13 May when it met Barbara Castle and presented her with an impressively researched document *The State of Nursing 1974*.[43] This suggested that while efficiency had improved as a result of fewer beds, a faster 'throughput' of patients and an increased workload in the community, this had not been reflected in better pay, nor had allowance been made for the growing complexity of treatment and care. The document expressed concern that the promised reform of nursing education outlined in the Briggs Report had not yet materialised. Quoting the DHSS's own figures it showed that more than half of nurses in the NHS earned less than £30 a week, and a quarter of them less then £22 a week. But the biggest stir was caused by the RCN's announcement to Mrs Castle that unless the government took 'effective steps' to set up a speedy inquiry into nurses' pay and conditions, its members would resign *en masse* from the NHS and offer their services back as an agency.[44] It was the closest it was prepared to go towards taking industrial action.

The unions were livid that Mrs Castle, a Labour Minister, had agreed to see the RCN first.[45] COHSE convened a special NEC meeting for 16 May determined that it would make a decisive intervention in the campaign. This meeting came under intense rank-and-file pressure with members from two branches – Lincoln Heath and Warley – demanding and winning the right to address it. Both called for a stronger lead on strike action from the NEC and threatened to secede from COHSE if their demands were not met. COHSE was due to see Harold Wilson on 20 May and Albert Spanswick issued a statement to the press in which he threatened industrial action unless at least £100 million was forthcoming. When this did not materialise, COHSE's contingency plans for industrial action from 23 May were put into force. There were six points: a ban on clerical duties, domestic duties, 'acting up' (filling in for seniors) and on all overtime; selected and short withdrawals of labour; ancillary staff were to refuse to perform domestic jobs usually carried out by nurses.

As well as these pressures COHSE organised massive demonstrations in major cities up and down the country. The RCN stood aloof from the demonstrations although it tactically supported the press sponsored 'Fair Play for Nurses' campaign until this was taken over by trades unionists and left-wing activists. In addition unofficial demonstrations were organised in many towns by spontaneously formed Nurses Action Committees, with student nurses as their driving force. COHSE, as the most militant nurses' union was particularly successful in attracting many of the nurses involved in these groups to join it. The NUGMW and NUPE had also stayed aloof from the demonstrations, at least at national level, largely because they did not want to embarrass the new Labour government which had been elected on a very slender majority. A notable feature of the campaign was the support received from the working class in general. Miners in South Wales briefly came out in support of nurses, as did 3,000 engineering workers at Automotive Products in Leamington Spa. There were sympathy strikes in Newcastle, Manchester and elsewhere. At the Whittington Hospital in North London patients went on hunger strike for a day in support of the nurses.[46]

COHSE's campaign continued throughout the summer of 1974, even though Barbara Castle had taken much of the heat out of the situation on 23 May, two days after COHSE had initiated industrial action and before the RCN's threat of mass resignations was due to take effect. She established an independent Committee of Inquiry into Nurses and Midwives Pay and Conditions, outside the Whitley Council system, under Lord Halsbury who chaired the Doctors and Dentists Standing Review Body. She hoped that this would defuse the growing militancy of nurses and that the energies of their organisations would be concentrated upon the gathering and presentation of evidence to it. All organisations suspended their actions with the exception of COHSE which was under considerable internal pressure and recruiting members so fast that its NEC was encouraged to continue with its militant position. It demanded an immediate interim payment to help hard-pressed nurses in advance of the Inquiry's findings. When this was not forthcoming it stepped up its action from 20 June, banning work with private patients, agency nurses and all non-emergency admissions. 200 wards had already been closed as a result of its existing industrial action. The banning of non-emergency patients began to have a telling effect, particularly in mental hospitals. Some psychiatrists sought to get round the ban by admitting all patients as 'emergencies' under the 1959 Mental Health Act. COHSE branches responded by setting up committees of trade unionists to vet all admissions, directly challenging medical prerogatives.

COHSE's campaign of industrial action did not succeed in its immediate objectives. An interim payment was not achieved, and the NEC managed only to extricate itself on 29 June by winning a commitment from the government to speed up the publication of a report and vague promises from Mrs Castle that she 'will consider' asking Halsbury 'to recommend an interim payment' if the report was unduly delayed.[47] The appointment of the Halsbury Committee had indeed taken the heat out of the situation, although increasingly Mrs Castle faced confrontation on other fronts, with radiographers angry over their pay and conditions – they were also given a committee of enquiry under Lord Halsbury – and action by ancillary workers and some nurses against private beds in NHS hospitals. However her action was successful in defusing the nurses' pay campaign. Most of the industrial action initiated by COHSE involved emergency cover and only occasionally did it go beyond the bounds set by the NEC. An isolated exception was at Highcroft Psychiatric Hospital, Birmingham, where 300 nurses belonging to both COHSE and NUPE walked out for a 24-hour period.

The actions of COHSE could be said to have increased pressure on the committee to produce a speedy report, which materialised on 17 September. The award amounted to 30 per cent overall with some groups of ward sisters and charge nurses receiving 58 per cent salary increases. The report argued that large increases were necessary to combat an estimated 20 per cent staff shortage and to create a more attractive career structure in anticipation of the reform of nursing education proposed by the Briggs Committee. The report's recommendations in detail covered a wide range of issues, from increased overtime pay to longer holidays, to the value of £170 million.[48] It did not recommend any reduction in the length of the working week and, as some have suggested, the report was generally unadventurous.[49] Even though its terms of reference covered the structure of nursing as well as pay and conditions, it made no recommendations which might have disturbed the traditional patterns of subordination to the medical profession – for example by calling for an enhanced clinical role for nurses.

Nevertheless the immediate outcome was very favourable, especially for COHSE. Despite protests to the contrary by Inquiry members themselves, the pay award was interpreted as a vindication of the principle that 'militancy pays'. The RCN could justifiably claim that in substantive terms its document *The State of Nursing* had enjoyed the greatest impact on 'official' opinion, although even the RCN had felt it necessary to back up its 'reasoned argument' with threats of resignation from the NHS. Yet among nurses at large the results of the Halsbury Report was identified as the products of militancy, and COHSE, as demonstrably the most militant organisation during the dispute, gained most through it. It was often able to embarrass other organisations at nurses' meetings and demonstrations, and recruit large numbers of nurses.

The year following the Halsbury Campaign was COHSE's most successful recruitment period ever, and the union achieved a rate of growth that has hardly ever been emulated elsewhere in the trade union movement. By 1979 membership had grown to 215,000, almost triple its 1970 figure. In the process COHSE was transformed from a relatively small organisation, influential mainly among psychiatric nurses, into the twelfth largest union in the TUC. It had achieved much greater coverage among general nurses, and for the first time had become a serious rival to the RCN for the leadership of the profession. As a result it could no longer be said that the typical nurse was not a trade unionist. During the 1974 pay dispute nurses shed their traditionally passive image in a long hot summer of protests and industrial action the like of which had never been seen before. COHSE, more than any other organisation, helped them to do it. Given that inflation rapidly eroded the value of the award itself, this change was the most lasting legacy of the 1974 dispute. As far as nurses' pay and conditions were concerned, it turned out to be only another staging post on the long march and not, as many thought at the time, the journey's end.

Notes

[1] General Whitley Council, *Circular 23* (1968).

[2] M.J. Carpenter, *The Development of Trade Union Activity Among Nurses in Britain 1910-76*, Ph.D Thesis, University of Warwick (1986).

[3] 'Way out of Turmoil', *HSJ*, October 1969.

[4] *HSJ*, November 1967.

[5] B. Robb, 'Sans Everything and After', *Nursing Times*, 24 April 1975.

[6] See R. Crossman, *The Diaries of a Cabinet Minister*, Vol. 3 (1973).

[7] 'What the Ely Report Did Not Say', *HSJ*, May 1969.

[8] See C. Ham, *Policy Making in the NHS* (1981), Ch. 5.

[9] HMSO, *Report of the Committee of Inquiry into Whittingham Hospital* (Payne), (1972), para. 110.

[10] E.K. Jerrome and P.L. Chubb, 'From Commitment to Conflict', *The Hospital*, February and March 1970.

[11] R. Dyson, *The Ancillary Staff Industrial Action* (1974).

[12] See T. Manson in M. Stacey (ed.), *Health and the Division of Labour* (1977).

[13] A. Coote and B. Campbell, *Sweet Freedom* (1982), p.17.

[14] For a more detailed account of these events, see L. Panitch, *Social Democracy and Industrial Militancy* (1976).

[15] As reported in *HSJ*, August-September 1967.

[16] NBPI, Report *No. 29* (1967).

[17] J, Mitchell *The National Board for Prices and Incomes* (1972), p.178.

[18] See Panitch, op.cit., pp.133-4.

[19] NBPI, *Report No. 166* (1971).

[20] *HSJ*, December 1969.

[21] NBPI, *Report No. 166*.

[22] *Health Services* (*HS* – COHSE's retitled official newspaper), April 1972.

[23] Article reprinted from *Sheffield Star*, in *HS*, May 1973.

[24] NBPI, *Report No. 60*.

[25] *Nursing Times*, 23 August 1968.

[26] *Daily Mail*, 16 May 1969.

[27] 'Unite and Fight', *Nursing Times*, 22 May 1969.

[28] Crossman, op.cit., p.450.

[29] *Daily Mail*, 8 April 1969.

[30] *News of the World*, 20 April 1969.

[31] 'Letters', *Nursing Times*, 17 April 1969.

[32] 'Raise the Roof!', ibid., 7 June 1968.

[33] See D. Widgery, *Health in Danger* (1979), p.112.

[34] See *The Times* and *Glasgow Herald* for 8 November 1969.

[35] 'Letters', *Guardian*, 7 January 1970.

[36] *Financial Times*, 19 February 1970.

[37] According to COHSE, *From Phase Three to Halsbury* (1974), p.2. See also 'Diary of a Campaign', *HS*, June 1974.

[38] B. Castle, *The Castle Diaries 1974-6* (1980), p.104.

[39] N. Bosanquet, 'Words Can Win More Pay', *Nursing Times*, 25 April 1974.

[40] 'RCN Demands Salary Talks', *Nursing Times*, 4 April 1974.

[41] *Nursing Times*, 9 May 1974.

[42] *From Phase Three to Halsbury*, p.5.

[43] As summarised in *Nursing Times*, 23 May 1974.

[44] Ibid.

[45] See *Castle Diaries*, p.104.

[46] *Red Weekly*, 6 June 1974.

[47] *Nursing Times*, 4 July 1974.

[48] HMSO, *Report of the Committee of Inquiry into the Pay and Related Conditions of Service of Nurses and Midwives* (Halsbury) (1974).

[49] For example, J. Berridge, *A Suitable Case for Treatment: A Case Study of Industrial Relations in the NHS* (1976), pp.46-7.

Chapter 21
The Spanswick Era, 1974-83

The years of Albert Spanswick's general secretaryship, which stretched from 1974 until his death in 1983, were some of the most eventful in the union's history, as they were in the NHS and society at large. The Spanswick era opened auspiciously in 1974 with the election of a Labour government and success for the union's Halsbury campaign. Unfortunately disappointment and disillusion were to follow as a result of NHS cuts, the 'Winter of Discontent' and the election of the Thatcher government in 1979. The era closed in 1983 with one of the most remarkable industrial disputes for a generation which, though not completely successful, demonstrated that health service trade unionism had come of age.

The Years of Expansion

In terms of recruitment, the mid-1970s were COHSE's most successful years, when membership was lifted to its present high plateau. Its militancy during the Halsbury campaign, as the only nurses' organisation which was prepared to take industrial action, struck the right chord with many health workers. Almost overnight the union rose to become the twelfth largest in the TUC. As we have seen, the years between 1970 and 1979 were those during which the membership boomed, a development which had a number of political consequences. Gone was much of the caution and conservatism of the past, and along with it the inward looking approach and narrow vision that had led it to be expelled from the TUC in 1972 for registering under the Conservatives' 1971 Industrial Relations Act. The union now faced outwards, and began to play a much fuller role in the broader labour movement.

Much of this change was indeed linked with Albert Spanwick's general secretaryship. One of his first acts was to take COHSE back into the TUC. By 1976 he had been elected to its General Council, the TUC's inner cabinet from which the union had been absent since Bartlett retired in 1963. Spanswick became an increasingly powerful figure in the TUC as unions in the public services began to wield a growing influence; he played a central role in the TUC's campaign against cuts in public expenditure after 1976, and chaired its Health Services Committee which was so influential in the 1982 pay dispute. In subsequent years other union officials followed his example. For example, David Williams, Spanswick's successor as General Secretary, was elected on to the Labour Party's National Executive Committee, followed by Sid Ambler, who retired as COHSE's president in 1986.

While individual union leaders can have a significant impact on the movement's fortunes, it would be wrong to place too much emphasis upon their influence in isolation from the wider environment in which they operate. COHSE's dynamism during the 1970s was part of a more general 'push from below' which many public sector unions experienced. It was carried forward by a variety of other influences including a rapid growth in the NHS labour force, growing competition among both unions and professional associations for membership, the spread of bonus incentive schemes, the erosion of low wages by rapid price rises and, following the election of a Labour government in 1974, employment legislation which gave further impetus to the spread of shop stewards and local bargaining. The social composition of the union also changed. Although male psychiatric nurses in their middle years still dominated many of the positions of influence in COHSE, there was an influx of younger, general trained nurses into the union, most of whom were women, many of them black. By the late 1970s there quarters of COHSE members were women, with only one other TUC affiliated union having a higher proportion. All these changes helped to create a more open industrial and political outlook within COHSE.

The larger and more confident union which emerged in the 1970s was much less head office and branch secretary dominated than before. Many new branches were created and old ones revitalised. Although branch secretaries and full-time officers remained powerful within it, the union's organisation now rested more often on a broader base of steward activists who were for the most part in closer contact with the membership as a whole. Albert Spanswick was not the only author of these changes, but he helped to push them along, at the same time taking the more traditionally minded members with him. Though politically on the right of the Labour Party, his style was nevertheless much more emphatic than most previous COHSE leaders, even at times aggressive. 'We are not any pseudo-professional body but a fully fledged trade union', he declared in an interview conducted shortly after he took office in 1974.[1]

The growth of the union led to important organisational changes. Head office expanded. The research and publicity department, and the journal, now became separated, and *Health Services* was launched as a much more 'up-front', campaigning tabloid newspaper, more fitting to the more dynamic organisation which COHSE had become. A proper library was established. More specialist staff were recruited in such areas as research, education, law, press and public relations, to advise the General Secretary and the other national officers. The officer force was also expanded in the regions, and boundaries were made largely coterminous with those established by the NHS reorganisation of 1974.

Labour Comes to Power

There was a new mood of optimism and self-confidence within COHSE, which was operating within what appeared to be an extremely favourable external environment. It has been claimed that the trade union movement has never enjoyed more power in Britain than in the years 1974-6.[2] Certainly a rising tide of militancy associated with an almost unprecedented growth in membership, had helped in 1974 to dispatch Ted Heath's Conservative Government, in an election called on the issue of union power. Instead a Labour Government was elected which seemed more radical than any since 1945, promising in its election manifesto to shift the balance of power in society 'irreversibly' in favour of working class people and their families. The new government certainly acted quickly during 1974 to repeal the 1971 Industrial Relations Act, and to bring in reforms such as the Employment Protection Act, Trade Union and Labour Relations Act, and the Health and Safety at Work Act, all of which appeared to establish a comprehensive network of employee and trade union rights.

Whatever might be said about the impact of the reforms in the private sector, where local union organisation was already on the whole well developed, they led in the public services to greatly improved recognition and an extension of bargaining rights at local level over a wide range of issues. Local managements were forced, often for the first time, to institute local industrial relations procedures, to recognise stewards and make provision for them to carry out their duties, and to provide them with access to bargaining information. The threat of external appeal, to industrial tribunals or the Arbitration and Conciliation Service (ACAS), put local managements on the defensive, making their personnel and industrial relations policies open to challenge as never before.

We must not exaggerate the extent of advantage gained by unions in the NHS. In most localities they did not become more than a countervailing power to administrators and senior professionals. It must also be remembered that professional associations were also able to take advantage of the employment legislation, by registering as trade unions to gain access to the newly established bargaining rights. Thus the RCN began to recover from the challenge mounted by COHSE during the Halsbury campaign, and regained the initiative during and after the 'Winter of Discontent', when the pendulum swung against the trade unions. COHSE had hoped that Lord McCarthy's review of the Whitley Council system might lead to action to enhance the position of unions in relation to professional associations. However his report in 1976 sanctioned the position of professional associations within the system.[3] There were also serious defects in some of the employment legislation as it applied to the NHS. For example, the Health and Safety at Work Act did not fully apply in the health service, which was granted 'crown immunity' from prosecution.

Even more disappointing was the decision of the incoming Labour government to implement the Tories' top-heavy bureaucratic reorganisation of the NHS, devised by Sir Keith Joseph in 1973, despite its manifesto commitment to create democratically elected health authorities. Barbara Castle, as Secretary of State for Health and Social Services, reasoned that

> It was too late to unscramble Sir Keith's eggs and another immediate reorganisation would have been disastrous for morale.[4]

While the new structure was one in which doctors now had to share power with administrators; users (through Community Health Councils) had only notional rights, and the majority of workers no formal means of influence at all. As Mrs Castle made only marginal adjustments to these arrangements, health workers realised that their only practical means of influencing decisions lay through their own collective strength. Labour's failure to reform the service on more socialist lines, helped to expose it to later Conservative attacks on the bureaucracy and inefficiency which they themselves had helped to create!

The reorganisation of the NHS at least brought some benefits to Northern Ireland, and success for COHSE's campaign for parity of wages and conditions with the rest of the UK. The new authorities in the province were now obliged to observe Whitley Council terms and conditions, and this provided a firm foundation for rapid growth of COHSE in Northern Ireland during the 1970s. In an area with extremely high rates of poverty and unemployment, the public services are especially vital, both to deal with the effects of appalling social deprivation, and in order to maintain levels of employment. COHSE has therefore been vigorous in defending services and in campaigning for economic justice for health workers in the province, at all times maintaining a strictly non-sectarian approach.

To be fair to Mrs Castle, it does seem from her *Diaries* that she fought to protect the NHS from the ever-tightening squeeze in spending, and to obtain improved pay for health service staff. Certainly the NHS fared better under her than under her successor, David Ennals, who replaced her in 1976 as Secretary of State for Health and Social Services. Yet there were signs of retreat prior to 1976, especially faced with a determined onslaught from the leaders of the medical profession, over their pay and the linked issue of pay beds. COHSE and other unions had campaigned for these to be removed from the NHS, in line with Labour's election manifesto, and some groups of members backed this up with industrial action at local level. The action taken at the new Charing Cross Hospital in London received most media attention, and generated most concern among consultants, because it was close to the centre of power within the profession. Meanwhile, negotiations with the hospital consultants over revisions to the contracts broke down. They also took industrial action over government proposals to pay higher salaries to those who were prepared to work full-time for the NHS and forgoe the opportunity to do part-time private work. The government sought to stabilise the situation in ways which reassured the consultants, but headed off the growing pressure for more fundamental reform of the NHS. Action on major questions concerning the functioning of the NHS was postponed by the appointment of a Royal Commission into the NHS, which did not report until shortly before Labour left office in 1979,[5] by which time any opportunity for radical reform had long passed. On pay beds Mrs Castle mysteriously decided to introduce legislation, rather than to use the powers she knew were already vested in her to eliminate them.[6] Under the deal worked out for the government between Lord Goodman and the British Medical Association (BMA), a Health Services Board would only eliminate pay beds at a rate sufficiently slow to enable consultants to set up alternative facilities in the private sector. Set up by the Health Service Act of 1976, it worked at a painfully slow rate, and was abolished after the Conservatives came to power in 1979.[7]

Fighting the Cuts

The Health Service Act failed also to check the growth of private medicine outside the NHS. Indeed it could be said to have quietly sanctioned it, rather conveniently for a Government which after 1976 was intent on cutting spending on the NHS, and public expenditure in general, as the price for securing a loan from the International Monetary Fund (IMF), to help the country out of its economic difficulties. The Labour Government under James Callaghan accepted almost without question the argument that public expenditure, previously seen as beneficial to the economy, was now at the root of the country's economic problems. By some unspecified process, it was said to have 'crowded out' private investment in Britain's manufacturing base. Other analyses were available, which took a much longer view of the problem, and suggested that industry and the city were more to blame for the failure to modernise the country's manufacturing base,[8] but these were not given serious attention. Instead a Labour government piloted policies which were to be implemented with whole-hearted enthusiasm by the Conservatives after 1979, such as: controls over the money supply, cash limits on public expenditure, cuts in public services, and permitting unemployment to rise.

All this was happening at a time when a 'Social Contract' operated between the Labour government and the trade union movement, when any sacrifices made by trade unionists and working class people in general, were supposed to be balanced by benefits. After 1976, it increasingly came to seem to many workers that only one side was keeping to the bargain. The flat rate £6 a week pay limit supervised through the TUC during 1975-6 to some extent favoured low paid workers, many of them to be found in the NHS. Their position began to deteriorate during the second year of restraint, however, and worsened still further during the third year of pay policy, when pay rises were limited (without the agreement of the TUC) to 10 per cent.

It was, however, the IMF imposed cuts in the planned growth of the NHS which had the most immediate impact. Even the much needed redistribution of finances that occurred between so-called 'well' (mainly southern) and 'less well' provided (mainly northern) regions, through the Resources Allocation Working Party (RAWP) formula, became – as COHSE protested – a mechanism for levelling down rather than lifting up standards. As early as November 1975 COHSE's NEC had warned of the damage cuts were having on the service, particularly in postponing overdue improvements, and the non-replacement of staff when they left. Many authorities foolishly cut back on student and pupil nurse training, a decision which had roll-on effects for years to follow. At the same time unemployment and poverty were on the increase, adding to the difficulties of health staff. As Sue Spilling, a COHSE health visitor put it at the time:

> How can you be expected to promote a healthy society with all the underlying problems of poverty and unemployment, quite apart from all the problems of bad housing and so on, imposed on so many families? Meanwhile we are facing cuts in our own staff and sharp increases in workload.

Many health workers could therefore see the direct damage that government policies were having on people's lives, and called on their unions to defend essential services.

COHSE sought constantly to bring the government to its senses, at first through behind the scenes pressure, but increasingly, as this had little effect, through public protest and action. At the 1976 Labour Party Conference Albert Spanswick moved a composite motion which advocated radical measures to defend and extend the NHS, not just to restore cuts, but also to nationalise the drugs industry, to end all health charges, expand health centres, and develop a comprehensive occupational health service. On November 17 of the same year, when 60,000 people demonstrated against the cuts in the streets of London. Albert Spanswick warned the government in plain words: 'Spurn these people at your peril'.

The most effective forms of resistance to the Government's measures were those which led to new alliances being formed between health unions and the wider local community. One of the most notable of these struggles, in which COHSE activists were involved, was the fight to maintain the precarious existence of the Elizabeth Garrett Anderson Hospital for Women situated next door to London's Euston station, on a prime redevelopment site. The fight highlighted many central issues, not least the lack of democracy and sensitivity of planners to the expressed needs of both staff and users, in a health service dominated by male administrators and consultants. By fighting together to 'Save the EGA', the campaigners were beginning to articulate the idea of an alternative health service, much closer to the people it purported to serve. This has often been a feature of many subsequent campaigns against closure.

Not all of these struggles were outright successes. Especially following the election of a Tory Government in 1979, local managements often felt able to take a more aggressive rather than conciliatory approach, and in a number of instances organised raiding parties to snatch patients away from hospitals where staff were 'working in' to keep services open, with the aid of police cordons and fleets of private ambulances. Many of these hospitals, such as St Benedict's hospital in Tooting, South London, were closed, never to reopen. But at Etwall in Derbyshire COHSE members refused to give up the fight and later succeeded in getting their hospital reopened. Although legal changes have now made occupations even more difficult to pursue, they remain an important option for activists to consider in the fight against closure. A COHSE working party has recently issued a set of *Guidelines*, which contains useful advice on the conduct of hospital occupations.

Success, however, can be measured in a number of ways. Undoubtedly, hospital occupations have served to rally opposition generally against attempts to run down the health service. Despite the set-backs there is no doubt that COHSE and other trade unionists' campaigns and struggles against the cuts had their impact, even after the Conservatives came to power. For example, Mrs Thatcher was forced to abandon, at least for the time being, plans for insurance funding of the NHS, and health service spending was maintained to a greater extent than other areas of social spending, and private medicine was not been encouraged to the extent that one might have expected. During the 1983 General Election she was forced to repudiate her own controversial 'Think Tank' proposals for the future of the welfare state and forced to promise that the NHS would be 'safe with us'.

Service and Professional Issues

The period from the late 1970s onwards was a time when COHSE found itself taking up a broad range of service and health-related issues other than cuts, and when the distinction between professional and trade union issues also became increasingly blurred. In the late 1970s COHSE found it had, for example, to: frame procedures for dealing with violent or potentially violent patients; formulate proposals to reform mental handicap nursing: define its policy in relation to moves to set up specialist secure units in psychiatric hospitals; and submit evidence to the Royal Commission on the NHS. In the early 1980s COHSE began to frame positive policies for the service, articulated in a series of well-researched documents in which the union's full-time officers and branch activists together played a key role. The pace of change was accelerating in the NHS in ways that were having a big impact on members' interests. The union needed to deal with these in such a way that the wider world was not given the impression that it was only concerned to defend its members' interests and job security by resisting all change.

This task became even more urgent under the Conservative government from 1979 which, at the same time as it formally maintained a commitment to the NHS, busily set about undermining its principles. COHSE closely analysed government policy statements, such as

Care in the Community (1981), and exposed the true and dangerous implications of the Government's apparently bland and innocuous proposals. Not the development of real community care services, which the union supports, but the abandonment of public responsibility to ensure adequate care for the elderly, mentally ill and handicapped, the chronically sick and the disabled. *Health Services* has also played a vital role in producing, with the help of activists, high quality investigations into the real impact of Government policies at local level. COHSE went on to utilise the wide experience of its members to articulate real alternatives, most impressively in its 1983 Working Party Report, *The Future of Psychiatric Services* (the Mallinson Report), which subsequently formed the basis for developing community care services in a number of districts. This reiterated COHSE's belief in the essential role the central-government funded NHS needs to play in the development of community services, given the uncertainties and limitations of local government services resulting from the Tories' rate-capping policies.

COHSE also became increasingly involved in campaigns on wider health issues, for example, against the Tory Government's attempts to suppress the 1980 Black Report, and its proposals to deal with health inequalities. It also subsequently affiliated to organisations such as the Campaign for Nuclear Disarmament and Greenpeace, taking stands on behalf of health workers on perhaps some of the most vital health questions of all. International issues increasingly figured highly in the union's work, from the support of trade unionists in South Africa and Chile, to campaigns to improve the health of Third World peoples.

At the same time COHSE could not afford to lose sight of the immediate material interests of its members, who have remained among the lowest paid in the community. Most of the gains made in 1974 were very rapidly eroded by inflation and yet another round of incomes policies. By 1978 the anger of COHSE members was mounting and in the autumn big claims for pay increases and reductions in hours were submitted to help health staffs keep abreast of rises in the cost of living. The Labour government of Jim

Callaghan would not initially budge from a 5 per cent offer in line with its income policy norms, but later marginally increased this to 8.8 per cent, with £3.50 a week to be made available for the lowest paid.

In January 1979 COHSE drew up guidelines for industrial action, and took a full part in the so-called 'Winter of Discontent', when low paid public sector workers revolted over their abysmal pay and conditions. COHSE's national guidelines gave advice on forms of action that could be taken – stoppages, work-to-rules, paperwork strikes etc – but emphasised that emergency cover was to be maintained at all times. These were not always followed to the letter by all branches, and some branches took forms of action which in hindsight are hard to justify, despite the understandable anger of low paid health staffs. Nevertheless, press reports greatly exaggerated the impact of industrial action on patient welfare. For example the TUC Report *A Cause for Concern* exposed among others a *Daily Mail* report of 29 January 1979 which had claimed that a woman was unable to receive hospital treatment because of the dispute. In fact she had already been waiting for two years for admission as a result of the cuts in public expenditure, which had been warmly applauded by the same newspaper.

The Labour Government eventually found a way out of the dispute through the appointment of the Clegg Commission, which was asked to compare pay levels of the public services with those outside. In the meantime, health workers received 9 per cent plus payments on account (for example, £2.50 for nurses, £1 for ambulance workers). The same year saw the defeat of the Labour Government and the action of public service workers has often been cited as one of the major reasons for Labour's defeat – as the public recoiled from the heartless face of trade unionism that it supposedly exposed. During the election the Tories said that they would not necessarily accept the Clegg Commission findings, but susbequently did so, despite the expense. This, and the shorter working week for nurses, accounts for quite a substantial part of the increased money the Conservatives claim to have spent on the health service. Nevertheless, though Clegg awarded much needed pay rises, he did little to solve the problem of low pay, for in line with the findings of the comparability exercise, he gave proportionately more to the higher paid. This was a background factor to the 1982 dispute.

Meanwhile, the Tories' restrictive employment legislation hit generally at trade unionists' rights to organise, and inside the service the government issued hard-line circulars such as *When Industrial Relations Break Down* in 1979, which urged management to take a much tougher line in local disputes. The General Nursing Council also disciplined a number of nurses for taking part in industrial action during the 'Winter of Discontent'. COHSE's policy then and since has been one of reluctance to take industrial action, but a defence of the right to use it as a last resort, provided patients' welfare is safeguarded. After 1979 COHSE's NEC responded defensively by issuing a revised set of guidelines to be followed for taking industrial action, including a Code of Conduct subsequently endorsed by COHSE Conference. The NEC was anxious both to protect members against possible disciplinary action, and to staunch the loss of some nursing members to the RCN over the industrial action issue. The Code insisted on the maintenance of emergency cover at all times, with the dignity and welfare of the patients being paramount.

The rapid growth of the RCN at this time was not only the result of its opposition to industrial action. It also gave considerable emphasis in recruitment to its indemnity insurance scheme, to nurses who were feeling in an increasingly vulnerable professional position. COHSE resisted the idea of offering a similar scheme for some considerable time, arguing that it was not needed, and that it might in fact encourage litigation against nurses. It eventually relented rather late in the day, in 1985, and now offers a scheme with similar coverage to that offered by the RCN but extended to all health staffs.

Trade union organisation in the NHS withstood this buffeting, and remained remarkably resilient. COHSE membership rose to a peak of 231,000 by 1982. Lessons were learnt from the Winter of Discontent, which in 1982 enabled COHSE and other NHS unions to mount and maintain a campaign of industrial action without significantly alienating public support, indeed mobilising it to an extent which seriously embarrassed the government. After receiving paltry increases for two years which were well below the rate of inflation, health staffs (along with other public sector workers) decided in the autumn of 1981 to combine forces. All major pay groups were now due, for the first time in the history of the NHS, to receive increases on the same date, 1 April 1982. The campaign was coordinated through the TUC Health Services Committee, chaired by Albert Spanswick, representing all NHS trade unions. The Committee drew up battle plans, setting the modest (perhaps on hindsight, too modest) target of a 12 per cent 'common core' claim for all major occupational groups, to compensate them for the rise in the cost of living. In response the Government only offered 6 per cent, though it gave the police 10 per cent and judges 18.6 per cent.

Before embarking on its campaign of industrial action, the TUC Health Services Committee went to see Patrick Jenkin, Secretary of State for Health and Social Services, in a vain last attempt to convince him of the justice of the health workers' case. This appeal fell on deaf ears, and the campaign to shift the Government's obstinacy by more direct pressure lasted through most of 1982. Thousands of health workers took industrial action which reduced 1,500 hospitals to an emergencies-only service. At the same time, public support magnified. Millions of trade unionists either demonstrated support or took sympathy strike action, in the largest show of working-class unity and solidarity since the General Strike of 1926. As Albert Spanswick proclaimed to COHSE's June 1982 Conference, at the height of the dispute:

> The battle for the hearts and minds of the nation's people has been won. They have judged the NHS staffs who have stood shoulder to shoulder with miners, steelworkers, dockers and thousands of other trade unionists, to be right in their struggle for pay justice and an end to low pay.

The campaign did have some effect on the Government, which increased its offer to nurses to 7.5 per cent, although some of the increase was expected to come from existing NHS funds, thus setting an ominous precedent for the future. The government also attempted to divide the unity of health staffs, by offering nurses, and subsequently professional and technical staff covered by the PT(A) Council (such as radiographers and physiotherapists) standing Pay Review Bodies (PRBs), on the lines long established for doctors and dentists.

Health workers fought on well beyond the autumn of 1982. In September Albert Spanswick received a standing ovation from delegates to the TUC Conference, until the whole Congress then turned to applaud and wave to the group of COHSE health staff from Ealing Hospital watching the debate in the public gallery. The Ealing workers then returned the waves in one of the most moving occasions in the recent history of the British labour movement. It seemed that day that working people as a whole were recovering their sense of oneness through the health workers' struggle for justice. In the words of the late Bill Dunn, an ambulance worker who was then COHSE branch secretary at Ealing, 'it was a tremendous experience'. The campaign culminated in the magnificent national day of action of 22 September 1982, when millions of workers took sympathy action, and 120,000 demonstrated in London in one of the largest trade union demonstrations ever seen. But no more concessions were forthcoming from the Government, whose general popularity had been boosted by the Falklands War.

The TUC did not know how to take the campaign forward after 22 September. To initiate more 'days of action' would likely lead to demoralisation, to wage all out industrial action might have lost public support, and to call a general strike would have led to accusations that the TUC was challenging the authority of a democratically elected government. It decided to do none of these things, but largely stood aside to let the dispute take its own course. The dispute dragged on until 14 December, when a special COHSE Delegate Conference decided to call it a day, after COHSE's NEC had put the limited options open to the membership. On the following day the TUC Health Services Committee terminated the campaign of industrial action.

The campaign was not an outright victory, and some have argued that errors were made.[9] It nevertheless showed that health service trade unionism was by no means a spent force and had, in fact, come for the first time to the forefront of the whole labour movement. Health workers had shown that they could maintain unity and collective discipline among themselves, and build powerful links with working class people outside the service. Health service trade unionism had indeed come of age.

Notes

[1] Quoted by R. Taylor, *The Fifth Estate*, 1978, p.353.

[2] P. Hain, *Political Strikes*, 1986.

[3] W. McCarthy, *Making Whitley Work*, 1976.

[4] B. Castle, *The Castle Diaries 1974-6*, 1980, p.142.

[5] HMSO, *Report of the Royal Commission on the NHS* (Merrison Report), 1979. 1980.

[6] See her *Diaries*, p.132.

[7] For a more detailed account of these events see B. Griffith et al, *Banking on Sickness*, 1987, Ch. 1.

[8] A. Gamble and P. Walton, *Capitalism in Crisis*, 1976.

[9] See, for example, the accounts of the dispute by G. Morris and S. Rydzkowski, 'Anatomy of a Dispute', *Health and Social Services Journal*, 12 April 1984; and D. Cook, 'Lessons of the NHS Dispute', *Marxism Today*, February 1983.

Chapter 22

'Hope and Optimism, in Spite of the Present Difficulties'[1]

The years following the 1982 pay dispute have proved to be some of the most testing the union has ever faced. Not only did COHSE face, from 1983, a Tory government with an increased majority entrenched in its second term of office, but it was also stunned by the death of two of its most experienced national officials, Albert Spanswick and Terry Mallinson – attributable in part at least to the strains of the 1982 pay campaign.

David Williams, who had proved his skills over the years as a behind-the-scenes Whitley Council negotiator and union administrator, succeeded Albert Spanswick as general secretary. He was immediately pitched as leader of the union into dealing with a rapidly changing as well as often hostile environment. He steered COHSE through largely by adopting a low-key approach. The union adapted itself remarkably well to the pressures on it, dealing with a stream of government mis-information about the NHS and its intentions towards it, and a plethora of policy initiatives which required rapid and decisive responses. By the end of April 1987, when Hector MacKenzie took over as General Secretary, COHSE had held its own, and the slight loss of membership since 1982 from 231,000 was stabilised at 212,000. This is no mean achievement at a time when job losses among ancillary workers have been severe, and when compared with the dramatic fall in trade union membership as a whole, of something in the order of 24 per cent since 1979.[2] Rather than rest on its laurels, however, there are clear signs

381

– of which we will hear more later – that a radical review of policies, priorities and organisation is now taking place within the union, just as it is in the movement as a whole.

The strains have been experienced by all sections of the union, who have struggled hard to maintain the membership, to defend the service and protect the living conditions of health workers. The union has had to respond to the demands of: changes in employment and industrial relations law; the Griffiths reorganisation of the NHS; the monitoring of health service cuts and the real effects of government 'community care' policies; the need to prove to the membership, prior to a ballot on the issue, the vital necessity of retaining a political fund; the enormous amount of evidence that must be collected for submission to the Pay Review Bodies established for nurses and PT(A) workers; the monitoring and co-ordination of local campaigns against privatisation of ancillary services; as well as policy discussion of a wide variety of service issues, from radical proposals to restructure nurse training, to suggesting ways of effectively responding to the threat of AIDS (Acquired Immune Deficiency Syndrome). These are just some of the issues which have confronted COHSE in the past four years. Any critical assessment made of the union's performance during the past four years, must also recognise how much has been achieved in very difficult circumstances.

Safe With Them?

The Government's claim that the NHS has been 'safe with us' rests primarily on its own statistics, which purport to show that it has increased spending on it at a time when public expenditure has generally been under pressure. Mrs Thatcher claims that 'the only cuts we have made are cuts in waiting lists'.[3] The argument about the validity of government statistics has often been heated, with COHSE has contending that the figures have been deliberately 'massaged'. The government's claim to have increased spending by 24 per cent in real terms after inflation is taken into account, has recently been disputed by a careful examination of the statistical evidence, which shows also that the number of beds available to the NHS has been falling, despite growing demands for care.[4] COHSE members themselves have been only too aware of the reality of cuts and closures, and lengthening waiting lists, and have alerted their union and the public at large to the effects.

COHSE's campaign against NHS cuts intensified in the run-up to the general election, through its 'No Cuts 87' campaign, which has combined vigorous local defence campaigns with national publicity based on grass roots collection of evidence through 'Carewatch'. *Health Services* and the union's publicity services have both played important roles in this campaign, for example by publicising successful campaigns such as those in Shropshire and South Wales, and in passing ammunition on to Labour MPs like Michael Meacher (who is sponsored by the union) to use in Parliament. The union's education services, which have become much more decentralised upon the regions, have also helped to equip activists – an increasing number of them women and ethnic minority members – for such campaigns. This is achieved not least by seeking to raise members' consciousness that something can be done, in a general atmosphere that all too easily could encourage despondency. The No Cuts 87 campaign yet again serves to highlight the importance of good communications between all sections of COHSE's organisation, and on the ability of the union to mobilise support outside the union. Without such defence campaigns as these, there is no doubt that the health and social services would be in an even worse state today. The union has more than played its part in keeping the state of the health service high on the political agenda.

Perhaps in the future the campaign against health cuts will be seen as marking the beginning of the recovery of the labour movement, following the tragic defeat of the miners in 1985. There had certainly been an enormous degree of moral and material support from within COHSE for the miners' magnificent stand. Members recognised that the ruthless logic of 'efficiency' which sought to grind the miners down, regardless of the social costs, was the same uncaring philosophy which lay behind attacks on the health service and the welfare state. The Conservative government was aware that the time was not yet ripe for such a direct assault on the NHS. This has been manifested less directly, in particular by the introduction of 'general management' into the NHS, and the attempt to privatise hospital ancillary and other vital support services.

The Conservative government quickly implemented the recommendations in 1983 of Roy Griffiths, Managing Director of Sainsbury's, that multi-disciplinary management teams, created in 1974, should be replaced at all levels by single 'general managers' who need not have any NHS let alone professional background.[5] While COHSE did not deny that improvements in management were necessary, it condemned Griffiths' promotion of a 'business ethos' in the NHS for being based on a 'mechanistic' and inappropriate notion of efficiency, as a prelude to eventual complete privatisaton. COHSE also highlighted the impact of the Griffiths reforms upon nursing management. Very few nurses have been appointed general managers, and many authorities have failed to appoint a Director of Nursing Services.

Ancillary Workers Fight Back

The campaign against the privatisation of ancillary services has proved difficult, not least because the government has increasingly resorted to central direction and threats of financial penalties in order to force compliance from recalcitrant health authorities. Its introduction after 1983 also came at a time when health workers were demoralised by the lack of success of the 1982 pay campaign, and by the election of another Conservative Government. There was thus little appetite among the members of COHSE or other health unions for a concerted national campaign of industrial action, and the fight against privatisation has largely been left to the initiative of local activists. So long as certain guidelines are followed, COHSE has automatically declared all local disputes official. There has been some attempt by unions to coordinate more regional and national support, for example through solidarity demonstrations in support of key struggles such as Hammersmith and Addenbrooks hospitals. There are signs that these battles are leading to increased cooperation between NHS unions. For example, the four ASC unions (COHSE, NUPE, TGWU and GMB), have recently appointed a joint privatisation campaign worker at national level.

Despite the difficulties COHSE and other unions face, the Government has by no means had all its own way. Many health authorities, particularly in the 'Celtic fringes' of Scotland, Wales and Northern Ireland have fought, often under pressure from unions, a concerted rearguard campaign against compliance with central government directives. Even when services have been put out to tender they have, in the vast majority of circumstances (82 per cent) so far been awarded to in-house bids from existing health staffs. This is 'victory' of a sorts, but the price is usually a deterioration in conditions and staffing levels, with no guarantee of overall security, as contracts are reviewed every three years. The threat of privatisation has therefore served as a powerful disciplinary weapon, eroding the ability of unions to protect health workers' conditions of employment. In only a few instances, such as Littlemore Hospital, Oxford, and Gateshead in north east England, have local campaigns of industrial action successfully defeated privatisation proposals – or succeeded in delaying the privatisation timetable. These have nevertheless been significant in maintaining workers' morale.

The fight is not over once the contract is awarded to an outside contractor. COHSE has constantly sought to expose the typically poor standards observed by contractors, and the ultimate effects upon standards of care. Once contracts have been awarded it has, however, usually proved difficult to get them revoked, partly because of the powerful political connections companies often have with Conservative MPs. Although only a small proportion of ancillary services have so far been privatised, often in cleaning services, there is no room for complacency. With the 1987 general election successfully behind them the Conservative Government, through John Moore, the Secretary of State for Social Services, has launched a new offensive on privatisation in the NHS. Developments like clinical budgeting, and the implementation of the unit level structure of Griffiths, are helping to make the NHS ripe for more general privatisation. So is growing concentration in the contracting industry, with firms like Pritchards (part of the giant Hawley group) now offering total health care packages, and increased agitation against the NHS by right wing pressure groups like the Institute of Economic Affairs.

As well as providing rich pickings and job opportunities for businessmen and officers from the armed forces, both privatisation and Griffiths are part of an ideological offensive against the health service, which seeks to undermine public faith in it. The underlying rationale, as Alan Walker puts it, is the 'public burden thesis', which assumes 'that the public sector is wasteful, inefficient and unproductive', a view for which, like it or not, there is considerable public support,[6] despite the fact that the NHS delivers a better standard of care, to more of the population, for less money, with less administrative overheads, than any free market system could.[7] That does not mean that there is no room for improvement, but COHSE has correctly insisted that questions of efficiency and democracy cannot be separated. The union argues that many of the problems associated with the NHS have been due to its lack of responsiveness to the needs of both users and rank-and-file health workers. In pursuit of its long-standing campaign to democratise the NHS, COHSE initiated discussions with the Socialist Health Association (SHA) and NUPE which recently resulted in a common policy of separate, elected health authorities with consumer, union and local authority representation. This was adopted by the TUC in 1986 and, at the time of writing, is still being discussed within the Labour Party.

What has tended to be obscured in all the arguments about structure, however, is discussion about what goals the NHS should be set, and how it might best achieve them. These are both very important issues which unions and the labour movement must face if they are to respond effectively to the threats posed by Griffiths and privatisation. Implicit in both are an attack on how the NHS has operated to date, particularly under a system of medical dominance, which COHSE has long fought. There is some substance to the criticisms, even though the proposed solutions – the increased use of business methods and resort to the market – would be disastrous. If current threats are to be averted, defence of the existing service is not enough. It is also necessary to articulate and more sharply define alternatives and positive policies for the service, and seek allies for them in the wider community.

The Conditions for Success

One of the prime lessons of all COHSE's campaigns of recent years is that the economistic trade union methods widely adopted during the 1970s, of simply trying to slog it out in a two-sided battle against the employers, do not now seem so effective in the NHS (or elsewhere, for that matter). The most successful campaigns of the 1980s have been those which have also politicised the issues involved, and so mobilised support beyond the NHS. They may have usually depended in the first instance on a high level of membership mobilisation, but even more crucial has been convincing a wider public that the issues at stake are ones that concern them, too. This is indeed what the union's campaigns over Griffiths and privatisation have not yet completely succeeded in doing.

A high level of internal membership mobilisation was certainly associated with COHSE's successful campaign in 1985 to convince members of the necessity of retaining a political fund. Normally sleepy branches were suddenly energised, and all levels of the organisation were mobilised into communicating the arguments to the members. The result was a massive 91 per cent vote in favour of a political fund, one of the highest in the trade union movement. The successful campaign, supported by COHSE, to reinstate Wendy Savage, the consultant obstetrician suspended because of her controversial methods (she had the audacity to take pregnant women's wishes into account when deciding on a course of treatment) showed how public support and action can result in victories. This has also been the case with the partially successful campaign to compel the Government to face up to its responsibilities in relation to the prevention and treatment of AIDS. At the same time the union itself was forced to define its own position on the wider issues linked to AIDS, and Conference in 1987 adopted a policy of total opposition to discrimination agianst lesbians and gay men.

The largely successful campaign against the 'crown immunity' of the NHS from prosecution in the courts, is an important illustration of the need for both union mobilisation and public support, backed up by effective political intervention at local and national levels. COHSE had campaigned against crown immunity ever since it was retained in the 1974 Health and Safety at Work Act. Then in 1984 19 patients died and 355 staff and patients were taken ill in an outbreak of food poisoning at Stanley Royd hospital in Yorkshire. The local COHSE branch, with the help of full-time officers, spearheaded a highly effective media campaign, which drew attention to appalling conditions and poor management of the hospital kitchens, showed how the problem was not an isolated one, and how crown immunity stood in the way of effective action to remedy it.

COHSE's campaign resulted in much-needed local improvements, though the union insists that these have not gone far enough. It is also concerned that the newly-installed 'cook-chill' systems might be hazardous, a view supported by the influential London Food Commission. The union's campaign also led within less than two years to significant legislative change: the 1986 National Health Service Amendment Act. This removed crown immunity from the NHS in regard to health and safety, even though the government had originally only intended to remove it from hospital kitchens alone. The Act was a very significant victory, even though crown immunity has not yet been entirely eliminated from the NHS. Its continued existence has hampered COHSE's efforts to protect resident health staffs' rights as tenants, threatened as a result of Health Circular (85) 19, which called on districts to remove most forms of hospital staff accommodation on 'economic' grounds. Nevertheless, spirited resistance by COHSE branches, backed up by information and support from head office, and pressure by COHSE-sponsored MPs in Parliament, has so far significantly reduced the impact of the Circular in many districts. The Circular had originated from a 'scrutiny' conducted by Sir Derek Rayner of Marks and Spencer.

The campaigns of the 1980s have thus reinforced the need for COHSE to look more generally outwards, and to link up with other pressure groups and unions, and gain favourable media coverage for its campaigns. This has also underlined the importance of the union's links with the Labour Party and its sponsored MPs in Parliament. COHSE has recently appointed a Parliamentary Liason Officer, to increase the effectiveness of this area of the union's work. The local level, however, is an equally important arena of intervention, where good links with other unions, outside pressure groups, sympathetic Community Health Council and health authority members, and the media, can make all the difference in waging successful campaigns.

Low Pay – the Fight Continues

Not only are these points valid over service issues, they seem also apply to what are regarded as the more traditional areas of union activity over pay and conditions, and help to explain the union's mixed degree of success, according to which occupational group one looks at. Nurses and PT(A) workers have done better than ancillary workers and NHS clerical workers, partly because they can more easily mobilise the support of a wider public and convince them also that their interests as patients are likely to be affected. The PRBs have also given nurses and professional staff as a whole greater increases than they could probably have otherwise obtained through collective bargaining. Whatever the government's original motives for establishing them, they have become bulwarks against any government attempt to scrap national pay and conditions (regionalisation of pay bargaining and merit payments are among the proposals being currently reviewed). The PRB system has also compelled unions to prepare their case much more thoroughly than was the case through over-the-table pay bargaining (though the Whitley Council remains an important area of bargaining over non-pay conditions of service). The PRB system has also promoted greater cooperation between staff side organisations, especially in order to respond to government interference in its affairs. Interference has included: behind-the-scenes pressure on the PRBs to limit the size of their awards; delays in implementation of awards; and a refusal to fully fund awards from central government finances.

COHSE continues to exercise considerable influence over the Nurses' and Midwives' Staff Side strategy, with Hector MacKenzie succeeding David Williams as its Chair. In 1987 the RCN even broke with previous tradition and accepted COHSE's case for flat rate pay increases to restore the position of the lowest paid nurses. The PRB Reports recommended increases of 9.5 per cent overall for nurses and PTA workers, and were implemented immediately by the government. The award hardly went any way, however, to remove the scourge of low pay, nor can it compensate nursing and PT(A) staff for the stress imposed by cuts and heavier workloads due to the increase in the numbers of patients treated.

Other health workers have been even less fortunate, partly because they have been less able to mobilise public sympathy, and have been wrongly regarded as less essential to the service. Ancillary workers in particular have been hit by severe job losses of the order of 19 per cent betwen 1978 and 1985.[8] An end to the chronic and worsening problem of low pay among ancillary workers is not yet in sight. As Colm O'Kane, COHSE's Assistant General Secretary pointed out when he was chief ancillary negotiator, ancillary staff are also the only major group in the NHS (apart from ambulance workers) still on a basic 40 hour week. On this as on so much else, they have lost considerable ground to other workers. The gap in average earnings between hospital ancillaries and manual workers generally has widened considerably since 1975, for both men and women. In April 1987, 50 per cent of men and 80 per cent of women ancillaries were earning less than the supplementary benefit levels for a small family of £123.61 a week.[9] There is thus an appalling concentration of poverty-level wages among them.

The majority of ancillaries – 67 per cent – are women, and an unknown but large number are from ethnic minorities. Many are also part-timers whose job and the income they derive from it is vitally important to themselves and their families. COHSE has recently put considerable emphasis in its strategy for improving the position of ancillary workers upon securing 'equal pay for work of equal value', in line with EEC directives. This has been because job segregation between men and women has been shown to be at the root of much of the low pay in the health service, and has been unaffected by the provisions of the 1970 Equal Pay Act. As the pursuit of individual 'equal value' claims through industrial tribunals has proved increasingly difficult, the union is now seeking to negotiate new grading structures which are fair to women. The employers have resisted this for some considerable time. Though there are some signs that this attitude is changing, the road to full equality is not likely to be an easy one. The cost to the employers would be high, at a time when they appear to be more interested in seeking greater 'flexibility' from workers within the existing wage and salary budgets.

The 'equal pay for equal value' issue is one that has potential ramifications far beyond the ancillary worforce. It calls into question the whole division of labour in health care in which the female (often black) majority who are supposedly assigned the caring and supportive tasks, are subordinated in terms of power and income to the minority (largely white) male elite who supposedly carry out curing and strategic administrative responsibilities. In practice the supposed distinctions are greatly exaggerated. Ancillary and supportive staff often find themselves providing the emotional and practical support to patients that professionals are too busy or sometimes not inclined to give. Nurses carry a wide range of diagnostic and treatment responsibilities, many of them performed by auxiliaries and nurses in training. Low paid women clerical workers also take on a wide number of the administrative responsibilities without which the high-flying male careers could not take off.[10] Is this not flexibility enough? 'Individually based equal opportunity' policies, important though they are, cannot fully remedy this situation, as by definition they can only project a few more women and black people up an already unfair hierarchy.

Project 2000 – the Issues at Stake

One of the most promising challenges to the subordination of women within the health system, but also one fraught with dangers, is the United Kingdom Central Council for Nursing' Midwifery and Health Visiting (UKCC) 'Project 2000' proposals for the restructuring of nurse education and training.[11] Its sweeping proposals for reorganising training are based on the assumption that in the future nursing care in institutional and non-institutional settings will be provided by fully trained and autonomous 'registered nurse practitioners', supervising 'helpers' who will have only received a limited on-the-job training. Other proposals include the creation of an advanced level of 'specialist practitioner' beyond registration, the phasing out of the 'second level' enrolled nurse, and full student status for nurses in training.

COHSE recognises the revolutionary nature of the proposals and supports the need for change. The proposals are likely, if implemented, to lead to much fuller recognition of the skills of registered nurses, and implicitly challenge the age-old subordination of nurses to the medical profession. Nurses are offered the prospect of a clinical road to career advancement, at a time when Griffiths has effectively closed off the managerial road to the top. COHSE has warned, however, that there will be losers as well as gainers, particularly present auxiliary and enrolled nurses, and it fears that nursing may increasingly become 'a white, middle class profession'.[12] COHSE's evidence in response to the UKCC's proposals therefore called for the retention of a second level 'practical' nurse, with proper training, in place of what it saw as the 'pure elitism' of the so-called helper grade, which would down-grade existing nursing auxiliaries. While agreeing with the shift to full student status for learners, the union insisted that the current training salary should not be replaced with lower grants. It was also concerned about the effect of genericist training upon certain sectors of nursing, such as midwifery and mental handicap care.

COHSE is putting increased resources into 'professional' work generally, for example, by organising discussions and seminars in the regions, and has created a new Professional Officer post at national level, with a brief for developing the union's work in this area. There is a realisation that, if it is to compete more effectively with the RCN, the union will need to take more professional initiatives of its own rather than having to respond to those developed elsewhere. Care will obviously have to be exercised to ensure that professional issues do not get 'hived off' from the mainstream of the union's work. After all, though sectionalism does have a presence within the union, COHSE's underlying philosophy of industrial unionism has always emphasised the importance of the whole health care team to patient and client welfare. This is a much broader and indeed more appropriate philosophy of health care than the often narrow, occupationally limited horizons of professionalism. Although this philosophy has deep roots in COHSE's history, it also better meets contemporary health care needs.

Back to Present-day Reality

Seemingly hopeful developments like Project 2000 are, however, no solution in themselves, unless they are implemented within the framework of a properly funded health service, one which provides health workers with guarantees of pay justice and the resources with which to develop their skills for the benefits of patients. Without such guarantees, the benefits of Project 2000 will at most accrue to a small elite of practitioners, while basic care will suffer, or even be casualised. Redefining basic care as the work of 'helpers' rather than 'nurses', makes such work more vulnerable not just to removal from the health service, but from the paid labour force altogether. In the dangerous days that lie ahead, it is vital that all health staff maintain a united front, as some of them may well be offered concessions, but in ways that contribute to the continued run-down of the NHS. The groups of patients who stand most to suffer from this are those whose most pressing need is often basic nursing care, such as the elderly and the chronically ill.

Yet though there are points of possible division, the conditions are also generally favourable for constructing a common front among health workers. In terms of pay, nurses and PT(A) staffs have not done that much better than super-exploited ancillary workers, despite the PRB system, which together with the effects of cuts, helps to explain why so many leave the service each year. Despite the high salaries earned by general managers, the majority of administrative and clerical workers (mainly women), are not fairly rewarded for the important contribution they make to the service. Indeed many of them exist on poverty-level wages. And all groups of staff are potentially united by the common knowledge that the gap between the possibility of improved standards of care, and the reality of worsening conditions, grows wider every day.

As one example, ambulance men and women are a group of health staff who seem to have made some headway. After much resistance from the employers, they have achieved a new grading structure which at last fully recognises their role as an emergency service. The reality on the ground, however, is that due to cuts many ambulance workers do not have the resources to carry out these responsibilities properly. For example, a Report in 1987 by Harriet Harman MP, in her role as the Labour Party main speaker on health issues, suggested that not one ambulance authority could meet official time-limits for answering emergency calls. Disturbing reports of increased stress on ambulance men and women are becoming commonplace, as they struggle at great cost to themselves and their familes to maintain a decent service.[13] The services for so-called 'walking' patients are also being decimated, as usual in the name of the great god 'efficiency', which means in plain English a worse service, or no service at all.

A similar story could be told about almost every other occupational group. A small minority of mainly senior personnel may be unsympathetic to, or even profiting from the crisis in the NHS.[14] Yet despite the very real divisions of occupation, class, gender and ethnic group, the majority of all grades of staff are potentially united by a widespread commitment to the health service, and an increasing sense of frustration that they are unable to give the best care that the nation's resources could provide. COHSE's traditions of industrial unionism and its campaigns of the 1980s have shown how this potential unity might be harnessed with wider public concern and action to fight more effectively for a better deal for both patients and staff. At a time of crisis in the trade union movement as a whole, COHSE has therefore been able to demonstrate in action one of the great potential strengths of public service unionism: its ability to bridge the artificial divide between workers and consumers, which has been exploited to such destructive effect by Thatcherism.

Facing the Future

There is thus every reason for, as the saying goes, 'hope and optimism, in spite of the present difficulties', that out of the forms of trade unionism now being pioneered by unions such as COHSE, might well come a renaissance of the ideals which inspired the NHS, in the service and out to the wider society. The future therefore holds possibilities as well as dangers, and COHSE has the sound financial and membership base from which it can seek to realise them. With an eye to the future, a COHSE Working Party is currently examining the whole question of the union's future organisation and priorities. Set up as a result of the union's 1986 Conference, one of the most forward looking in COHSE's history, it is deliberating at a time when much that was long taken for granted inside both the NHS and the labour movement, is now being scrutinised. This does not mean that all traditional values and approaches need be abandoned, but at the very least they require fresh justification, rather than simply being restated as articles of faith.

One problem which is bound to occupy the attention of the Working Party is that, like it or not, the traditional strongholds of the union, the mental hospitals, are no longer the backbone from which the union can safely organise. Care is shifting out into 'the community', and many of the old hospitals will close. Ever since the Mallinson Report, COHSE has in fact sought less to defend institutions, more to promote a positive notion of community care which is far removed from the government's 'care on the cheap' version. There is a growing realisation among members that properly resourced and well organised community care holds many potential benefits for staff and users. Services are organised on much less hierarchial lines than previously. Staff have to develop a much more negotiated relationship with clients and their relatives, but they also find that they have more independance in relation to managers and the medical profession. There are fewer unbending rules and procedures to follow, much more discretion and judgement to exericse.

The ground on which the NHS as a whole rests, and its existing system of collective bargaining, is not much steadier. The dangers are obvious for those who care to notice: more widespread privatisation, increased charges for NHS services, the erosion if not the ending of nationally negotiated pay and conditions, and the possible shift of community care outside the framework of the NHS and local government. It is only right that COHSE sounds alarms about such possibilities as they are unlikely to be implemented in ways beneficial to either staff or users.

Yet it makes no sense, having tried without success to hold back the waves, to continue standing in their way. As COHSE has increasingly shown in response to the government's initiatives on community care, much better to use the strength one has, to divert or even rechannel the impact of change in the most positive possible directions.

Thus COHSE, while fighting privatisation, has tried its utmost to make sure contracts are awarded in-house. Though an end to nationally negotiated pay and conditions in NHS would unquestionably be a retrograde step, it would in some sense create new possibilities for local union organisation. This, if no other, is one reason why the government will hesitate before moving in such a direction.[15] COHSE campaigns for NHS control of community care, but recognises the vital role of local authorities and increasingly seeks to organise staff in local authoroity social services. It condemns the spread of private medicine and the residential homes for the elderly 'industry', but is now seeking to organise them, for as Hector MacKenzie put it to me: 'staff in the private sector are working people, too'.[16] The effect of such changes in recruiting strategy will be to shift the union's identity as an industrial union. Already COHSE now publicly describes itself as 'the health care' rather than, as formerly, 'the health service' union. It will continue to fight to maintain the NHS and health care services, but will also seek to follow health workers and organise them, wherever they may be employed.

The implications for the future are clear: COHSE needs to maintain an open, flexible approach towards policies, union structure and methods of organising in order to seize the opportunities open to it – as of course does the trade union movement as a whole. Unions are of necessity 'secondary' organisations, whose structure and organisation must to some extent be shaped by the contours of the principal outside organisations, the employers, whom they exist to influence.[17] If these contours change, then unions must also adapt or face the consequences. Their efficiency and effectiveness now more than ever depends upon creating a structure which promotes good and continuous communications between all sections of the organisation, to enable a rapid response to changing demands. COHSE has shown how this can be achieved for one-off campaigns, such as the campaign in favour of a political fund, and the No Cuts '87 campaign. In future it will need to incorporate the processes developed during such campaigns more permanently into its methods of organising.

For much of the twentieth century, centralisation has

been the dominant principle in the British trade union movement, as unions have sought to concentrate and mobilise power in relation to increasingly monopolistic employers, and an ever-expanding central government machinery. In such circumstances bureaucracy was almost bound to take precedence over democracy. In the 1960s and 70s, the base of the movement was significantly broadened out to include stewards and activists, but on the whole the membership remained passive, or only intermittently active, and often did not regard the union as 'their' property. Thatcherism has of course exploited this situation to the full. The established and indirect lines of communication within COHSE, up from the branch, to the region and then the NEC, have been fractured by the most recent employment legislation, with which Conference in 1987 decided to comply, which provides for direct membership elections to the NEC. The onus is now on the trade union movement to prove, in a more substantial way than this, that they, rather than the government, will be seen to 'give the unions to the members'. The decentralisation of power which this will involve, will also equip the union better to deal with the new environment of health care which appears to be in the process of emergence, namely one in which the union is likely to face a more powerful local management in the NHS, and a plurality of employers outside it.

Of course, effective national leadership will be just as necessary in the days that lie ahead. Thatcherism's emphasis on decentralisation and the granting of more 'power to the people' is not complete rhetoric, but the overall reality is more often one in which central government is seeking to exercise increasingly dictatorial powers, as it tries to impose the changes which it wishes to see implemented. The extent to which this has already occurred over the privatisation of ancillary services, is only a prelude to what can be expected in future. Health workers will therefore need to muster the maximum possible unity, and particularly need to overcome the sectionalism that has weakened them for so long. Although this is unlikely to come in the immediate future from a merger between COHSE and other organisations, given the union's strong financial and membership position, and determination to maintain an independent, viable union, this does not rule out better cooperation with other health unions. As we have seen this has already been manifested in, for example, the campaign against privatisation, and resistance to government attempts to interfere in the work of the PRB.

One of the most important developments of all, and perhaps the key to success on all other fronts, is growing pressure from within the union to alter that fact that it remains a union which is dominated at all levels by 'middle of the road', middle aged, middle position, white male psychiatric nurses. In recent years, COHSE has campaigned vigorously to improve women's rights in general and their participation in the union. At the 1986 Labour Party Conference, the union led the call for a special government Ministry for Women to become Labour Party policy, and the male bastion of the TUC has recently accepted suggestions of COHSE and other unions that it set up an Equal Rights Department, concentrating mainly on women's issues. COHSE has also brought out a growing amount of publicity material aimed at women, recently issuing a booklet, *Equality Action*, as a guide to branches for negotiating equal opportunities for women, and ethnic minority and disabled staff. This emphasises that it is vital to involve such staff fully in the negotiations which take place, as implementing such policies over their heads defeats the object. Making certain that such laudable policies are followed through in practice will require a massive effort from the union as a whole, involving a much wider awareness of the pernicious effects of racism, sexism and discrimination on the grounds of disability. This, too, depends also on a broadening of branch organisation out from the officers and stewards, to the membership as a whole, and the rooting out of all such inequalities at every level of COHSE's structure.

Such developments would give real meaning to the idea of the union as a 'confederation' for mutual support between all the groups which belong to it. Combined with the greater openness associated with campaigns since the 1980s, when the union has more confidently sought wider public support for its campaigns, this will continue to make COHSE a force to be reckoned with. The union has learnt that organisations representing user groups, such as CHCs, trades councils, and other pressure groups, can be partners in a common struggle against a health service which is often unresponsive to the needs of both workers and users. Such campaigns will intensify in the future, given the threat the health service now faces, and it is certainly possible that through them COHSE and its allies will begin to anticipate practical alternatives to the existing health service, as well as the one which the Conservative government is seeking to impose on us.

It can be achieved. This history has many times demonstrated the boundless energy and creativity that has existed among generations of health workers, as they have battled to secure fair remuneration, decent conditions, and a service which matches their ideals. There is nothing new about present difficulties. Health workers have always faced an uphill struggle, but their sense of possibility, that things *could* be different, has never been defeated. It remains a potent force, which COHSE is well placed to harness in the future, for the benefit of health workers and society as a whole. There could be no better challenge for the future.

Notes

[1] A slogan of the Namibia liberation movement.

[2] 'TUC reveals 24% membership drop', *Guardian*, 25 June 1987.

[3] Quoted by Radical Statistics Health Group, *Facing the Figures*, 1987, p.36.

[4] ibid, especially Chapter 3.

[5] DHSS, *Report of the NHS Management Inquiry*, 1983. For a critical study of this system in operation see N. Davidson, *The Question of Care*, 1987.

[6] A. Walker, 'The Political Economy of Privatisation', in J. Le Grand and R. Robinson (eds), *Privatisation and the Welfare State*, 1984, pp 19-44.

[7] See B. Abel-Smith, *Value for Money in Health Services*, 1976.

[8] COHSE, *NEC Report*, 1987, para. 147.

[9] Trade Union Side of Ancillary Staffs Council, *Claim for Improvements in Pay and Conditions of Ancillary Staff*, 1987.

[10] For example, for nurses see Low Pay Unit/NUPE, *Nursing a Grievance*, 1987, and clerical workers see Economic and Social Research

Council (ESRC), *Processes of Discrimination*, 1987.

[11] UKCC, *Project 2000: A New Preparation for Practice*, 1986.

[12] COHSE, *Project 2000: It Affects You!*, 1987.

[13] See reports in *Health Services*, March and September 1987.

[14] Such as the hospital consultants who are suspected of deliberately maintaining long NHS waiting lists, in order to encourage patients to see them privately. See the evidence presented in J. Yates, *Why Are We Waiting?*, 1987.

[15] See the advice to government proffered by R. Dyson, in 'Pay Bargaining and the Patient', *Health Services Journal*, 9 October 1986.

[16] While private hospitals generally observe Whitley Council rates of pay and conditions, these are often disregarded by owners of residential homes, whose treatment of their staff often leaves a great deal to be desired, according to the small-scale investigation by R. Winney, *Health Service Workers, Union Organisation, and the Threat of Privatisation* (unpublished dissertation, University of Warwick), 1987.

[17] R. Hyman and R. Fryer, 'Trade Unions', in R. McKinlay (ed), *Processing People*, 1975, pp. 150-213.

Index